MW00380320

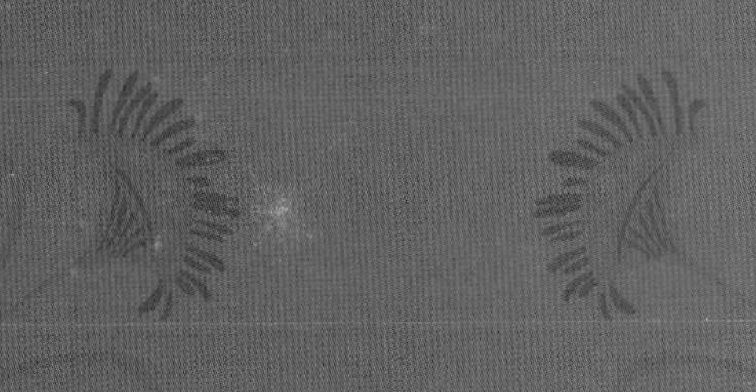

DERMAL NEEDLING THERAPY

皮肤针疗法

Project Editors: Shen Cheng-ling & Liu Shui

Copy Editor: Zhao Hai-bin

Book Designer: Dai Shan-shan

Cover Designer: Dai Shan-shan

Typesetter: Wei Hong-bo

DERMAL NEEDLING THERAPY

皮肤针疗法

▸ **Zhang Xue-li**

Professor & Chief Physician

▸ **Liu Ying**

Associate Chief Physician

Acupuncture and Moxibustion Department,
Dongzhimen Hospital Affiliated to
Beijing University of Chinese Medicine,
Beijing, China

Chief Translaters

Ji Bo, Ph. D. TCM
Associate Research Fellow,
Beijing University of Chinese Medicine

Wang Meng-qiong, M. S. TCM
College of Traditional Chinese Medicine,
Capital Medical University, Beijing, China

Fu Ai-zhen
Beijing University of Chinese Medicine

Translaters

Chen Qian-yi **Du Li-lan** **Gao Yuan** **Li Fang** **Li Lin**
Qi Hui-fang **Wang Chun-yang** **Wang Jing-xia**
Wang Yan **Yao Ke-yu** **Zeng Guang**

Edited by

Fang Ting-yu
Professor, Beijing University of Chinese Medicine
Dorothy Wong
Acupuncturist (USA)

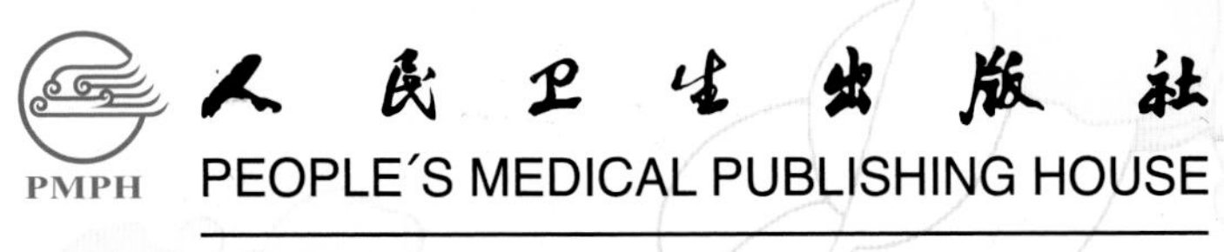

人民卫生出版社
PEOPLE´S MEDICAL PUBLISHING HOUSE
BEIJING • LONDON • NEW YORK

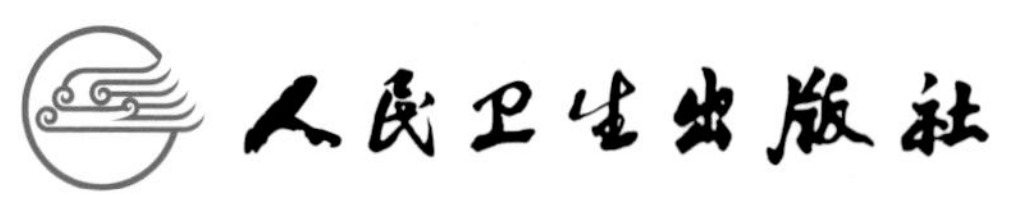

PMPH PEOPLE´S MEDICAL PUBLISHING HOUSE

Website: http://www.pmph.com

Book Title: Dermal Needling Therapy
皮肤针疗法

Contact address: Bldg 3, 3 Qu, Fangqunyuan, Fangzhuang, Beijing 100078, P.R. China, phone/fax: 8610 6769 1034, E-mail: pmph@pmph.com

For text and trade sales, as well as review copy enquiries, please contact PMPH at pmphsales@gmail.com

Disclaimer

This book is for educational and reference purposes only. In view of the possibility of human error or changes in medical science, neither the author, editor, publisher, nor any other party who has been involved in the preparation or publication of this work guarantees that the information contained herein is in every respect accurate or complete. The medicinal therapy and treatment techniques presented in this book are provided for the purpose of reference only. If readers wish to attempt any of the techniques or utilize any of the medicinal therapies contained in this book, the publisher assumes no responsibility for any such actions.

It is the responsibility of the readers to understand and adhere to local laws and regulations concerning the practice of these techniques and methods. The authors, editors, and publishers disclaim all responsibility for any liability, loss, injury, or damage incurred as a consequence, directly or indirectly, of the use and application of any of the contents of this book.

First published: 2008
ISBN: 978-7-117-10636-8/R · 10637

Cataloguing in Publication Data:
A catalog record for this book is available from the CIP-Database China.

Printed in The People's Republic of China

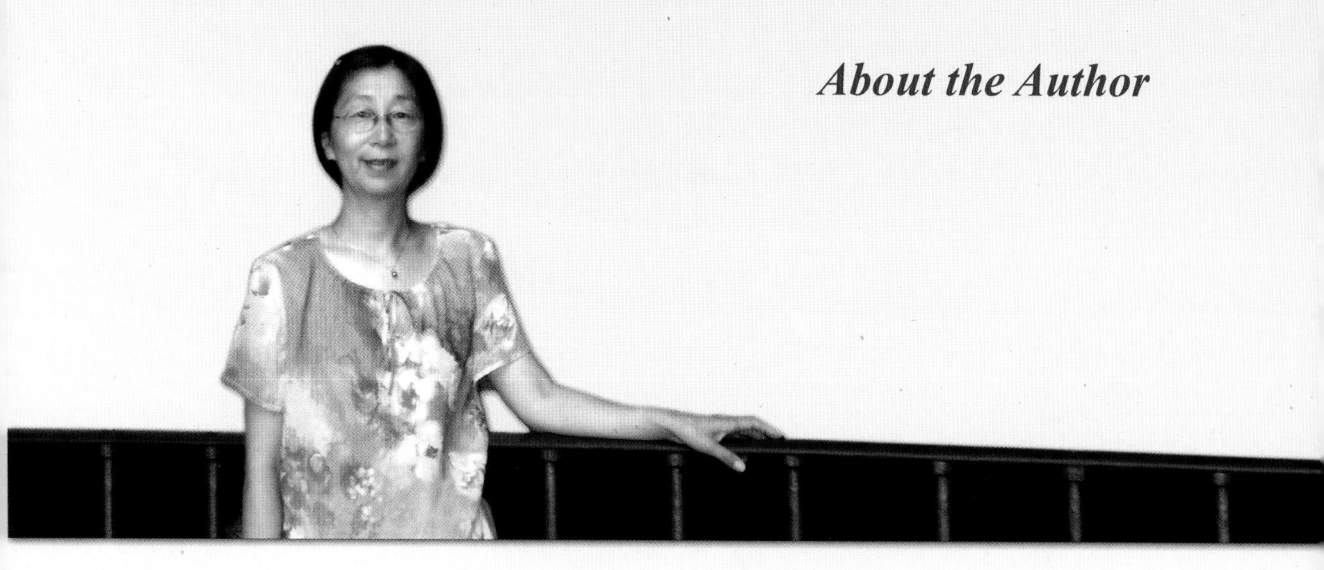

About the Author

Zhang Xue-li, a professor & chief physician of Acupuncture and Moxibustion Department of Dongzhimen Hospital Affiliated to Beijing University of Chinese Medicine. Professor Zhang is also an Honorary Professor of Chinese Medical Institute & and Register of London, England.

Dr. Zhang has 24 years of experience in clinical practice, teaching and research. She has taught students from over 40 countries and many diverse cultures. She specializes in treating facial paralysis, acne, chloasma, digestive disorders and chronic pain syndrome with acupuncture, plum blossom needles and timing acupuncture.

Dr. Zhang has taught acupuncture and moxibustion in the UK, Switzerland and Italy. She has published over 20 papers and 4 books.

DERMAL NEEDLING THERAPY
皮肤针疗法

Preface

Dermal needling is an external therapy used for palliative or treatment purposes by tapping on the surface of certain points or areas of the body with a dermal needle. It is frequently used in clinic and characterized by its extensive indication uses, conspicuous therapeutic efficacy, convenient operation, economics and safety, etc. With about 20 years' clinical experience, the author has taken the quintessential data from its masses and assembled various specialists' distillation of researches to compile this book—*Dermal Needling Therapy*.

This book is composed of two parts: Part 1 is about dermal needling and its principles of treatment, characteristics, operation, tapping areas, indications, management and precautions for abnormal occurrences during treatment. For the readers' convenience, it also supplies the locations of acupuncture points and their indications along with features of anatomy according to the fourteen channels. Part 2 gives an introduction to the principle of differentiating syndromes, treatment, point combination and point selection together with 86 common diseases in fields of internal medicine, external trauma and orthopedics, gynecology and pediatrics dermatology, and otolaryngology. Each disease includes such parts as overview, cause and mechanism of disease, types of syndrome and treatment. In the part about treatment principles, it introduces a variety of point combination to give the readers more choices in treatment planning. In order to avoid a wrong diagnosis, there is a specific reference section about differential diagnosis of commonly misinterpreted diseases. The theories of nurse support and early prevention of each disease are provided to help recover early.

The point combination without reference is all from the author's clinical experience, otherwise others footnoted. Although the author has done the best he can, there is possible editing errors and oversights. We hereby request our readers to contribute their suggestions and comments.

Zhang Xue-li & Liu Ying

Department of Acupuncture and Moxibustion,
Dongzhimen Hospital Affiliated to
Beijing University of Chinese Medicine
May 2008

Table of Contents

Part 1 The Outline

Chapter 4

Chapter 5

Part 2 The Clinical Practice

Chapter 1

Chapter 2

Treatment 112/

Part 1 The Outline

Chapter 1

An Introduction to the Dermal Needling Therapy

Dermal needling therapy is an important part of Chinese acupuncture. It is performed by the superficial insertion of several short needles put together to tap certain areas or points of the body to treat disorders. It is characterized by a wide scope of functions, evident curative effect, easy operation, cost effectiveness and safety of use. It plays an important role in the health care system.

Dermal needling derives from ancient techniques called "half needling", "surrounding shallow needling", and "skin needling," as recorded in *The Inner Classic* (*Nèi Jīng*, 内经). For example, in *The Treatise on Needle in Formal Use in Miraculous Pivot* (*Líng Shū · Guān Zhēn*, 灵枢 · 官针), it says, "*There are nine needling techniques applied to cope with nine different diseases…the seventh is named the 'shallow needling'.*" It also says, "*There are twelve needling techniques used for various diseases of the twelve main channels, …the fifth is the 'shallow needling', a method in which the needles are inserted to five spots with one in the center and the four scattered around it. It is applied to treat arthralgia due to superficial cold which involves a large area.*" This arrangement of the five needles is the core concept of dermal needling. *The Treatise on Essential Techniques of Needle Insertion in Basic Questions* (*Sù Wèn · Cì Yào Lùn*, 素问 · 刺要论) says, "*Since disease is located in superficial or deep portions, shallow or deep acupuncture can be applied. Each follows the rule-differed depth of needle .insertion for different conditions.*" *The Treatise on Needle in Formal Use in Miraculous Pivot* describes, "*There are five needling techniques used to treat diseases associated with the five zang organs. One is called 'half needling,' i.e. the swift and shallow insertion of a needle and immediate withdrawal of it without any injury to the muscle. It resembles the action of pulling out a single strand of hair.*" All of these records indicate that needling insertion techniques should be divided into superficial and deep types. As illustrated, the history of dermal needling originates from the aspect of an ancient superficial needling technique.

1. The Structure of the Dermal Needle

Since it only penetrates through the epidermis, the needle used in this technique is named the dermal needle. As *The Treatise on the Prescribed Depth of Needle Insertion in Basic Questions* (*Sù Wèn · Cì Qí Lùn*, 素问 · 刺齐论) says, "*The needle only pricks the skin and it doesn't injure the muscle.*" It has a hammer-like head fixed with short stainless steel needles. In the shape of a lotus, its handle is 15~19cm in length. It has a variety of names respective to the specific types of needles. The kind that is made of five needles arranged in the shape of plum blossom is called the plum blosom needle (see Fig. 1, Fig. 2, Fig. 3); the one composed of seven needles is known as the seven-star needle (see Fig. 4); the one with eighteen needles embedded in a bamboo stick is named the arhat needle. The latter type causes little pain in treatment in which children accept it willingly, so it is called the "child needle". If electricity is connected to a plum-blossom needle, it is called the electric plum blossom needle. Recently, there is a newly developed roller needle, which is a cylinder-shaped dermal needle. In general, all the types of needles mentioned above are different types of dermal needle.

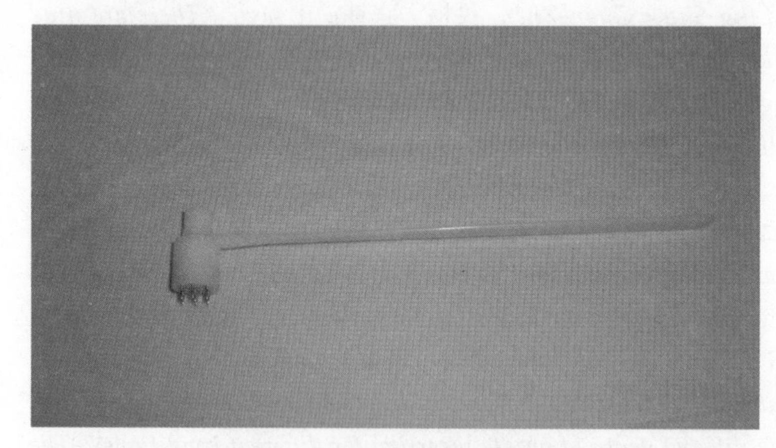

Fig. 1 Plum blossom needle (1)

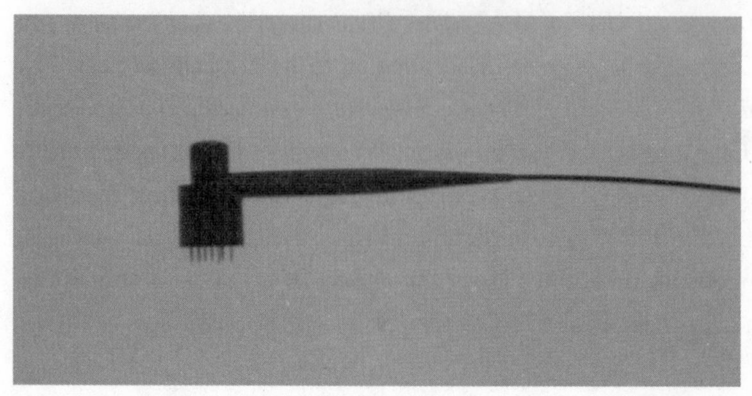

Fig. 2 Plum blossom needle (2)

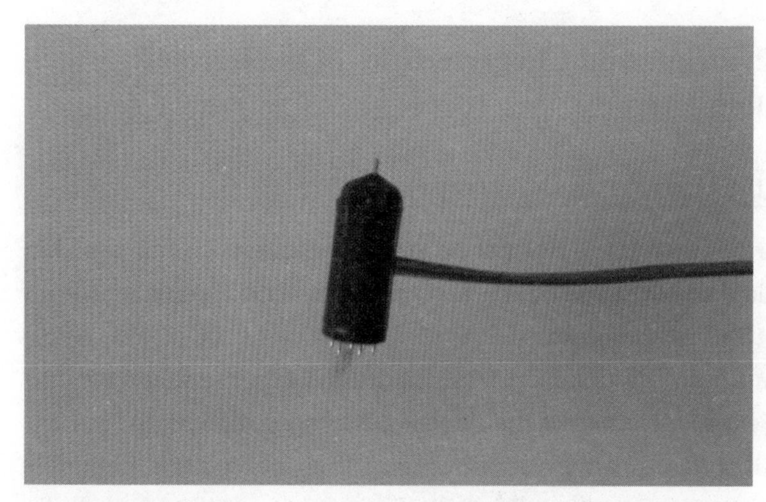

Fig. 3 Plum blossom needle (3)

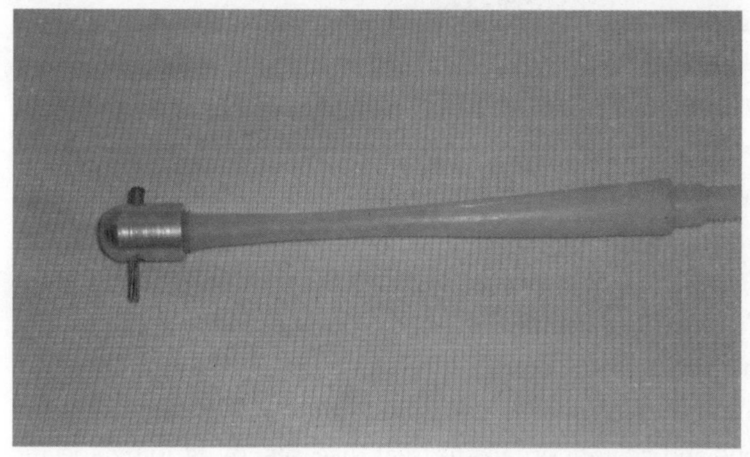

Fig. 4 Seven-star needle

2. Storage and Sterilization of the Dermal Needle

It is important to prevent the needle tip from getting rusted and hooked. To have a needle in good condition, the tip must not collide against hard surfaces. Dirt such as scab, scurf, etc. is adhered to the needle tip, so it must be thrown away or sterilized after each use. After sterilization, the needle should stay dry and bound with sterilized absorbent cotton and put in a dry place to prevent the needle tips from damage or getting rusty.

The dermal needle is usually soaked in 75% alcohol for sterilization for 30 minutes, or boiled in water, or put in an autoclave.

Section 1 The Principle and Characteristics of the Dermal Needling Therapy

1. The Principle of the Dermal Needle Therapy

The treatment principle for the dermal needle technique is to tap the skin to trigger and regulate the function of the *zang-fu* organs and channels. It is an approach to prevent and treat diseases.

The therapy is based on the philosophy of traditional Chinese medicine and its channel theory, especially that of the twelve cutaneous regions, which are the areas of the skin reflecting the functioning of the twelve main channels respectively. *The Treatise on Cutaneous Region in Basic Questions* (*Sù Wèn · Pí Bù Lùn*, 素问 · 皮部论) says "*Cutaneous regions are part of the twelve channels located in the superficial layers of the body. That is why they are attacked first by pathogenic factors. Thus, they are located at the most superficial part of the body with the responsibility for protecting the body.*" Invasion of the body by pathogenic factors begins from the skin and hair, subsequently affecting the *zang-fu* organs via the channels and collaterals. *The Collected Treatises of Zhang Jing-yue* (*JǐngYuè Quán Shū*, 景岳全书) says, "*Internal diseases may have manifestations on the exterior.*" Therefore, the cutaneous regions function to safeguard the body, resist exogenous pathogenic factors and reflect the diseased condition.

The dermal needling therapy makes use of the transmitting effect between the cutaneous regions and *zang-fu* organs to treat diseases. By tapping specific regions of the body, points or reaction spots, dermal needling eliminates disease, regulates the deficiency and excess conditions of the *zang-fu* organs to restore normal functioning, balancing yin and yang, and clearing the channels and collaterals to restore free flow of qi and blood.

2. The Characteristics of the Dermal Needling Therapy

(1) Wide Scope of Indications

Remarkable curative effect has been found in treatment of internal, external, gynecological, pediatric, ENT and dermal conditions. It can not only treat chronic but also acute diseases.

(2) Remarkable Curative Effect

It is not only effective to functional disorders, but also to some organic diseases. For some diseases there is a distinct curative effect within a short course of treatment. In addition, if the patient gets continuous treatment for some chronic diseases, good result is shown.

(3) Easy Operation

It is simple to learn how to perform the techniques of the dermal needling therapy, so it has been popular among doctors in different medical departments, upon the increasing number of patients who like this therapy. It is versatile in its uses such that people who are not knowledgeable of Chinese medicine use it to treat a variety of diseases, while those who have little medical knowledge can also use it for promotion of health.

(4) Economics and Safety

The use of a single needle during treatment, the simple structure of this instrument, its low cost and easy operation without complicated assistance allow for economic relief of the manufacturers and patients. Since the dermal needle only penetrates the epidermis and doesn't go deep into muscles, there is no risk in treatment. Even inexperienced beginners do not cause accidents as long as the manipulation is mild.

With the advantages mentioned above, the dermal needling therapy is popular among people and well received by acupuncturists. However, if it is a severe case, it alone cannot bring effect, so the addition of other interventions must be combined.

Section 2 Operation

1. Operation

The operation is divided into two types according to the needles chosen, ie. tapping and roller needling.

(1) Tapping

Sterilize the sites for tapping with 75% alcohol. One end of a sterilized dermal needle is held in the right hand of the operator, fixed in the small red and white skin of the palm with the ring finger and little finger. This end exposes 1~1.5cm. It is supported by the middle finger and thumb and the index finger extends straight, similar to stabilizing and keeping a gun down. Tap the skin repeatedly with the needles in a perpendicular angle to the skin. The elastic force of the wrist is used. When the needle tips touch the skin, immediately lift the needle. Aiming at the target, the intensity of tapping is even. The needle is swiftly lifted and one may hear "da, da," a clear and melodious sound during treatment. Different sites and stimulus intensity are selected according to the condition. The frequency of stimulation is usually 70~90 taps/min. (see Fig. 5~Fig. 13)

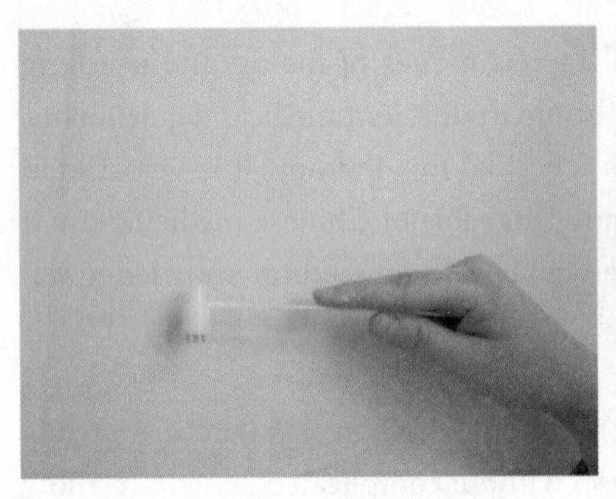

Fig. 5 Posture of holding the needle (1)

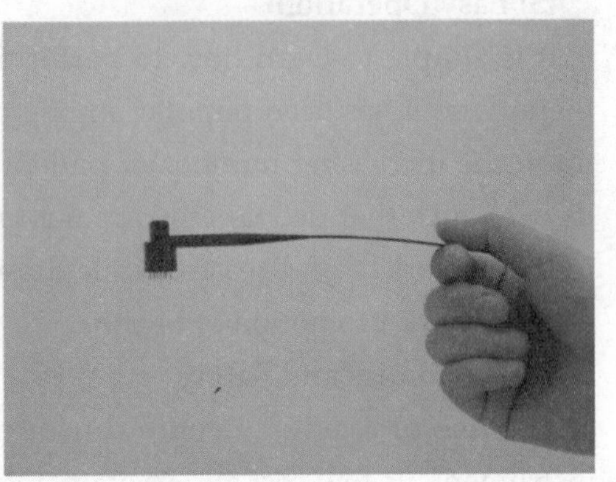

Fig. 6 Posture of holding the needle (2)

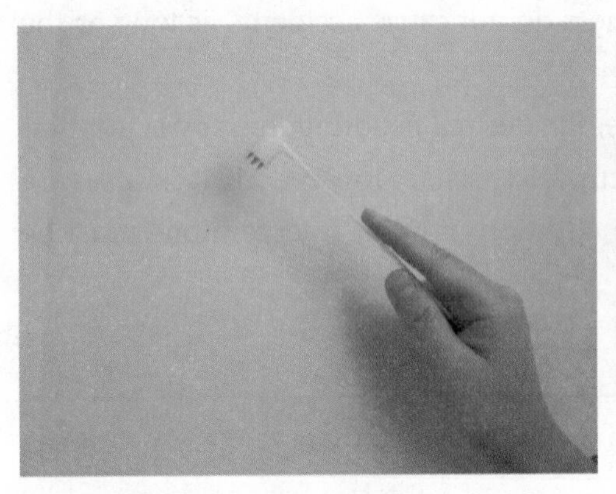

Fig. 7 Tapping process (1)-a

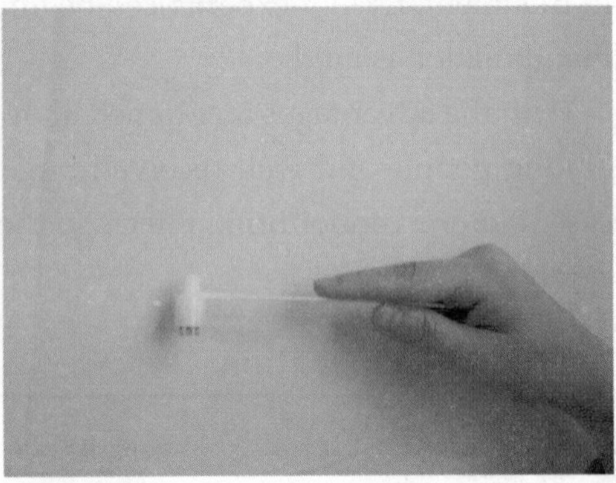

Fig.8 Tapping process (1)-b

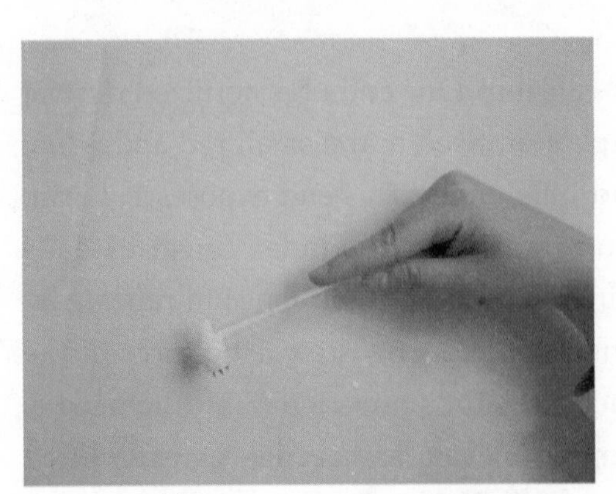

Fig. 9 Tapping process (1)-c

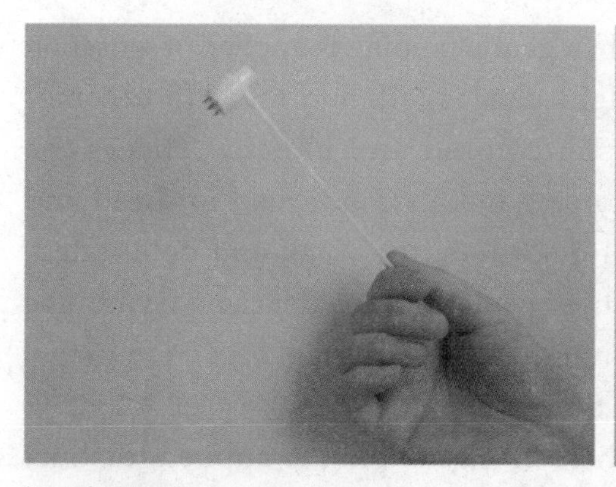

Fig. 10 Tapping process (2)-a

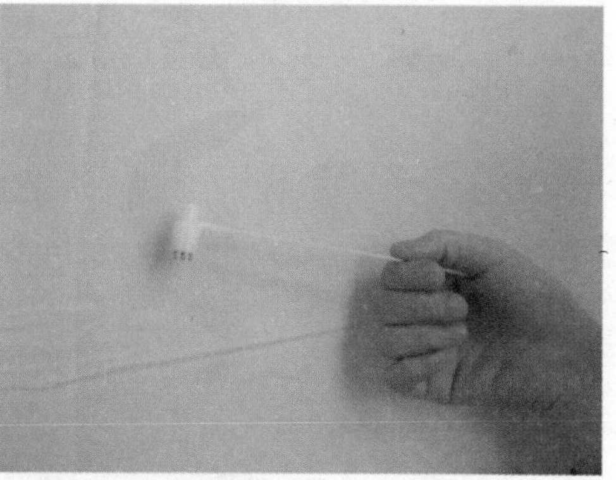

Fig. 11 Tapping process (2)-b

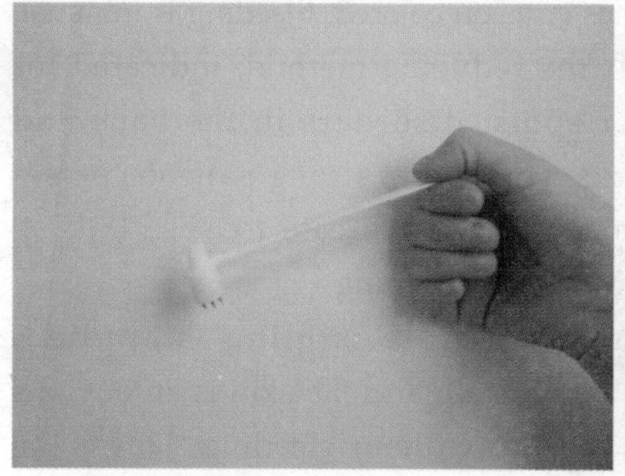

Fig. 12 Tapping process (2)-c

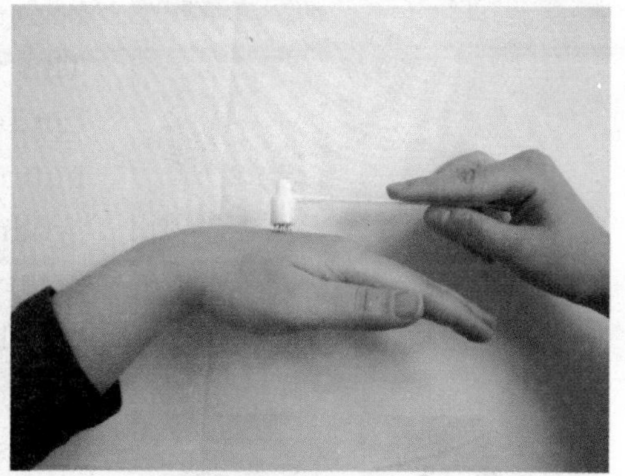

Fig. 13 The angle (90°) formed by the needle and the surface of skin

Pain or bleeding may occur if one of these incidents happens: the elastic force of the wrist is failed to use, the needle tips are not perpendicular to the skin, the needle is lifted slowly, or use hooked needle tips.

(2) Roller Needling

It is a specifically made device in the shape of a cylinder. After sterilization with 75% alcohol, hold the handle and make it roll back and forth on the body. A long and narrow surface or a patch of skin is stimulated.

2. Stimulus-Intensity and Course of Treatment

The stimulus-intensity is decided by the disease and health condition of the patient and the site to be treated. In general, it is usually performed in gentle, moderate and strong manipulations. It uses the fundamental concepts of the reinforcing and reducing methods. In most cases, gentle tapping is the reinforcing method, strong tapping is the reducing method and moderate tapping is the even method.

(1) Gentle Tapping

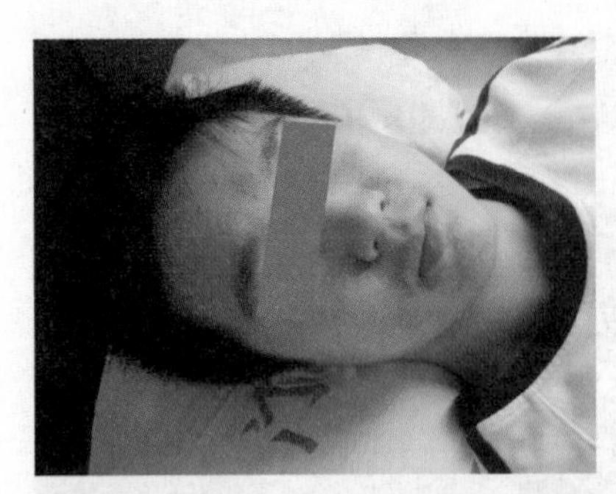
Fig. 14 Gentle tapping (right lips)

When gentle tapping is applied, a sensation of slight pain is felt, and the skin becomes crimson colored and blotchy. This is the reinforcing method, indicated for head and facial disorders, the weak and debilitated, geriatrics, pediatrics, and deficiency syndrome or chronic diseases. (see Fig. 14)

(2) Strong Tapping

When strong tapping is applied, distinct pain is felt, but it is tolerable, and the skin becomes crimson colored. Bleeding is minimal. This is the reducing method, indicated for tender spots, disorders in the back and buttocks, young and strong patients, excess syndrome and acute disease. (see Fig. 15)

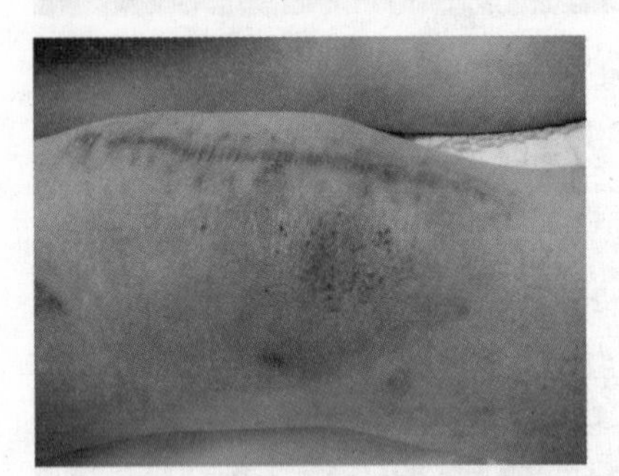
Fig. 15 Strong tapping (right knee)

(3) Moderate Tapping

When moderate tapping is applied, slight pain is felt, and the skin is an obvious crimson color without bleeding. This is the even method, indicated for mild conditions. In addition, the pain threshold should be concerned when the extent of stimulus-intensity is chosen. Proper regulation is applied based on the patient's dullness of the skin. (see Fig. 16)

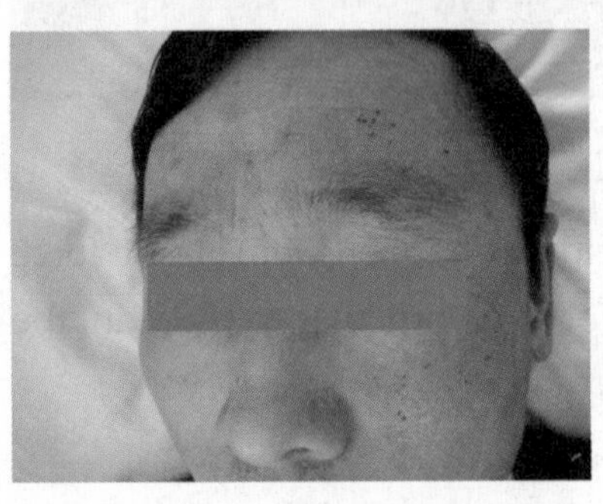
Fig. 16 Moderate tapping (left forehead and cheek)

Treatment is given once a day or every other day, 10 treatments make one course, and there is an interval of 3~5 days between each course of treatment if resumed.

Section 3 Sites for Tapping

According to the theory of channels, there are three modes of tapping: tapping in line with corresponding channels, point tapping and tropical tapping. Tapping can also be applied to both sides of the vertebral column in light of the neural segment domination.

1. Tapping in Line with Corresponding Channels

It is usually applied to the limbs where the twelve main channels pass, nape, back and lumbo-sacral region where the *DU* Vessel and Bladder Channel of Foot *Taiyang* pass. Since the twelve main channels connect with the *zang-fu* organs internally and externally with the limbs, skeleton, five sense organs and nine orifices, the coordination of the human body is harmonized. Obvious pathologic changes in the passageway of the channels occur in a disease state. The dermal needling therapy performed along the traveling course of channels regulates the *zang-fu* organs and clears channels as the *zang-fu* organs, channels and collaterals and skin are closely related. The *Du* Vessel described as "the sea of the yang channels" can regulate yang qi of the whole body, and the Back-*Shu* points all distribute on the first line of the Bladder Channel on the back. Thus, various disorders are treated when it is applied to the posterior *Du* Vessel and Bladder Channel.

2. Point Tapping

It is based on the therapeutic effect of points. Clinically, the following specific points are selected, i.e. extra points like EX-B2 (*huá tuó jiá jǐ*) and *ashi* points. The *yuan*-source points, the *luo*-connecting points, the *xi*-cleft points are distributed on the channels superior to the elbow and knee. They are used to treat disorders related to the corresponding *zang-fu* organs, channels and collaterals. The selection of points is according to the following principles:

(1) Local Point Selection

It refers to the selection of points directly in the diseased areas or adjacent spots. For example, LI 20 (*yíng xiāng*) is selected for nose disorders, ST 6 (*jiá chē*) and ST 4 (*dì cāng*) for deviation of the mouth, RN 12 (*zhōng wǎn*) and ST 21 (*liáng mén*) for stomachache, EX-LE5 (*xī yǎn*) for knee pain. Tapping is also applied to the tender spots or positive reactive spots known as the "*ashi* points".

(2) Distal Point Selection

It refers to points selected far from the diseased area or points located below the elbow and knee. But they are on the traveling course of the related channels. For instance, LI 4 (*hé gǔ*), ST 44 (*nèi tíng*) are selected for toothache, LU 5 (*chǐ zé*) for cough, ST 36 (*zú sān lǐ*) for stomachache, and BL 40 (*wěi zhōng*) for pain in the lower back. In practice, points on paired channels or other related channels can be selected. For example, ST 36 (*zú sān lǐ*) or SP 4 (*gōng sūn*) is selected in the treatment of stomachache.

(3) Selection of Points according to Syndromes

It refers to selection of points according to symptoms or cause of disease and mechanism, known as empirical points. For instance, DU 14 (*dà zhuī*) is selected for high fever, DU 26 (*shuǐ gōu*) for coma, HT 6 (*yīn xì*) and KI 3 (*tài xī*) for night sweating. For diseases due to disorder of qi movement, RN 17 (*dàn zhōng*) and RN 6 (*qì hǎi*) are selected. SP 10 (*xuè hǎi*), BL 17 (*gé shù*) are selected in blood disorders.

The above points can be used alone or in combination. For example, RN 17 (*dàn zhōng*), LU 1 (*zhōng fǔ*), LU 5 (*chǐ zé*), LU 7 (*liè quē*) are selected for asthma of the excess type. Among them, LU 1 (*zhōng fǔ*) is an adjacent point, LU 5 (*chǐ zé*) and LU 7 (*liè quē*) are distant point, while RN 17 (*dàn zhōng*) is selected according to syndromes.

(4) Selection of Points according to Modern Medical Theory

Modern anatomical knowledge is often used in the selection of points, eg selection of the extra points of EX-B2 (*huá tuó jiá jǐ*). They are the correspondent spots to segmental distribution of nerves, so they are selected for head and facial disorders. EX-B2 (*huá tuó jiá jǐ*) points located between C5 and T8 are selected for disorders of the respiratory and cardiovascular systems or upper limbs, and those between T6 and L5 are used for digestive diseases, and extra points EX-B2 (*huá tuó jiá jǐ*) points between L1 and S2 are used for urinary diseases or conditions of the lower limbs.

3. Local Tapping

It refers to tapping applied to the diseased area. For instance, round or scattered tapping is applied to the red swelling and painful place due to sprain or obstinate tinea. Tapping is also applied to the skin lesion in dermal disease.

Chapter 2

Indications and Precautions

Section 1 Indications

Dermal needling is widely used among a variety of indications such as hypertension, headache, migraine, facial and peripheral neuroparalysis, stomachache, abdominal pain, neurosthenia, cough, asthmatic bronchitis, menstrual irregularities, dysfunctional uterine bleeding, climacteric syndrome, pediatric indigestion, enuresis, pediatric cerebral palsy, acute mastitis, varicosity, folliculitis, stiff neck,Ganglionic Cyst, tennis elbow, alopecia, nervous dermatitis, acne, rhinitis, toothache, myopia, stye, etc., resulting in good outcomes.

Section 2 Precautions

Although it is safe in treatment, bear in mind the following key notes.

1. Check the needles frequently to see if the needle tips are hooked or rusted, or if the shaft is smooth. Always have the needles sterilized and the operator's hands washed thoroughly before practice.

2. Gentle and vertical tapping is given to lessen the pain. No bleeding is caused. In addition, a proper sequence and direction should be maintained.

3. If there is ulceration or trauma on the skin, do not use this therapy, along with cases due to acute infectious diseases and acute abdomen disorders.

4. If localized minimal bleeding is called for, it is essential to give strict sterilization, and the interval between treatments is properly prolonged to keep away infection.

5. When the roller needling is used, one must check to see if the roller is moving freely. Do not apply it along the border of the bone in order to avoid pain or bleeding.

Chapter 3

Management and Prevention of Accidents

Although it is safe, some accidents may occur in treatment if the operator is careless, or has a lack of anatomical knowledge, or fails to see the particularities of patients. Once an accident happens, the practitioner should properly handle the problem or patients may suffer from the therapy. Therefore, it is necessary to prevent accidents from happening at any given time.

Section 1 Syncope during Acupuncture

Cause: It is usually seen in patients who receive this therapy for the first time often due to nervous tension, general debilities, fatigue, hunger, too many stimulated points, or too strong manipulations.

Manifestations: Patients suddenly suffer from dizziness, vertigo, pallor, nausea, vomiting, palpitations, shortness of breath, cold sweating. In severe cases, there may be cold limbs, drop of blood pressure, thready pulse and even loss of consciousness.

Management: Cease treatment immediately, and ask the patients to lie flat, lower his head, loosen his clothes and keep warm. For mild cases, give him some hot tea, warm or sugar water. Usually spontaneous recovery is seen. For severe cases, besides the above management, acupressure is applied to DU 26 (*shuǐ gōu*), LI 4 (*hé gǔ*) or ST 36 (*zú sān lǐ*).

Prevention: For those who receive this therapy for the first time or are mental stress, it is imperative to reason him out of his fears and tension. For first-time sensitive patients, do not tap too forcefully and avoid stimulate sensitive parts. For hungry or over-tired patients, advise them to take food or restore their health first before starting the therapy.

Section 2 Hematoma

A hematoma is subdermal bleeding in the local area resulting from an injury to the bigger blood vessels as a result of tapping. Initially, there is swelling with distending pain, followed by appearance of skin discoloration in the localized area. It is unnecessary to manage this kind of bruise since it is due to minimal capillary bleeding. If there is severe painful swelling and the discoloration is larger, a cold compress is applied first, followed by hot compress 24~48 hours later to propel the dissipation and absorption of the local congestion.

Section 3 Allergic Reaction to the Skin

Some patients may have small skin irritation like pimples and itching in the treating area as a result of dermal needling. It is unnecessary to deal with it if the symptoms are mild, considering these are normal and distinctive reactions upon successive treatments. If there are hives with severe itching, cease treatment, and apply some hormonal ointment to the affected skin.

Section 4 Pneumatothorax

Generally speaking, the dermal needling therapy is safe, but there are reports about pneuomothorax in cases of application to the back of the body after an emphysema condition. This is possibly due to rupture and fusion of the alveolar wall which is very thin, resulting from strong tapping. Although such accidents are seldom seen, it deserves a great deal of concern to avoid unnecessary sufferings. Gentle tapping is applied to the back of a patient with emphysema to ensure that no pneuomothorax occurs.

Chapter 4

The Points of the Fourteen Channels

Section 1 The Lung Channel of Hand *Taiyin*

1. LU 1 (*zhōng fŭ*) Front-*Mu* Point

[Location] In the superior lateral part of the anterior thoracic wall, 1 *cun* below LU 2 (*yún mén*), on the level of the 1st intercostal space, 6 *cun* lateral to the anterior midline.

[Anatomy]

(1) Layer of needling: Skin-subcutaneous tissue-greater pectoral muscle-smaller pectoral muscle-short head of the biceps brachii muscle-coracobrachial muscle.

(2) Innervation and vasculature: In the superficial layer, there are the cephalic vein, intermediate supraclavicular nerve, lateral cutaneous branches of the 1st intercostal nerve. In the deeper layer, there are the medial branches of the anterior thoracic nerves, the thoracoacromial artery and vein, the medial and lateral thoracic artery.

[Indications] Cough, shortness of breath, distending pain and fullness in the chest, shoulder and back pain.

[Operation] Puncture obliquely 0.5~0.8 *cun*. Never puncture deeply to prevent injury to the lung.

2. LU 4 (*xiá bái*)

[Location] On the medial side of the upper arm and on the radial border of the biceps brachii muscle, 4 *cun* below the anterior end of the axillary fold, or 5 *cun* above the cubital crease.

[Anatomy]

(1) Layer of needling: Skin-subcutaneous tissue-long head of the muscle-brachial muscle.

(2) Innervation and vasculature: In the superficial layer, there are the cephalic vein and the lateral brachial cutaneous nerve. In the deeper layer, there are the musculocutaneous nerve and the brachial artery.

[Indications] Cough, shortness of breath, dry vomiting, fullness in the chest, pain in the medial part of the upper arm.

[Operation] Puncture perpendicularly 0.5~1 *cun*.

3. **LU 5 (*chǐ zé*)** *He*-Sea Point

[Location] In the cubital crease, in the depression of the radial side of the tendon of the biceps brachii muscle.

[Anatomy]

(1) Layer of needling: Skin-subcutaneous tissue-brachioradial muscle-brachial muscle.

(2) Innervation and vasculature: In the superficial layer, there are the lateral cutaneous nerves of the forearm. In the deeper layer, there are the radial nerve trunk, deep branches of the radial nerves, the muscular branches of the musculocutaneous nerves, the anterior branches of the radial collateral artery (the branches of the deep brachial artery).

[Indications] Cough, shortness of breath, hemoptysis, hectic fever, sore throat, distension and fullness in the chest, infantile convulsion, vomiting and diarrhea, spasmodic pain in the elbow and arm.

[Operation] Puncture perpendicularly 0.8~1.2 *cun*, or prick to bleed.

4. **LU 6 (*kǒng zuì*)** *Xi*-Cleft Point

[Location] On the radial side of the palmar surface of the forearm and on the line connecting LU 5 (*chǐ zé*) and LU 9 (*tài yuān*), 7 *cun* above the cubital crease.

[Anatomy]

(1) Layer of needling: Skin-subcutaneous tissue-branchioradial muscle-radial flexor muscle of the wrist-round pronator muscle-long flexor muscle of the thumb.

(2) Innervation and vasculation: In the superficial layer, there are the cephalic vein and the lateral cutaneous nerve of the forearm. In the deep layer there are the superficial branches of the radial artery, the medial nerve muscle branches, the deep branches of the radial artery and the radial recurrent artery.

[Indications] Cough, shortness of breath, hemoptysis, sore throat, spasmodic pain in the elbow and arm, hemorrhoids.

[Operation] Puncture perpendicularly 0.5~1.2 *cun*.

5. **LU 7 (*liè quē*)** *Luo*-Connecting Point; Confluent Point That Links the *Ren* Vessel

[Location] On the radial side of the forearm, proximal to the styloid process of the radius, 1.5 *cun* above the cubital crease, between the brachioradial muscle and the long abductor muscule of the thumb.

[Anatomy]

(1) Layer of needling: Skin-subcutaneous tissue-long abductor muscle of the thumb-tendon of the brachioradial muscle-quadrate pronator muscle.

(2) **Innervation and vasculature:** In the superficial layer, there are the lateral cutaneous nerve of the forearm and the superficial branches of the radial nerve. In the deep layer, there are the deep branches of the radial artery, the muscular branches of the median nerve and radial artery.

[Indications] Cough, shortness of breath, sore throat, hemiplegia, deviation of the eye and mouth, migraine, pain and stiffness in the neck, toothache.

[Operation] Puncture superiorly or inferiorly and obliquely 0.3~0.8 *cun*.

6. LU 8 (*jīng qú*) *Jing*-River Point

[Location] On the radial side of the palmer surface of the forarm, in the depression between the radial artery and the styloid process of the radius, 1 *cun* above the cubital crease.

[Anatomy]

(1) **Layer of needling:** Skin-subcutaneous tissue-between the radial flexor muscle of the wrist and the long abductor muscle of the thumb-quardrate pronator muscle.

(2) **Innervation and vasculature:** In the superficial layer, there is the lateral cutaneous nerve of the forearm. In the deep layer, there are the muscular branches of the median nerve, the deep branches of the radial nerve and the radial artery.

[Indications] Cough, shortness of breath, sore throat, wrist and hand pain.

[Operation] Puncture perpendicularly 0.3~0.5 *cun*.

7. LU 9 (*tài yuān*) *Shu*-Stream Point; *Yuan*-Source Point; Influential Point

[Location] At the radial end of the transverse crease of the wrist, where the pulsation of the radial artery is palpable.

[Anatomy]

(1) **Layer of needling:** Skin-subcutaneous tissue-between the radial flexor muscle or the wrist and the long abductor muscle of the thumb.

(2) **Innervation and vasculature:** In the superficial layer, there are the lateral cutaneous nerve of the forearm. In the deep layer, there are the radial artery and vein, the muscular branches of the medial nerve and the branches of the radial nerve.

[Indications] Cough, shortness of breath, hemoptysis, chest pain, sore throat, absence of pulse, pain in the wrist.

[Operation] Avoid the radial artery. Puncture perpendicularly 0.3~0.5 *cun*.

8. LU 10 (*yú jì*) *Ying*-Spring Point

[Location] In the depression proximal to the 1st metacarpophalangeal joint, on the radial side of the midpoint of the 1st metacarpal bone and on the junction of the red-white boundary of the hand.

[Anatomy]

(1) Layer of needling: Skin-subcutaneous tissue-short abductor muscle of the thumb-opponens muscle of the thumb-short flexor muscle of the thumb.

(2) Innervation and vasculature: In the superficial layer, there are the cutaneous branches of the median nerve and the superficial branches of the radial nerve. In the deeper layer, there are the muscular branches of the median and ulnar nerves, the muscular branches of the ulnar nerve and the main arteries of the thumb.

[Indications] Cough, hemoptysis, fever, painful and swollen throat and pharynx, aphonia, mammary pain, heat in the center of the palm.

[Operation] Puncture perpendicularly 0.5~1 *cun*.

9. LU 11 (*shào shāng*) *Jing*-Well Point

[Location] On the radial side of the distal segment of the thumb, 0.1 *cun* from the corner of the finger nail.

[Anatomy]

(1) Layer of needling: Skin-subcutaneous tissue.

(2) Innervation and vasculature: There are the superficial branches of the radial nerve, the dorsal digital branches of the proper palmar digital nerve (branches of the median nerve) and the main arteries of the thumb.

[Indications] Sore throat, apoplectic coma, vomiting due to summer heat, infantile convulsion, mania, cough, epistaxis.

[Operation] Puncture perpendicularly 0.1 *cun*, or 0.2~0.3 *cun* horizontally towards the wrist.

Section 2 The Large Intestine Channel of Hand *Yangming*

1. LI 1 (*shāng yáng*) *Jing*-Well Point

[Location] On the radial side of the distal segment of the index finger, 0.1 *cun* from the corner of the finger nail.

[Anatomy]

(1) Layer of needling: Skin-subcutaneous tissue.

(2) Innervation and vasculatur: There are the dorsal digital branches of the proper palmar digital nerve and the dorsal metacarpal artery.

[Indications] Sore throat, tinnitus and deafness, apoplexy, coma, absence of sweating in febrile diseases, toothache, bluish blindness.

[Operation] Puncture 0.1 *cun*.

2. LI 2 (*èr jiān*) *Ying*-Spring Point

[Location] In the depression of the radial side, distal to the 2nd metacarpophalangeal joint when a loose fist is made.

[Anatomy]

(1) Layer of needing: Skin-subcutaneous tissue-lumbrical muscle tendon.

(2) Innervation and vasculature: In the superficial layer, there are the dorsal digital nerve of the radial nerve,the proper palmar digital nerve of the median nerve, and the dorsal digital artery.

[Indications] Toothache, sore throat, deviation of the eye and mouth, eye pain, febrile disease.

[Operation] Puncture perpendicularly 0.2~0.4 *cun*.

3. LI 4 (*hé gŭ*) *Yuan*-Source Point

[Location] On the back of the hand, between the 1st and 2nd metacarpal bones and on the radial side of the midpoint of the 2nd metacarpal bone.

[Anatomy]

(1) Layer of needling: Skin-subcutaneous tissue-1st dorsal interosseous muscle-abductor muscle of the thumb.

(2) Innervation and vasculature: In the superficial layer, there are the branches of the radial nerve, the dorsal vein network of the hand and the dorsal metacarpal artery. In the deep layer, there are the deep branches of the ulnar nerve and the radial artery of the index finger.

[Indications] Headache, toothache, painful conjunctival congestion, sore throat, aphonia, deviation of the eye and mouth, hemiplegia, mumps, furuncle, amenorrhea, abdominal pain, lockjaw, infantile convulsion, epistaxis, tinnitus and deafness, fever with chills, absence of sweating, profuse sweating, hives, malaria.

[Operation] Puncture perpendicularly 0.5~1 *cun*.

4. LI 5 (*yáng xī*) *Jing*-River Point

[Location] On the radial side of the crease of the wrist, in the depression between the short extensor and long extensor muscles of the thumb when it is tilted upward.

[Anatomy]

(1) Layer of needling: Skin-subcutaneous tissue-extensor retinaculum of the hand, (between the short and long extensor muscles of the thumb).

(2) Innervation and vasculature: In the superficial layer, there are the branches of the superficial branches of the radial nerve and the cephalic vein. In the deep layer, there are the posterior interosseous nerve and artery.

[Indications] Headache, tinnitus and deafness, sore throat, wrist and hand pain, toothache.

[Operation] Puncture perpendicularly 0.5~0.8 *cun*.

5. LI 6 (*piān lì*) *Luo*-Connecting Point

[Location] When the elbow is flexed, on the radial side of the dorsal surface of the forearm and on the line linking LI 5 (*yáng xī*) and LI 11 (*qū chí*), 3 *cun* above the crease of the wrist.

[Anatomy]

(1) Layer of needling: Skin-subcutaneous tissue-short extensor muscle of the thumb-long radial extensor muscle of the wrist-long abductor muscle of the thumb.

(2) Innervation and vasculature: In the superficial layer, there are the lateral cutaneous nerve of the forearm and the superficial branches of the radial nerve and the cephalic vein. In the deep layer, there are the muscular branches of the radial nerve and radial artery.

[Indications] Tinnitus, deafness, conjunctival congestion, epistaxis, painful throat, aching pain in the arm.

[Operation] Puncture perpendicularly 0.3~0.5 *cun* or obliquely 1 *cun*.

6. LI 10 (*shǒu sān lǐ*)

[Location] On the radial side of the dorsal surface of the forearms and on the line linking LI 5 (*yáng xī*) and LI 11 (*qū chí*), 2 *cun* below the elbow.

[Anatomy]

(1) Layer of needling: Skin-subcutaneous tissue-long radial extensor muscle of the wrist-short radial extensor muscle of the wrist-supinator muscle.

(2) Innervation and vasculature: In the superficial layer, there are the lateral cutaneous nerves of the forearm. In the deep layer, there are the branches of the radial nerve, the muscular branches of the radial nerve and radial recurrent artery.

[Indications] Elbow pain, paralysis and numbness of the upper limbs, abdominal pain, diarrhea, abdominal distension, toothache, aphonia.

[Operation] Puncture perpendicularly 0.8~1.2 *cun*.

7. LI 11 (*qū chí*) *He*-Sea Point

[Location] At the lateral end of the cubital crease, and with the elbow flexed, at the midpoint of the line linking LU 5 (*chǐ zé*) and the external humeral epicondyle.

[Anatomy]

(1) Layer of needling: Skin-subcutaneous tissue-long radial extensor muscle of the wrist and short radial extensor muscle of the wrist-brachioradial muscle-

anconeus muscle.

(2) Innervation and vasculature: In the superficial layer, there is the posterior cutaneous. nerve of the forearm. In the deep layer, there are the radial nerve trunk and the muscular branches of the radial nerve and the muscular cutaneous nerve, radial collateral artery (deep branches of the humeral artery) and the radial recurrent artery.

[Indications] Febrile disease, hemiplegia, rubella, pain, swelling and weakness of the upper limbs, sore throat, toothache, painful conjunctival congestion, abdominal pain with vomiting and diarrhea, dysentery, hypertension, scrofula, mania.

[Operation] Puncture perpendicularly 1~1.5 *cun.*

8. LI 12 (*zhǒu liáo*)

[Location] With the elbow flexed,on the lateral side of the upper arm, 1 *cun* above LI 11 (*qū chí*), on the border of the humerus.

[Anatomy]

(1) Layer of needling: Skin-subcutaneous tissue-brachioradial muscle-brachial triceps muscle.

(2) Innervation and vasculature: In the superficial layer, there is the posterior cutaneous nerve of the forearm. In the deep layer, there are the muscular branches of the radial nerve and deep humeral artery.

[Indications] Pain, numbness and contracture in the elbow and arm, somnolence.

[Operation] Puncture perpendicularly 0.5~1 *cun.*

9. LI 14 (*bì nào*)

[Location] On the lateral side of the upper arm, at the insertion of the deltoid muscle and on the line linking LI 11 (*qū chí*) and LI 15 (*jiān yú*), 7 *cun* above LI 11 (*qū chí*).

[Anatomy]

(1) Layer of needling: Skin-subcutaneous tissue-deltoid muscle.

(2) Innervation and vasculature: In the superficial layer, there are the lateral cutaneous nerve of the arm and posterior cutaneous nerve of the arm. In the deep layer, there are the muscular branches of the axillary nerve and the thoracoacromial artery.

[Indications] Scrofula, painful shoulder and arm, eye disease, muscular contracture of the neck.

[Operation] Puncture perpendicularly 0.8~1.5 *cun* or superiorly and obliquely 0.8~1.5 *cun.*

10. LI 15 (*jiān yú*)

[Location] On the shoulder, superior to the deltoid muscle, in the depression anterior and inferior to the acromion when the arm is abduced or stretched on the level of the shoulder.

[Anatomy]

(1) Layer of needling: Skin-subcutaneous tissue-deltoid muscle-subdeltoid bursa-suprapinous muscle.

(2) Innervation and vasculature: In the superficial layer, there are the lateral branches of the supraclavicular nerve and the muscular branches of the cutaneous axillary nerve. In the deep layer, there are the muscular branches of the axillary nerve, thoracoacromial artery and supinator humeral artery.

[Indications] Painful shoulder and arm, hemiplegia, contracture of the elbow and arm, hives, scrofula.

[Operation] Puncture perpendicularly 0.8~1.5 *cun* or inferiorly and obliquely 0.8~1.5 *cun*.

11. LI 16 (*jù gŭ*)

[Location] On the shoulder, in the depression between the scapular extremity of the clavical and the spine of the scapula.

[Anatomy]

(1) Layer of needling: Skin-subcutaneous tissue-clavicular ligament-tendon of the supraspinatus muscle.

(2) Innervation and vasculature: In the superficial layer, there are the lateral branches of the supraclavicular nerve. In the deep layer, there are the suprascapular nerve and artery.

[Indications] Pain in the shoulder, back and the upper arm, motor impairment of the upper limbs, scrofula, goiter.

[Operation] Puncture perpendicularly 0.4~0.6 *cun*. Never puncture deeply to prevent injury to the lung and trigger pneumatothorax.

12. LI 19 (*kŏu hé liáo*)

[Location] On the upper lip, just below the lateral border of the nostril, on the level of DU 26 (*shuĭ gōu*)

[Anatomy]

(1) Layer of needling: Skin-subcutaneous tissue-orbicular muscle of the mouth.

(2) Innervation and vasculature: In the superficial layer, there is the infraorbital nerve (branches of the axillary nerve). In the deep layer, there are the facial nerve and the artery of the upper lip (branches of the facial nerve).

[Indications] Stuffy mouth and nose, epistaxis.

[Operation] Puncture perpendicularly 0.5~0.8 *cun.*

13. LI 20 (*yíng xiāng*)

[Location] Between the naso-labial groove, at the midpoint of the outer border of the nasal ala, just in the naso-labial groove.

[Anatomy]

(1) Layer of needling: Skin-subcutaneous tissue-levator muscle of the upper lip.

(2) Innervation and vasculature: In the superficial layer, there is the infraorbital nerve. In the deep layer, there are the buccal and zygomatic branches of the facial nerve and the facial artery.

[Indications] Stuffy nose, mouth bleeding, epistaxis, face itching, nasal polyp.

[Operation] Puncture perpendicularly 0.2~0.5 *cun* or superiorly and obliquely 0.2~0.5 *cun*.

Section 3 The Stomach Channel of Foot *Yangming*

1. ST 1 (*chéng qì*)

[Location] On the face, directly below the pupil, between the eyeball and the infraorbital ridge.

[Anatomy]

(1) Layer of needling: Skin-subcutaneous tissue-orbicular muscle of the eye-intraorbital inferior straight and oblique muscles.

(2) Innervation and vasculature: In the superficial layer, there is the infraorbital nerve. In the deep layer, there are the zygomatic branches of the facial nerve and infraorbital artery. In the orbit there are the ophthalmic nerve and ophthalmic artery.

[Indications] Twitching of eyelid, epistaxis, toothache, painful face.

[Operation] Puncture perpendicularly 0.3~0.7 *cun* along the infraorbital ridge. It is advisable to insert the needle slowly and never do the lifting and thrusting manipulations to prevent injury to the blood vessels and induce intraorbital bleeding.

2. ST 2 (*sì bái*)

[Location] On the face, directly below the pupil, in the depression of the infraorbital foramen.

[Anatomy]

(1) Layer of needling: Skin-subcutaneous tissue-orbicular muscle of the eye, levator muscle of the upper lip-infraorbital foramen.

(2) Innervation and vasculature: In the superficial layer, there is the infraorbital nerve. In the deep layer,there are the infraorbital nerve and artery, and the branches of the zygomatic nerve.

[Indications] Painful conjunctival congestion, cloudiness of the cornea, twitching of the eyelid, tears running irritated by wind, headache and painful face, deviation of the eye and mouth.

[Operation] Puncture perpendicularly 0.2~0.4 *cun.*

3. ST 3 (*jù liáo*)

[Location] On the face, directly below the pupil, on the level of the lower end of the nasal ala, beside the nasolabial groove.

[Anatomy]

(1) Layer of needling: Skin-subcutaneous tissue-levator muscle of the upper lip.

(2) Innervation and vasculature: In the superficial layer, there is the infraorbital nerve. In the deep layer, there are the buccal branches of the facial nerve and facial artery.

[Indications] Deviation of the eye and mouth, twitching of the eyelid, epistaxis, toothache, painful face.

[Operation] Puncture perpendicularly 0.3~0.6 *cun.*

4. ST 4 (*dì cāng*)

[Location] On the face, beside the mouth corner, directly below the pupil.

[Anatomy]

(1) Layer of needling: Skin-subcutaneous tissue-orbicular muscle of the mouth-buccal muscle.

(2) Innervation and vasculature: In the superficial layer, there are the infraorbital nerve and mental nerve (branches of the mandible nerve). In the deep layer, there are the buccal branch of the facial nerve and facial artery.

[Indications] Deviation of the eye and mouth, tic of the mouth corner, toothache, tears running, unclosed mouth.

[Operation] Puncture horizontally 0.5~1 *cun* towards ST 6 (*jiá chē*).

5. ST 6 (*jiá chē*)

[Location] On the cheek, one (middle) finger breadth anterior and superior to the mandibular angle, in the depression when the masseter muscle is prominent on chewing.

[Anatomy]

(1) Layer of needling: Skin-subcutaneous tissue-risorius muscle-masseter muscle.

(2) Innervation and vasculature: In the superficial layer, there is the great auricular nerve (branch of the mandibular nerve). In the deep layer, there are the mandibular branches of the facial nerve, the masseter muscle of the mandibular nerve and facial artery.

[Indications] Deviation of the eye and mouth, swollen cheeks, toothache, lockjaw, facial tic.

[Operation] Puncture perpendicularly 0.3~0.5 *cun* or obliquely towards ST 4 (*dì cāng*).

6. ST 7 (*xià guān*)

[Location] On the face, anterior to the ear, in the depression between the zygomatic arch and the mandibular notch.

[Anatomy]

(1) Layer of needling: Skin-subcutaneous tissue-masseter muscle-lateral pterygoid muscle.

(2) Innervation and vasculature: In the superficial layer, there are the great auricular nerve and the auriculotemporal nerve. In the deep layer, there are the zygomatic branches of the facial nerve and the muscular branches of the mandibular nerve and the superficial temporal artery. In the deeper layer, there is the mandibular nerve trunk at the foramen ovale.

[Indications] Lockjaw, painful jaw and face, toothache, tinnitus, deafness.

[Operation] Puncture perpendicularly 0.5~1.2 *cun*.

7. ST 8 (*tóu wéi*)

[Location] On the lateral side of the head, 0.5 *cun* above the anterior hairline at the corner of the forehead, 4.5 *cun* lateral to the midline of the head.

[Anatomy]

(1) Layer of needling: Skin-subcutaneous tissue-galea aponeurotica.

(2) Innervation and vasculature: In the superficial layer, there are the superaorbital nerve (the branches of the ophthalmic nerve) and the auriculotemporal nerve.

[Indications] Headache, dizziness, tears running irritated by wind, twitching eyelid, blurred vision, eye pain.

[Operation] Puncture 0.5-1 *cun* along the scalp with the tip of the needle directed horizontally and posteriorly.

8. ST 9 (*rén yíng*)

[Location] On the neck, beside the Adam's apple, on the anterior border of the ternocleidomastoid muscle where the pulsation of the common carotid artery is palpable.

[Anatomy]

(1) **Layer of needling:** Skin-subcutaneous tissue-platysma-uppermost belly of the omohyoid muscle.

(2) **Innervation and vasculature:** In the superficial layer, there are the transverse nerve of the neck, the cervical branches of the facial nerve and anterior jugular vein. In the deep layer,there are the collearal nerve, the hypoglossal nerve, the superior thyroid artery. In the deeper layer, there are the cervical vagina vasorum (in which there are the internal carotid artery and vein, and the vagal trunk), and the cervical sympathetic trunk posterior to the vagina vasorum.

[Indications] Sore throat, hypertension, headache, scrofula, dysphagia, fullness in the chest, shortness of breath.

[Operation] Puncture perpendicularly 0.2~0.4 *cun*. Avoid the common carotid artery.

9. ST 18 (*rŭ gēn*)

[Location] On the chest, directly below the nipple, on the lower border of the breast, in the 5th intercostal space, 4 *cun* lateral to the anterior midline.

[Anatomy]

(1) **Layer of needling:** Skin-subcutaneous tissue-great pectoral muscle-external intercostal muscle-internal intercostal muscle.

(2) **Innervation and vasculature:** In the superficial layer, there are the lateral cutaneous branches of the intercostal nerve and the thoraco-epigastric vein. In the deep layer, there are the anterior thoracic nerve, intercostal nerve and artery.

[Indications] Mastitis, hypogalactia, pain in the chest, cough, hiccups.

[Operation] Puncture obliquely along the intercostal space 0.5~0.8 *cun*, or puncture perpendicularly 0.4 *cun*.

10. ST 20 (*chéng măn*)

[Location] On the upper abdomen, 5 *cun* above the centre of the umbilicus, 2 *cun* lateral to the anterior midline.

[Anatomy]

(1) **Layer of needling:** Skin-subcutaneous tissue-anterior sheath of the rectus muscle of the abdomen-rectus muscle of the abdomen.

(2) **Innervation and vasculature:** In the superficial layer,there are the lateral and anterior cutaneous branches of the anterior branches of the 6th to 8th thoracic nerves and the superficial epigastric vein. In the deep layer, there are the branches or tributaries of the superior epigastric artery and vein and the

muscular branches of the anterior branches of the 6th to 8th thoracic nerves.

[Indications] Stomachache, vomiting, abdominal distension, borborygmus, poor appetite.

[Operation] Puncture perpendicularly 0.5~0.8 *cun*.

11. ST 21 (*liáng mén*)

[Location] On the upper abdomen, 4 *cun* above the centre of the umbilicus, 2 *cun* lateral to the anterior midline.

[Anatomy]

(1) Layer of needling: Skin-subcutaneous tissue-anterior sheath of rectus muscle of the abdomen-rectus muscle of the abdomen.

(2) Innervation and vasculature: In the superficial layer, there are the lateral and anterior cutaneous branches of the anterior branches of the 6th to 8th thoracic nerves and the superficial epigastric vein. In the deep layer, there are the branches or tributaries of the superior epigastric artery and vein and the muscular branches of the anterior branches of the 6th to 8th thoracic nerves.

[Indications] Stomachache, vomiting, abdominal distension, poor appetite, loose stools.

[Operation] Puncture perpendicularly 0.5~0.8 *cun*.

12. ST 24 (*huá ròu mén*)

[Location] On the upper abdomen, 1 *cun* above the centre of the umbilicus, 2 *cun* lateral to the anterior midline.

[Anatomy]

(1) Layer of needling: Skin-subcutaneous tissue-anterior sheath of the rectus muscle of the abdomen-rectus muscle of the abdomen.

(2) Innervation and vasculature: In the superficial layer, there are the lateral and anterior cutaneous branches of the anterior branches of the 6th to 8th thoracic nerves and the superficial epigastric vein. In the deep layer,there are the branches or tributaries of the superior epigastric artery and vein and the muscular branches of the anterior branches of the 6th to 8th thoracic nerves.

[Indications] Mania, vomiting, restlessness, abdominal distension.

[Operation] Puncture perpendicularly 0.5~0.8 *cun*.

13. ST 25 (*tiān shū*)

[Location] On the middle of the abdomen, 2 *cun* lateral to the centre of the umbilicus.

[Anatomy]

(1) Layer of needling: Skin-subcutaneous tissue-anterior rectus sheath of the abdomen-posterior rectus sheath of the abdomen.

(2) **Innervation and vasculature:** In the superficial layer, there are the anterior cutaneous branches of the intercostal nerve, superficial epigastric artery and vein. In the deep layer, there are the intercostal nerve and artery, and the superior and interior epigastric artery.

[Indications] Abdominal distending pain, diarrhea, dysentery, constipation, acute appendicitis, febrile disease, hernia, edema, menstrual irregularity.

[Operation] Puncture perpendicularly 0.8~1.2 *cun*.

14. ST 26 (*wài líng*)

[Location] On the lower abdomen, 1 *cun* below the centre of the umbilicus, 2 *cun* lateral to the anterior midline.

[Anatomy]

(1) **Layer of needling:** Skin-subcutaneous tissue-anterior rectus sheath of the abdomen-posterior rectus sheath of the abdomen.

(2) **Innervation and vasculature:** In the superficial layer, there are the anterior cutaneous branches of the intercostal nerve and the superficial epigastric artery and vein. In the deep layer, there are the intercostal nerve and artery, and the inferior epigastric artery.

[Indications] Abdominal pain, hernia, dysmenorrhea.

[Operation] Puncture perpendicularly 1~1.5 *cun*.

15. ST 28 (*shuǐ dào*)

[Location] On the lower abdomen, 3 *cun* below the centre of the umbilicus, 2 *cun* lateral to the anterior midline.

[Anatomy]

(1) **Layer of needling:** Skin-subcutaneous tissue-anterior rectus sheath of the abdomen-straight muscle of the abdomen.

(2) **Innervation and vasculature:** In the superficial layer, there are the anterior lateral cutaneous branches of the intercostal nerve and the superficial epigastric artery and vein. In the deep layer, there are the intercostal nerve and artery, and the inferior epigastric artery.

[Indications] Distension and fullness of the lower abdomen, abdominal pain, dysmenorrhea, dysuria.

[Operation] Puncture perpendicularly 0.8~1.2 *cun*.

16. ST 29 (*guī lái*)

[Location] On the lower abdomen, 4 *cun* below the centre of the umbilicus, 2 *cun* lateral to the anterior midline.

[Anatomy]

(1) **Layer of needling:** Skin-subcutaneous tissue-anterior rectus sheath of the

abdomen-straight muscle of the abdomen.

(2) Innervation and vasculature: In the superficial layer, there are the inferior iliac nerve and the inferior epigastric artery and vein. In the deep layer,there are the intercostal nerve and the inferior epigastric artery and vein.

[Indications] Pain in the lower abdomen, amenorrhea, dysmenorrhea, uterine prolapse, morbid leucorrhea, hernia, pain inside the penis, dysuria.

[Operation] Puncture perpendicularly 0.8~1.2 *cun*.

17. ST 31 (*bì guān*)

[Location] On the anterior side of the thigh, on the line linking the anterior-superior iliac spine and the superior-lateral corner of the patella, on the level of the perineum when the thigh is flexed, in the depression lateral to the sartorius muscle.

[Anatomy]

(1) Layer of needling: Skin-subcutaneous tissue-fascia lata-tensor muscle of the fascia lata-musculus rectus femoris-musculus vastus lateralis.

(2) Innervation and vasculature: In the superficial layer, there is the lateral cutaneous nerve of the thigh. In the deep layer, there are the the superior gluteal nerve and the cutaneous branches of the femoral nerve, the lateral femoral circumflex artery and vein.

[Indications] Atrophy and impediment of the thigh, motor difficulties of the lower limbs, lower back and leg pain.

[Operation] Puncture perpendicularly 0.8~1.2 *cun*.

18. ST 32 (*fú tù*)

[Location] On the anterior side of the thigh, on the line linking the anterior-superior iliac spine and the superior-lateral corner of the patella, 6 *cun* above this corner.

[Anatomy]

(1) Layer of needling: Skin-subcutaneous tissue-fascia lata-musculus rectus femoris-musculus vastus intermedius.

(2) Innervation and vasculature: In the superficial layer, there are the anterior cutaneous branches of the femoral nerve (branches of the femoral nerve) and the lateral cutaneous femoral nerve. In the deep layer, there are the cutaneous branches of the femoral nerve and the lateral femoral circumflex artery.

[Indications] Leg pain, motor difficulties of the lower limbs, beriberi, hernia, abdominal distension.

[Operation] Puncture perpendicularly 1~2 *cun*.

19. ST 34 (*liáng qiū*)

[Location] With the knee flexed, on the anterior side of the thigh, on the line linking the anterior superior iliac spine and the superior-lateral corner of the patella, 2 *cun* above this corner.

[Anatomy]

(1) Layer of needling: Skin-subcutaneous tissue-fascia lata-lateral femoral muscle.

(2) Innervation and vasculature: Same as ST 32 (*fú tù*).

[Indications] Stomachache, painful swollen knee joint, motor difficulties, mammary pain.

[Operation] Puncture perpendicularly 1~1.5 *cun*.

20. ST 35 (*dú bí*)

[Location] With the knee flexed, in the lateral depression between the patella and its ligament.

[Anatomy]

(1) Layer of needling: Skin-subcutaneous tissue-capsule of knee joint-alar folds.

(2) Innervation and vasculature: In the superficial layer, there are the lateral cutaneous nerve of the calf and the anterior femoral nerve. In the deep layer,there are the peroneal nerve, the knee joint of the common peroneal nerve and the arterial network of the knee joint.

[Indications] Knee joint pain, motor difficulties, beriberi.

[Operation] Puncture obliquely 0.8~1.5 *cun* with the needle tip directed slightly towards the medial side.

21. ST 36 (*zú sān lǐ*) *He*-Sea Point

[Location] On the anteriolateral side of the leg, 3 *cun* below ST 35 (*dú bí*), one (middle) finger breadth from the anterior crest of the tibia.

[Anatomy]

(1) Layer of needling: Skin-subcutaneous tissue-anterior tibial muscle-long extensor muscle of the toe-interosseous membrane of the leg-posterior tibial muscle.

(2) Innervation and vasculature: In the superficial layer, there is the lateral cutaneous nerve of the artery. In the deeper layer of the interosseous membrane of the leg, there are the tibial nerve and the posterior tibial artery.

[Indications] Stomachache, vomiting, abdominal distension, borborygmus, dyspepsia, atrophy and impediment of the lower limbs, diarrhea, constipation, dysentery, malnutrition in children due to improper feeding, mania, beriberi, edema, palpitation, shortness of breath, consumptive disease, or serving to improve health.

[Operation] Puncture perpendicularly 1~2 *cun*.

22. ST 37 (*shàng jù xū*) Lower *He*-sea Point of the Large Intestine Channel

[Location] On the anteriolateral side of the leg, 6 *cun* below ST 35 (*dú bí*), one (middle) finger breadth from the anterior crest of the tibia.

[Anatomy] Same as ST 36 (*zú sān lǐ*).

[Indications] Abdominal distending pain, dysentery, constipation, acute appendicitis, paralysis caused by wind-stroke, beriberi, atrophy-flaccidity of the lower limbs.

[Operation] Puncture perpendicularly 1~1.5 *cun*.

23. ST 38 (*tiáo kǒu*)

[Location] On the anteriolateral side of the leg, 8 *cun* below ST 35 (*dú bí*), one (middle) finger breadth from the anterior crest of the tibia.

[Anatomy] Same as ST 36 (*zú sān lǐ*).

[Indications] Motor impairment of the shoulder and arm, cold and painful lower limbs, dysentery, swollen feet, systremma.

[Operation] Puncture perpendicularly 1~1.5 *cun*.

24. ST 39 (*xià jù xū*) Lower *He*-Sea Point of the Small Intestine Channel

[Location] On the anteriolateral side of the leg, 9 *cun* below ST 35 (*dú bí*), one (middle) finger breadth from the anterior crest of the tibia.

[Anatomy] Same as ST 36 (*zú sān lǐ*).

[Indications] Pain in the lower abdomen, lumbovertebral pain with the testis involved, acute mastitis, atrophy-impediment of the limbs, diarrhea, bloody purulent stools.

[Operation] Puncture perpendicularly 1~1.5 *cun*.

25. ST 40 (*fēng lóng*) *Luo*-Connecting Point

[Location] On the anteriolateral side of the leg, 8 *cun* above the tip of the external malleolus, two (middle) finger breadth from the crest of the tibia.

[Anatomy]

(1) Layer of needling: Skin-subcutaneous tissue-long extensor muscle of the toe-interosseous membrane of the leg-posterior tibial muscle.

(2) Innervation and vasculature: In the superficial layer, there is the lateral cutaneous nerve of the calf. In the deep layer, there are the nerve of the calf and the anterior tibial artery, and the tibial nerve and artery of the calf in the deep interosseous membrane of the leg.

[Indications] Profuse sputum, asthma, cough, pain in the chest, headache, painful and swollen throat and pharynx, constipation, mania, epilepsy, atrophy-impediment of the lower limbs, vomiting.

[Operation] Puncture perpendicularly 1~1.5 *cun*.

26. ST 41 (*jiě xī*) *Jing*-River Point

[Location] In the central depression of the transverse crease between the instep of the foot and leg, between the long extensor muscle of the great toe and the long extensor muscle of the toe.

[Anatomy]

(1) Layer of needling: Skin-subcutaneous tissue-between the long extensor muscle of the great toe and the long extensor muscle of the toe.

(2) Innervation and vasculature: In the superficial layer, there are the medial dorsal cutaneous nerve (the branches of the superficial peroneal nerve). In the deep layer, there are the deep peroneal nerve and the anterior tibial artery.

[Indications] Headache, dizziness and vertigo, mania, abdominal distension, constipation, atrophy-impediment of the lower limbs, conjunctival congestion, delirium caused by stomach fire.

[Operation] Puncture perpendicularly 0.5~1 *cun*.

27. ST 43 (*xiàn gǔ*) *Shu*-Stream Point

[Location] On the instep of the foot, in the depression distal to the junction of the 2nd and 3rd metatarsal bones.

[Anatomy]

(1) Layer of needling: Skin-subcutaneous tissue-long extensor muscle of the toe-2nd dorsal interosseous muscle-oblique head of the adductor of the great toe.

(2) Innervation and vasculature: In the superficial layer, there are the medial dorsal cutaneous nerve. In the deep layer, there are the deep peroneal nerve, lateral planter nerve and dorsal pedal artery.

[Indications] Facial edema, borborygmus, diarrhea, painful and swollen instep of the foot, febrile disease, painful conjunctival congestion.

[Operation] Puncture perpendicularly 0.3~0.5 *cun*.

28. ST 44 (*nèi tíng*) *Ying*-Spring Point

[Location] On the instep of the foot, at the junction of the red and white skin proximal to the margin of the web between the 2nd and 3rd toes.

[Anatomy]

(1) Layer of needling: Skin-subcutaneous tissue-between the long and short extensor muscles of the 2nd and 3rd toes.

(2) Innervation and vasculature: In the superficial layer, there are the dorsal digital nerve (the branches of the deep peroneal nerve). In the deep layer, there are the deep peroneal nerve and the dorsal artery of the foot.

[Indications] Toothache, laryngalgia, epistaxis, abdominal distension, dysentery, diarrhea, painful swollen dorsum of the foot, febrile disease, stomachache, casting up of gastric acid.

[Operation] Puncture perpendicularly 0.3~0.5 *cun*.

Section 4 The Spleen Channel of Foot *Taiyin*

1. SP 1 (*yǐn bái*) *Jing*-Well Point

[Location] On the medial side of the distal segment of the great toe, 0.1 *cun* from the corner of the toe nail.

[Anatomy]

(1) Layer of needling: Skin-subcutaneous tissue-root of the nail.

(2) Innervation and vasculature: There are the medial dorsal cutaneous nerve of the foot, the dorsal digital nerve and the dorsal digital artery of the foot.

[Indications] Abdominal distension, hematochezia, hematuria, metrorrhagia or metrostaxis, menorrhagia, mania, dream-disturbed sleep, infantile convulsion, syncope, pain in the chest.

[Operation] Puncture 0.1 *cun*.

2. SP 3 (*tài bái*) *Shu*-Stream Point; *Yuan*-Source Point

[Location] On the medial border of the foot, posterior and inferior to the 1st metatarsal phalangeal joint, in the depression of the junction of the red and white skin.

[Anatomy]

(1) Layer of needling: Skin-subcutaneous tissue-short abductor muscle of the thumb.

(2) Innervation and vasculature: In the superficial layer, there are the medialdorsalcutaneous nerve of the foot. In the deep layer, there are the common digital plantar nerves and the plantar metatarsal arteries.

[Indications] Stomachache, abdominal distending pain, borborygmus, vomiting, diarrhea, constipation, dysentery, hemorrhoids, beriberi, sluggishness.

[Operation] Puncture perpendicularly 0.8~1 *cun*.

3. SP 4 (*gōng sūn*) *Luo*-Connecting Point; Confluent Point That Links the Thoroughfare Vessel

[Location] On the medial border of the foot, anterior and inferior to the proximal end of the 1st metatarsal bone.

[Anatomy]

(1) Layer of needling: Skin-subcutaneous tissue-short abductor muscle of the toe-short flexor muscle of the toe.

(2) Innervation and vasculature: In the superficial layer, there are the dorsal cutaneous nerve of the foot and the saphenous nerve. In the deep layer, there are the medial plantar nerve and artery.

[Indications] Stomachache, vomiting, indigestion, borborygmus and abdominal distending pain, constipation, diarrhea, restlessness, insomnia, edema, mania, somnolence, beriberi.

[Operation] Puncture perpendicularly 0.5~1 *cun*.

4. SP 5 (*shāng qiū*) *Jing*-River Point

[Location] In the depression, anterior and inferior to the medial malleolus, at the midpoint of the line linking the tuberosity of the navicular bone and the tip of the medial malleolus.

[Anatomy]

(1) Layer of needling: Skin-subcutaneous tissue-triangular ligament.

(2) Innervation and vasculature: In the superficial layer, there are the saphenous nerve and the great saphenous vein. In the deep layer, there are the medial anterior malleolar artery.

[Indications] Abdominal distension, borborygmus, diarrhea, dysentery, indigestion, jaundice, somnolence, mania, infantial epilepsy, cough, pain in the foot and malleolus, hemorrhoids.

[Operation] Puncture perpendicularly 0.5~0.8 *cun*.

5. SP 6 (*sān yīn jiāo*) Crossing Point that links the Liver, Spleen and Kidney Channels

[Location] On the medial side of the leg, 3 *cun* directly above the tip of the medial malleolus, posterior to the medial side of the tibia.

[Anatomy]

(1) Layer of needling: Skin-subcutaneous tissue-long flexor muscle of the toe-posterior tibial muscle-long flexor muscle of the great toe.

(2) Innervation and vasculature: In the superficial layer, there are the saphenous nerve and the great saphenous vein. In the deep layer, there are the tibial nerve and the branches of the posterior tibial artery.

[Indications] Diarrhea, abdominal distension, indigestion, menstrual, irregularity metrorrhagia or metrostaxis, morbid leucorrhea, prolapse of the uterus, amenorrhea, dysmenorrhea, dystocia, postpartum fainting, lochiorrhea, spermatorrhea, impotence, premature ejaculation, pain of the penis, hernia, edema, dysuria, enuresis, impediment and pain of the lower limbs, beriberi, insomnia, eczema, urticaria, hypertension, neurodermatitis, infertility.

[Operation] Puncture perpendicularly 1~1.5 *cun*. It is contraindicated in pregnancy women.

6. **SP 8 (*dì jī*)** *Xi*-Cleft Point

[Location] On the medial side of the leg, on the line that links the tip of the medial malleolus and SP 9 (*yīn líng quán*), 3 *cun* below SP 9 (*yīn líng quán*).

[Anatomy]

(1) Layer of needling: Skin-subcutaneous tissue-soleus muscle.

(2) Innervation and vasculature: In the superficial layer, there are the saphenous nerve and the great saphenous vein. In the deep layer, there are the tibial nerve and the branches of the posterior tibial artery.

[Indications] Abdominal pain, diarrhea, dysuria, edema, menstrual, irregularity spermatorrhea, motor impairment of the lower back, poor appetite.

[Operation] Puncture perpendicularly 1~1.5 *cun.*

7. **SP 9 (*yīn líng quán*)** *He*-Sea Point

[Location] On the medial side of the leg, in the depression posterior and inferior to the medial condyle of the tibia.

[Anatomy]

(1) Layer of needling: Skin-subcutaneous tissue-semitendinous muscle-medial head of the gastrocnemius muscle.

(2) Innervation and vasculature: In the superficial layer, there are the saphenous nerve and the great saphenous vein. In the deep layer, there are the branches of the deep medial inferior genicular artery and muscle of the tibial nerve. In the deeper layer there are the tibial nerve trunk and arterial trunk.

[Indications] Abdominal distension, edema, dysuria or incontinence of urine, pain in the penis, vaginal pain, spermatorrhea, knee pain, jaundice.

[Operation] Puncture perpendicularly 1~2 *cun.*

8. **SP 10 (*xuè hǎi*)**

[Location] With the knee flexed, on the medial side of the thigh, 2 *cun* above the superior medial corner of the patella, on the prominence of the medial head of the quadriceps muscle of the thigh.

[Anatomy]

(1) Layer of needling: Skin-subcutaneous tissue-medial femoral muscle.

(2) Innervation and vasculature: In the superficial layer, there are the anterior cutaneous branches of the femoral nerve and the great saphenous vein. In the deep layer, there are the muscular branches of the femoral nerve and the medial superior genicular artery.

[Indications] Menstrual irregularity, dysmenorrhea, amenorrhea, metrorrhagia or metrostaxis, hives, cutaneous pruritus, erysipelas, dribbling urination, pain in the medial side of the thigh.

[Operation] Puncture perpendicularly 1~1.2 *cun*.

9. SP 14 (*fù jié*)

[Location] On the lower abdomen, 1.3 *cun* below SP 15 (*dà héng*), 4 *cun* lateral to the anterior midline.

[Anatomy]

(1) Layer of needling: Skin-subcutaneous tissue-external oblique muscle of the abdomen-internal oblique muscle of the abdomen –transverse muscle of the abdomen.

(2) Innervation and vasculature: In the superficial layer, there are the lateral cutaneous branches of the 11th intercostal nerve and the branches of the thoraco-epigastric artery. In the deep layer, there are the 11th intercostal nerve and artery.

[Indications] Abdominal pain, diarrhea, constipation.

[Operation] Puncture perpendicularly 1~1.5 *cun*.

10. SP 15 (*dà héng*)

[Location] On the middle abdomen, 4 *cun* lateral to the centre of the umbilicus.

[Anatomy]

(1) Layer of needling: Skin-subcutaneous tissue-external oblique muscle of the abdomen-internal oblique muscle of the abdomen-transverse muscle of the abdomen.

(2) Innervation and vasculature: In the superficial layer, there are the lateral cutaneous branches of the 10th intercostal nerve. In the deep layer, there are the intercostal nerve and artery.

[Indications] Abdominal pain, diarrhea, constipation.

[Operation] Puncture perpendicularly 1~1.5 *cun*.

Section 5 The Heart Channel of Hand *Shaoyin*

1. HT 5 (*tōng lǐ*) *Luo*-Connecting Point

[Location] On the palmar side of the forearm, on the radial side of the ulnar flexor muscle of the wrist, 1 *cun* proximal to the cresae of the wrist.

[Anatomy]

(1) Layer of needling: Skin-subcutaneous tissue-between the ulnar flexor muscle of the wrist and superficial flexor muscle of the finger-deep flexor muscle of the finger.

(2) Innervation and vasculature: In the superficial layer, there are the medial cutaneous nerve of the forearm. In the deep layer, there are the branches of the ulnar nerve, artery and the ulnar nerve and artery trunks.

[Indications] Sudden aphonia, stiff tongue, palpitation, pain in the wrist and arm.

[Operation] Puncture perpendicularly 0.2~0.5 *cun*.

2. HT 6 (*yīn xì*) *Xi*-Cleft Point

[Location] On the palmar side of the forearm, on the radial side of the ulnar flexor muscle of the wrist, 0.5 *cun* proximal to the cresae of the wrist.

[Anatomy]

(1) Layer of needling: Skin-subcutaneous tissue-radial border of the ulnar flexor muscle of the wrist-deep flexor muscle of the finger.

(2) Innervation and vasculature: In the superficial layer, there are the medial cutaneous nerve of the forearm. In the deep layer, there are the branches of the ulnar nerve and artery, and the ulnar nerve and artery trunks.

[Indications] Heart pain, panic, palpitation, hematemesis, epistaxis, aphasia, steaming bone disorder and night sweating.

[Operation] Puncture perpendicularly 0.2~0.5 *cun*.

3. HT 7 (*shén mén*) *Shu*-Stream Point; *Yuan*-Source Point

[Location] On the wrist, at the ulnar end of the crease of the wrist, in the depression of the radial side of the ulnar flexor muscle of the wrist.

[Anatomy]

(1) Layer of needling: Skin-subcutaneous tissue-radial border of the ulnar flexor muscle of the wrist.

(2) Innervation and vasculature: In the superficial layer, there are the medial cutaneous nerve of the forearm. In the deep layer, there are the ulnar nerve and artery trunks.

[Indications] Heart pain, restlessness, amnesia, insomnia, palpitation, dementia, mania, epilepsy, icteric sclera, hypochondriac pain, feverish sensation in the palms, hematemesis, headache, dizziness, aphonia.

[Operation] Puncture perpendicularly 0.2~0.5 *cun*.

4. HT 8 (*shào fŭ*) *Ying*-Spring Point

[Location] In the palm, between the 4th and 5th metacarpal bones, at the spot of the palm where the little finger touches when a fist is made.

[Anatomy]

(1) Layer of needling: Skin-subcutaneous tissue-palmar aponenurosis-4th lumbrical muscle.

(2) Innervation and vasculature: In the superficial layer, there are the palmar branches of the ulnar nerve. In the deep layer, there are the common palmar nerve and artery and the palmar metacarpal artery.

[Indications] Palpitation, chest pain, dysuresia, enuresis, pruritus vulvae, vaginal pain, contracture of the little finger, feverish sensation in the palms, being easily frightened.

[Operation] Puncture perpendicularly 0.3~0.5 *cun*.

Section 6 The Small Intestine Channel of Hand *Taiyang*

1. SI 1 (*shào zé*) *Jing*-Well Point

[Location] On the ulnar side of the distal segment of the little finger, 0.1 *cun* posterior to the corner of the nail.

[Anatomy]

(1) Layer of needling: Skin-subcutaneous tissue-root of the nail.

(2) Innervation and vasculature: There are the proper palmar digital nerve and artery.

[Indications] Headache, nebula, sore throat, acute mastitis, hypogalactia, coma, febrile disease, deafness, pain in the posterior lateral part of the arm and shoulder.

[Operation] Puncture obliquely 0.1 *cun*.

2. SI 3 (*hòu xī*) *Shu*-Stream Point; Confluence Point that links the *Du* Vessel

[Location] On the ulnar side of the palm, when a hollow fist is made, proximal to the 5th metacarpophalangeal joint, at the end of the transverse crease and the junction of the red and white skin.

[Anatomy]

(1) Layer of needling: Skin-subcutaneous tissue-abductor muscle of the little finger-short flexor muscle of the little finger finger.

(2) Innervation and vasculature: In the superficial layer, there are the dorsal branches of the ulnar nerve and the dorsal metacar artery. In the deep layer, there are the deep branch of the ulnar nerve and the palmar nerve of the little finger.

[Indications] Pain and rigidity of the neck, deafness, febrile disease, malaria, night sweating, dizziness, conjunctival congestion, sore throat.

[Operation] Puncture perpendicularly 0.5~1 *cun*.

3. SI 4 (*wàn gŭ*) *Yuan*-Source Point

[Location] On the ulnar side of the hand, in the depression between the base of the 5th metacarpal bone and the hamate bone, and at the junction of the red and white skin.

[Anatomy]

(1) Layer of needling: Skin-subcutaneous tissue-abductor muscle of the little finger.

(2) **Innervation and vasculature:** In the superficial layer, there are the dorsal branches of the ulnar nerve and the dorsal artery of the hand. In the deep layer, there are the deep branches of the ulnar nerve and the ulnar artery.

[Indications] Headache, rigidity of the neck, tinnitus, deafness, nebula, contracture of the fingers, febrile disease without sweating, malaria, hypochondriac pain.

[Operation] Puncture perpendicularly 0.3~0.5 *cun.*

4. SI 6 (*yǎng lǎo*) *Xi*-Cleft Point

[Location] On the ulnar side of the posterior surface of the forearm, in the depression proximal to and on the radial side of the ulnar head.

[Anatomy]

(1) **Layer of needling:** Skin-subcutaneous tissue-between the ulnar extensor muscle of the wrist and the extensor muscle of the little finger.

(2) **Innervation and vasculature:** In the superficial layer, there are the posterior cutaneous nerve of the forearm and the bisilic vein. In the deep layer, there are the branches of the posterior interosseous nerve and artery.

[Indications] Headache, dizziness, tinnitus, deafness, febrile disease, mania, pain in the wrist.

[Operation] Puncture perpendicularly or obliquely 0.5~0.8 *cun.*

5. SI 8 (*xiǎo hǎi*) *He*-Sea Point

[Location] On the medial side of the elbow, in the depression between the olecranon of the ulna and the medial epicondyle of the humerus.

[Anatomy]

(1) **Layer of needling:** Skin-subcutaneous tissue-groove of the ulnar nerve.

(2) **Innervation and vasculature:** In the superficial layer, there are the branches of the medial cutaneous nerve of the forearm and the basilic vein. In the deep layer, there is the ulnar nerve trunk of the superior ulnar collateral artery.

[Indications] Pain in the elbow and arm, epilepsy, tinnitus, deafness.

[Operation] Puncture perpendicularly 0.3~0.5 *cun.*

6. SI 9 (*jiān zhēn*)

[Location] Posterior and inferior to the shoulder joint, 1 *cun* above the posterior end of the axillary fold when the arm is adducted.

[Anatomy]

(1) **Layer of needling:** Skin-subcutaneous tissue-long head of the brachial triceps muscle-teres major muscle.

(2) **Innervation and vasculature:** In the superficial layer, there are the lateral cutaneous branches of the 2nd intecostal nerve, ie the interostobrachial nerve. In

the deep layer, there are the axillar nerve, radial nerve and the branches of the posterior humeral circumflex artery.

[Indications] Pain in the scapular region, numb and painful hand and arm, motor impairment of the forearm, supraclavicular fossa pain.

[Operation] Puncture perpendicularly 1~1.5 *cun*.

7. SI 11 (*tiān zōng*)

[Location] On the scapular, in the depression of the centre of the infrascapular fossa, on the level of the 4th thoracic vertebra.

[Anatomy]

(1) Layer of needling: Skin-subcutaneous tissue-infraspinous muscle.

(2) Innervation and vasculature: In the superficial layer, there are the cutaneous branches of the posterior branches of the 5th thoracic nerve. In the deep layer, there are the branches of the suprascapular nerve and the scapular arterial network.

[Indications] Shoulder and arm pain, pain in the lateroposterior elbow and arm, asthma, acute mastitis.

[Operation] Puncture perpendicularly or obliquely 0.5~1 *cun*.

8. SI 12 (*bǐng fēng*)

[Location] In the centre of the suprascapular fossa, directly above SI 11 (*tiān zōng*), in the depression found when the arm is raised.

[Anatomy]

(1) Layer of needling: Skin-subcutaneous tissue-trapezius muscle-supraspinous muscle.

(2) Innervation and vasculature: In the superficial layer, there are the supraclavicular nerve. In the deep layer,there are the branches of the suprascapular nerve, collateral nerve and the suprascapular artery.

[Indications] Shoulder and arm pain, numbness and aching pain of the upper limbs.

[Operation] Puncture perpendicularly 0.5~1 *cun*.

9. SI 14 (*jiān wài shù*)

[Location] On the back, below the spinous process of the 1st thoracic vertebra, 3 *cun* lateral to the posterior midline.

[Anatomy]

(1) Layer of needling: Skin-subcutaneous tissue-trapezius muscle-rhomboid muscle.

(2) Innervation and vasculature: In the superficial layer, there are the cutaneous branches of the posterior branches of the 1st thoracic nerve. In the deep layer, there are the branches of the accessory nerve, the dorsal scapular nerve and artery.

[Indications] Shoulder and back pain, pain and rigidity of the neck.

[Operation] Puncture perpendicularly 0.5~0.8 *cun*.

10. SI 15 (*jiān zhōng shù*)

[Location] On the back, below the spinous process of the 7th thoracic vertebra, 2 *cun* lateral to the posterior midline.

[Anatomy]

(1) Layer of needling: Skin-subcutaneous tissue-trapezius muscle-rhomboid muscle- splenius muscle of the head.

(2) Innervation and vasculature: In the superficial layer, there are the cutaneous branches of the posterior branches of the 8th cervical nerve and the accompanying artery and vein. In the deep layer, there are the branches of the accessory nerve, the dorsal scapular nerve and the transverse cervical artery.

[Indications] Shoulder and back pain, cough, asthma.

[Operation] Puncture perpendicularly 0.5~0.8 *cun*.

11. SI 17 (*tiān róng*)

[Location] On the lateral side of the neck, posterior to the mandibular angle, in the depression of the anterior border of the sternocleidomastoid muscle.

[Anatomy]

(1) Layer of needling: Skin-subcutaneous tissue-parotid gland-posterior belly of the digastric muscle.

(2) Innervation and vasculature: In the superficial layer, there are the great auricular nerve and the external jugular vein. In the deep layer, there are the muscular branches of the facial nerve, posterior auricular artery, occipital artery, carotid and the vagus nerve trunk, where deep insertion of the needle is forbidden.

[Indications] Tinnitus, deafness, sore throat, aching pain and rigidity of the neck.

[Operation] Puncture perpendicularly 0.5~1 *cun*.

12. SI 18 (*quán liáo*)

[Location] On the face, directly below the outer canthus, in the depression below the zygomatic bone.

[Anatomy]

(1) Layer of needling: Skin-subcutaneous tissue-zygomatic muscle-masseter muscle-temporal muscle.

(2) Innervation and vasculature: In the superficial layer, there is the infraorbital nerve. In the deep layer, there are the the zygomatic branches of the facial nerve and the muscular branches of the mandibular nerve.

[Indications] Deviation of the eye and mouth, twitching of eyelids, toothache, swollen lips.

[Operation] Puncture perpendicularly 0.3~0.5 *cun* or obliquely 0.5~1 *cun.*

13. SI 19 (*tīng gōng*)

[Location] On the face, anterior to the tragus and posterior to the mandibular condyloid process, in the depression found when the mouth is open.

[Anatomy]

(1) Layer of needling: Skin-subcutaneous tissue-parotid gland-external auditory cartilage.

(2) Innervation and vasculature: There are the auriculotemporal nerve and the branches of the superficial temporal artery. In the deep layer there are the branches of the facial nerve.

[Indications] Tinnitus, deafness, ear pain, toothache, mania.

[Operation] Puncture perpendicularly 0.5~1 *cun* while the mouth is open.

Section 7 The Urinary Bladder Channel of Foot *Taiyang*

1. BL 1 (*jīng míng*)

[Location] On the face, in the depression slightly above the inner canthus.

[Anatomy]

(1) Layer of needling: Skin-subcutaneous tissue-orbicular muscle of the eye-adpose body of the orbit-internal rectus.

(2) Innervation and vasculature: In the superficial layer, there are the supratrochlear nerve of the branches of the inner canthus artery. In the deep layer, there are the temporal branches of the facial nerve, the oculomotor nerve, the supratrochlear and infratrochlear nerves and artery.

[Indications] Red swollen painful eyes, tears running irritated by wind, pterygium, blurred vision, nearsightedness, night blindness, color blindness, nebula.

[Operation] Ask the patient to close his eyes. Push the eyeball outward gently and let it stay there. Inseret the needle perpendicularly 0.3~0.5 *cun* along the orbital wall. Bleeding is often caused, so after withdrawl of the needle press the needle hole with a sterilized absorbent cotton wool for some minutes.

2. BL 2 (*cuán zhú*)

[Location] On the face, in the depression of the medial end of the eyebow, at the supraorbital notch.

[Anatomy]

(1) Layer of needling: Skin-subcutaneous tissue-orbicular muscle of the eye-superciliary corrugator muscle.

(2) Innervation and vasculature: In the superficial layer, there are the branches of the supratrochlear nerve and artery. In the deep layer, there are the temporal branches of the facial nerve and the temporal artery.

[Indications] Pain in the forehead and the supraorbital region, blurred vision, red swollen painful eyes, nearsightedness, twitching of eyelid, deviation of the eye and mouth.

[Operation] Puncture horizontally 0.5~0.8 *cun*.

3. BL 7 (*tōng tiān*)

[Location] On the head, 4 *cun* directly above the midpoint of the anterior hairline, 1.5 *cun* lateral to the midline.

[Anatomy]

(1) Layer of needling: Skin-subcutaneous tissue-epicranial aponeurosis.

(2) Innervation and vasculature: In the superficial layer, there are the superficial temporal artery and the branches of the auriculotemporal nerve.

[Indications] Headache, heaviness of the head, giddiness, stuffy nose, nasosinusitis.

[Operation] Puncture horizontally 0.5~0.8 *cun*.

4. BL 10 (*tiān zhù*)

[Location] On the nape, in the depression of the lateral side of the trapezius muscle, 1.3 *cun* lateral to the midpoint of the posterior hairline.

[Anatomy]

(1) Layer of needling: Skin-subcutaneous tissue-trapezius muscle-semispinal muscle of the head.

(2) Innervation and vasculature: In the superficial layer, there are the posterior branches of the 3rd cervical nerve and the branches of the occipital artery. In the deep layer, there are the greater occipital nerve and the occipital artery trunk.

[Indications] Headache, stiff neck, giddiness, red swollen and painful eye, pain in the shoulder and back, stuffy nose.

[Operation] Puncture perpendicularly or obliquely 0.5~0.8 *cun*.

5. BL 11 (*dà zhù*) Influential Point of Bone

[Location] On the back, below the spinous process of the 1st thoracic vertebra, 1.5 *cun* lateral to the posterior midline.

[Anatomy]

(1) Layer of needling: Skin-subcutaneous tissue-trapezius muscle-rhomboid

muscle-superior posterior serratus muscle.

(2) **Innervation and vasculature:** In the superficial layer, there are the medial cutaneous branches of the posterior branches of the 1st and 2nd thoracic nerves and the accompanying artery and vein. In the deep layer,there are the accessory nerve, the branches of the dorsal nerve and artery of the scapula.

[Indications] Cough, fever, headache, shoulder and back pain, pain and rigidity of the neck.

[Operation] Puncture obliquely 0.5~0.8 *cun*. It is advisable not to apply deep insertion to the points on the back where the present channel passes to avoid injury to the internal organs.

6. BL 12 (*fēng mén*)

[Location] On the back, below the spinous process of the 2nd thoracic vertebra, 1.5 *cun* lateral to the posterior midline.

[Anatomy]

(1) **Layer of needling:** Skin-subcutaneous tissue-trapezius muscle-rhomboid muscle-superior posterior serratus muscle-erector spinal muscle.

(2) **Innervation and vasculature:** In the superficial layer, there are the cutaneous branches of the posterior branches of the 2nd and 3rd thoracic nerves and the accompanying artery and vein. In the deep layer, there are the accessory nerve, the dorsal nerve of the scapula, the posterior branches of the 2nd and 3rd thoracic nerves and the branches of the dorsal artery of the scapula.

[Indications] Cold, cough, fever and headache, blurred version, stiff neck, pain in the chest and back, stuffy nose.

[Operation] Puncture obliquely 0.5~0.8 *cun.*

7. BL 13 (*fèi shù*) Back-*Shu* Point of the Lung Channel

[Location] On the back, below the spinous process of the 3rd thoracic vertebra, 1.5 *cun* lateral to the posterior midline.

[Anatomy]

(1) **Layer of needling:** Skin-subcutaneous tissue-trapezius muscle-superior posterior-serratus muscle-erector spinal muscle.

(2) **Innervation and vasculature:** In the superficial layer, there are the cutaneous branches of the posterior branches of the 3rd and 4th thoracic nerves and the accompanying artery and vein. In the deep layer, there are the accessory nerve, dorsal nerve of the scapula, the muscular branches of the posterior branches of the 3rd and 4th thoracic nerves and the branches of the dorsal artery of the scapula.

[Indications] Cough, shortness of breath, fullness in the chest, back pain, hectic fever, night sweating, bone steaming disorder, hematemesis, stuffy nose.

[Operation] Puncture obliquely 0.5~0.8 *cun*.

8. BL 14 (*jué yīn shù*) Back-*Shu* Point of the Pericardium Channel

[Location] On the back, below the spinous process of the 4th thoracic vertebra, 1.5 *cun* lateral to the posterior midline.

[Anatomy]

(1) Layer of needling: Skin-subcutaneous tissue-trapezius muscle-rhomboid muscle-erector spinal muscle.

(2) Innervation and vasculature: In the superficial layer, there are the cutaneous branches of the posterior branches of the 4th and 5th thoracic nerves and the accompanying artery and vein. In the deep layer, there are the accessory nerve, the dorsal nerve of the scapula, the muscular branches of the posterior branches of the 4th and 5th thoracic nerves and the branches of the dorsal artery of the scapula.

[Indications] Heart pain, palpitation, constriction in the chest, cough, vomiting.

[Operation] Puncture obliquely 0.5~0.8 *cun*.

9. BL 15 (*xīn shù*) Back-*Shu* Point of the Heart Channel

[Location] On the back, below the spinous process of the 5th thoracic vertebra, 1.5 *cun* lateral to the posterior midline.

[Anatomy]

(1) Layer of needling: Skin-subcutaneous tissue-trapezius muscle-inferior border of the rhomboid muscle-erector spinal muscle.

(2) Innervation and vasculature: In the superficial layer, there are the cutaneous branches of the posterior branches of the 5th and 6th thoracic nerves and the accompanying artery and vein. In the deep layer, there are the accessory nerve, the muscular branches of the posterior branches of the 5th and 6th thoracic nerves and the dorsal branches of the artery of the scapula.

[Indications] Mania, epilepsy, palpitation, insomnia, restlessness, cough, hematemesis, noctural emission, heart pain, pain in the chest and back.

[Operation] Puncture obliquely 0.5~0.8 *cun*.

10. BL 16 (*dū shù*)

[Location] On the back, below the spinous process of the 6th thoracic vertebra, 1.5 *cun* lateral to the posterior midline.

[Anatomy]

(1) Layer of needling: Skin-subcutaneous tissue-trapezius muscle-broadest muscle of the back-erector spinal muscle.

(2) Innervation and vasculature: In the superficial layer, there are the cutaneous branches of the posterior branches of the 6th and 7th thoracic nerves and the accompanying artery and vein. In the deep layer, there are the accessory nerve, the muscular branches of the posterior branches of the 6th and 7th thoracic nerves and the branches of the dorsal branches of the artery of the scapula.

[Indications] Heart pain, abdominal distending pain, borborygmus, hiccups.

[Operation] Puncture obliquely 0.5~0.8 *cun*.

11. BL 17 (*gé shù*) Influential Point of Blood

[Location] On the back, below the spinous process of the 7th thoracic vertebra, 1.5 *cun* lateral to the posterior midline.

[Anatomy]

(1) Layer of needling: Skin-subcutaneous tissue-trapezius muscle-broadest muscle of the back-erector spinal muscle.

(2) Innervation and vasculature: In the superficial layer, there are the cutaneous branches of the posterior branches of the 7th and 8th thoracic nerves and the accompanying artery and vein. In the deep layer, there are the muscular branches of the posterior branches of the 7th and 8th thoracic nerves and the branches of the dorsal branches of the artery of the scapula.

[Indications] Pain in the epigastric region, vomiting, hiccups, difficulty in swallowing, cough, hematemesis, hectic fever, night sweating.

[Operation] Puncture obliquely 0.5~0.8 *cun*.

12. BL 18 (*gān shù*) Back-*Shu* Point of the Liver Channel

[Location] On the back, below the spinous process of the 9th thoracic vertebra, 1.5 *cun* lateral to the posterior midline.

[Anatomy]

(1) Layer of needling: Skin-subcutaneous tissue-trapezius muscle-broadest muscle of the back-erector spinal muscle.

(2) Innervation and vasculature: In the superficial layer, there are the cutaneous branches of the posterior branches of the 9th and 10th thoracic nerves and the accompanying arteries and veins. In the deep layer, there are the muscular branches of the posterior branches of the 9th and 10th thoracic nerves and the branches or tributaries of the related posterior intercostal arteries and veins.

[Indications] Jaundice, pain in the hypochondriac region, red eyes, blurred vision, night blindness, mania, epilepsy, back pain.

[Operation] Puncture obliquely 0.5~0.8 *cun*.

13. BL 19 (*dăn shù*) Back-*Shu* Point of the Gallbladder Channel

[Location] On the back, below the spinous process of the 10th thoracic vertebra, 1.5 *cun* lateral to the posterior midline.

[Anatomy]

(1) Layer of needling: Skin-subcutaneous tissue-broadest muscle of the back-erector spinal muscle.

(2) Innervation and vasculature: In the superficial layer, there are the cutaneous branches of the posterior branches of the 10th and 11th thoracic nerves and the accompanying artery and vein. In the deep layer, there are the muscular branches of the posterior branches of the 10th and 11th thoracic nerves and the branches of the related posterior intercostal artery and vein.

[Indications] Jaundice, pain in the hypochondriac region, vomiting, indigestion, bitter taste in the mouth.

[Operation] Puncture obliquely 0.5~0.8 *cun*.

14. BL 20 (*pí shù*) Back-*Shu* Point of the Spleen Channel

[Location] On the back, below the spinous process of the 11th thoracic vertebra, 1.5 *cun* lateral to the posterior midline.

[Anatomy]

(1) Layer of needling: Skin-subcutaneous tissue-broadest muscle of the back-inferior posterior serratus muscle-erector spinal muscle.

(2) Innervation and vasculature: In the superficial layer, there are the cutaneous branches of the posterior branches of the 11th and 12th thoracic nerves and the accompanying artery and vein. In the deep layer, there are the muscular branches of the posterior branches of the 11th and 12th thoracic nerves and the branches of the related posterior intercostal and infracostal arteries and veins.

[Indications] Abdominal distension, diarrhea, vomiting, stomachache, indigestion, edema, back pain, jaundice.

[Operation] Puncture perpendicularly 0.5~1 *cun*.

15. BL 21 (*wèi shù*) Back-*Shu* Point of the Stomach Channel

[Location] On the back, below the spinous process of the 12th thoracic vertebra, 1.5 *cun* lateral to the posterior midline.

[Anatomy]

(1) Layer of needling: Skin-subcutaneous tissue-broadest muscle of the back-inferior posterior serratus muscle-erector spinal muscle.

(2) Innervation and vasculature: In the superficial layer, there are the cutaneous branches of the posterior branches of the 12th thoracic and 1st lumbar nerves and the accompanying artery and vein. In the deep layer, there are the muscular branches of the posterior branches of the 12th thoracic and 1st lumbar nerves and the dorsal branches of the related intercostal artery.

[Indications] Pain in the epigastric region, abdominal distension, vomiting, borborygmus, pain in the chest and hypochondriac region.

[Operation] Puncture perpendicularly 0.5~1 *cun*.

16. BL 22 (*sān jiāo shù*) Back-*Shu* Point of the *Sanjiao* Channel

[Location] On the lower back, below the spinous process of the 1st lumbar vertebra, 1.5 *cun* lateral to the posterior midline.

[Anatomy]

(1) Layer of needling: Skin-subcutaneous tissue-broadest muscle of the back-inferior posterior serratus muscle-erector spinal muscle.

(2) Innervation and vasculature: In the superficial layer, there are the cutaneous branches of the posterior branches of the 1st and 2nd lumbar nerves and the accompanying artery and vein. In the deep layer, there are the muscular branches of the posterior branches of 1st and 2nd lumbar nerves and the related dorsal branches of the lumbar artery.

[Indications] Pain in the epigastric region, abdominal distension, vomiting, borborygmus, pain in the chest and hypochondriac region.

[Operation] Puncture perpendicularly 0.5~1 *cun*.

17. BL 23 (*shèn shù*) Back-*Shu* Point of the Kidney Channel

[Location] On the lower back, below the spinous process of the 2nd lumbar vertebra, 1.5 *cun* lateral to the posterior midline.

[Anatomy]

(1) Layer of needling: Skin-subcutaneous tissue-superficial layer of the thoracolumbar fascia-erector spinal muscle.

(2) Innervation and vasculature: In the superficial layer, there are the cutaneous branches of the posterior branches of the 2nd and 3rd lumbar nerves and the accompanying artery and vein. In the deep layer, there are the muscular branches of the posterior branches of the 2nd and 3rd lumbar nerves and the dorsal branches of the related lumbar artery and vein.

[Indications] Seminal emission, impotence, premature ejeculation, sterility, infertility, enuresis, menstrual irregularity, morbid leucorrhea, lower back pain, dizziness, tinnitus, deafness, dysuresia, edema, shortness of breath and cough.

[Operation] Puncture perpendicularly 0.5~1 *cun*.

18. BL 25 (*dà cháng shù*) Back-*Shu* Point of the Large Intestine Channel

[Location] On the lower back, below the spinous process of the 4th lumbar vertebra,1.5 *cun* lateral to the posterior midline.

[Anatomy]

(1) Layer of needling: Skin-subcutaneous tissue-superficial layer of the thoracolumbar fascia-erector spinal muscle.

(2) Innervation and vasculature: In the superficial layer, there are the cutaneous branches of the posterior branches of the 4th and 5th lumbar nerves and the accompanying artery and vein. In the deep layer, there are the muscular branches of the posterior branches of 4th and 5th lumbar nerves and the dorsal branches of the related lumbar artery and vein.

[Indications] Lumbovertebral pain, abdominal distending pain, diarrhea, constipation, dysentery.

[Operation] Puncture perpendicularly 0.5~1.2 *cun*.

19. BL 26 (*guān yuán shù*)

[Location] On the lower back, below the spinous process of the 5th lumbar vertebra, 1.5 *cun* lateral to the posterior midline.

[Anatomy]

(1) Layer of needling: Skin-subcutaneous tissue-superficial layer of the thoracolumbar fascia-erector spinal muscle.

(2) Innervation and vasculature: In the superficial layer, there are the cutaneous branches of the posterior branches of the 5th lumbar and 1st sacral nerves and the accompanying artery and vein. In the deep layer, there are the muscular branches of the posterior branches of 5th lumbar nerves and the dorsal branches of the lowest lumbar artery.

[Indications] Abdominal distension, diarrhea, constipation, dysuresia, enuresis, wasting and thirst disorder, lower back pain.

[Operation] Puncture perpendicularly 0.5~1.2 *cun*.

20. BL 27 (*xiǎo cháng shù*) Back-*Shu* Point of the Small Intestine Channel

[Location] On the sacrum, on the level of the 1st posterior sacral foramen, 1.5 *cun* lateral to the median sacral crest.

[Anatomy]

(1) Layer of needling: Skin-subcutaneous tissue-great gluteal muscle-erector spinal muscle.

(2) Innervation and vasculature: In the superficial layer, there are the middle clunial nerves. In the deep layer, there are the branches of the inferior gluteal nerve and the muscular branches of the posterior branches of the 1st sacral nerve.

[Indications] Seminal emission, enuresis, morbid leucorrhea, lower abdominal distending pain, diarrhea, dysentery, lower back and leg pain.

[Operation] Puncture perpendicularly 0.8~1.2 *cun*.

21. BL 28 (*páng guāng shù*) Back-*Shu* Point of the Urinary Bladder Channel

[Location] On the sacrum, on the level of the 2nd posterior sacral foramen, 1.5 *cun* lateral to the median sacral crest.

[Anatomy]

(1) Layer of needling: Skin-subcutaneous tissue-greatest gluteal muscle-erector spinal muscle.

(2) Innervation and vasculature: In the superficial layer, there are the middle clunial nerves. In the deep layer, there are the branches of the inferior gluteal nerve and the muscular branches of the posterior branches of the inferior and superior gluteal nerves.

[Indications] Seminal emission, enuresis, dysuresia, diarrhea, pain in the lower back and sacral region.

[Operation] Puncture perpendicularly 0.8~1.2 *cun*.

22. BL 29 (*zhōng lǚ shù*)

[Location] On the sacrum, on the level of the 3rd posterior sacral foramen, 1.5 *cun* lateral to the median sacral crest.

[Anatomy]

(1) Layer of needling: Skin-subcutaneous tissue-greatest gluteal muscle-sacrotuberous ligament.

(2) Innervation and vasculature: In the superficial layer, there are the middle clunial nerves. In the deep layer, there are the branches of the inferior gluteal nerve and the superior gluteal artery.

[Indications] Pain in the lower back and sacral region, wasting and thirst disorder, dysentery.

[Operation] Puncture perpendicularly 0.8~1.2 *cun*.

23. BL 30 (*bái huán shù*)

[Location] On the sacrum, on the level of the 4th posterior sacral foramen, 1.5 *cun* lateral to the median sacral crest.

[Anatomy]

(1) Layer of needling: Skin-subcutaneous tissue-greatest gluteal muscle-piriform muscle.

(2) Innervation and vasculature: In the superficial layer, there are the middle clunial nerves. In the deep layer, there are the branches of the inferior gluteal nerve and artery.

[Indications] Lower back and leg pain, morbid leucorrhea, seminal emission, menstrual irregularity.

[Operation] Puncture perpendicularly 0.8~1.2 *cun*.

24. **BL 31** (*shàng liáo*)

[Location] On the sacrum, at the midpoint between the posteriosuperior iliac spine and the posterior midline, just at the 1st posterior sacral foramen.

[Anatomy]

(1) Layer of needling: Skin-subcutaneous tissue-superficial layer of the thoracolumbar fascia-erector spinal muscle.

(2) Innervation and vasculature: In the superficial layer, there are the branches of the middle clunial nerve. In the deep layer, there are the branches of the lateral sacral nerve and the muscular branches of the posterior branches of the 1st sacral nerve.

[Indications] Lower back pain, menstrual irregularity, morbid leucorrhea, seminal emission, impotence, difficult bowels movement and dysuresia.

[Operation] Puncture perpendicularly 1~1.5 *cun*.

25. **BL 32** (*cì liáo*)

[Location] On the sacrum, medial and inferior to the posteriosuperior iliac spine, just at the 2nd posterior sacral foramen.

[Anatomy]

(1) Layer of needling: Skin-subcutaneous tissue-superficial layer of the thoracolumbar fascia-erector spinal muscle.

(2) Innervation and vasculature: In the superficial layer, there is the middle clunial nerve. In the deep layer, there are the posterior branches of the 2nd sacral nerve and the lateral sacral artery and vein.

[Indications] Lower back pain, menstrual irregularity, dysmenorrhea, dysuria, nocturnal emission, enuresis, pain, numbness and motor impairment of the lower limbs.

[Operation] Puncture perpendicularly 1~1.5 *cun*.

26. **BL 33** (*zhōng liáo*)

[Location] On the sacrum, medial and inferior to the posteriosuperior iliac spine, just at the 3rd posterior sacral foramen.

[Anatomy]

(1) Layer of needling: Skin-subcutaneous tissue-superficial layer of the thoracolumbar fascia-erector spinal muscle.

(2) Innervation and vasculature: In the superficial layer, there is the middle clunial nerve. In the deep layer, there are the branches of the lateral sacral artery and the muscular branches of the posterior branches of the 3rd sacral nerve.

[Indications] Lower back pain, menstrual irregularity, dysuresia, multicolor morbid leucorrhea, constipation.

[Operation] Puncture perpendicularly 1~1.5 *cun*.

27. BL 34 (*xià liáo*)

[Location] On the sacrum, medial and inferior to the posteriosuperior iliac spine, just at the 4th posterior sacral foramen.

[Anatomy]

(1) Layer of needling: Skin-subcutaneous tissue-superficial layer of the thoracolumbar fascia-erector spinal muscle.

(2) Innervation and vasculature: In the superficial layer, there is the middle clunial nerve. In the deep layer, there are the branches of the lateral sacral artery and the muscular branches of the posterior branches of the 4th sacral nerve.

[Indications] Lower back pain, dysuresia, borborygmus, constipation, lower abdominal pain.

[Operation] Puncture perpendicularly 1~1.5 *cun*.

28. BL 36 (*chéng fú*)

[Location] On the posterior side of the thigh, at the midpoint of the inferior gluteal crease.

[Anatomy]

(1) Layer of needling: Skin-subcutaneous tissue-greater gluteal muscle-between the long head of the biceps muscle of the thigh and the semitendinous muscle.

(2) Innervation and vasculature: In the superficial layer, there are the branches of the posterior femoral cutaneous nerve. In the deep layer, there are the branches of the inferior gluteal nerve and artery, the trunk of the sciatic nerve and the posterior cutaneous nerve of the thigh.

[Indications] Pain in the lower back, the sacral region and the gluteal region, hemorrhoids.

[Operation] Puncture perpendicularly 1~2.5 *cun*.

29. BL 39 (*wěi yáng*) Lower *He*-Sea Point of the *Sanjiao* Channel

[Location] At the lateral end of the popliteal crease, medial to the tendon of the biceps muscle of the thigh.

[Anatomy]

(1) Layer of needling: Skin-subcutaneous tissue-lateral head of the gastronemius muscle.

(2) Innervation and vasculature: In the superficial layer, there is the posterior femoral cutaneous nerve. In the deep layer, there are the branches of the tibial nerve and the external artery of the knee, and the common peroneal nerve trunk.

[Indications] Distension and fullness of the lower abdomen, dysuresia, regidity and pain of the lower back, cramp of the leg and foot.

[Operation] Puncture perpendicularly 1~1.5 *cun*.

30. BL 40 (*wěi zhōng*) *He*-Sea Point; Lower *He*-Sea Point of the Bladder Channel

[Location] At the midpoint of the popliteal crease, between the tendons of the biceps muscle of the thigh and the semitendinosus muscle.

[Anatomy]

(1) Layer of needling: Skin-subcutaneous tissue-between the medial and lateral heads of the gastrocnemius muscle-cavity lipid.

(2) Innervation and vasculature: In the superficial layer, there are the posterior femoral cutaneous nerve. In the deep layer, there are the starting point of the medial cutaneous nerve of the calf, the tibial nerve trunk, artery and vein.

[Indications] Lower back pain, pain numbness and motor impairment of the lower limbs, coma in wind-stroke, hemiplegia, abdominal pain, vomiting, diarrhea, dysuresia, enuresis, erysipelas.

[Operation] Puncture perpendicularly 1~1.5 *cun*.

31. BL 42 (*pò hù*)

[Location] On the back, below the spinous process of the 3rd thoracic vertebra, 3 *cun* lateral to the posterior midline.

[Anatomy]

(1) Layer of needling: Skin-subcutaneous tissue-trapezius muscle-rhomboid muscle-superior posterior serratus muscle-erector spinal muscle.

(2) Innervation and vasculature: In the superficial layer, there are the cutaneous branches of the posterior branches of the 3rd and 4th thoracic nerves and the accompanying artery and vein. In the deep layer, there are the accessory nerve, dorsal scapular nerve, the posterior branches of the 3rd and 4th thoracic nerves and the branches of the dorsal scapular artery, the scapular nerve and artery.

[Indications] Cough, shortness of breath, pulmonary tuberculosis, pain in the shoulder and back.

[Operation] Puncture obliquely 0.5~0.8 *cun*.

32. BL 43 (*gāo huāng*)

[Location] On the back, below the spinous process of the 4th thoracic vertebra, 3 *cun* lateral to the posterior midline.

[Anatomy]

(1) Layer of needling: Skin-subcutaneous tissue-trapezius muscle-rhomboid muscle-erector spinal muscle.

(2) **Innervation and vasculature:** In the superficial layer, there are the cutaneous branches of the posterior branches of the 4th and 5th thoracic nerves and the accompanying artery and vein. In the deep layer, there are phrenic nerve, dorsal scapulacostal nerve, the muscular branches of the posterior branches of the 4th and 5th thoracic nerves and branches of the dorsal nerve and artery of the scapula.

[Indications] Cough, shortness of breath, hematemesis,night sweating, pulmonary tuberculosis, poor memory, seminal emission, pain in the shoulder, scapular region and the lower back.

[Operation] Puncture obliquely 0.5-0.8 *cun*.

33. BL 44 (*shén táng*)

[Location] On the back, below the spinous process of the 5th thoracic vertebra, 3 *cun* lateral to the posterior midline.

[Anatomy]

(1) **Layer of needling:** Skin-subcutaneous tissue-trapezius muscle-rhomboid muscle-erector spinal muscle.

(2) **Innervation and vasculature:** In the superficial layer, there are the cutaneous branches of the posterior branches of the 5th and 6th thoracic nerves and the accompanying artery and vein. In the deep layer, there are the phrenic nerve, the dorsal scapulocostal nerve, the muscular branches of the posterior branches of the 5th and 6th thoracic nerves and branches of the dorsal scapular artery.

[Indications] Cough, shortness of breath, constriction in the chest, back pain.

[Operation] Puncture obliquely 0.5-0.8 *cun*.

34. BL 46 (*gě guān*)

[Location] On the back, below the spinous process of the 7th thoracic vertebra, 3 *cun* lateral to the posterior midline.

[Anatomy]

(1) **Layer of needling:** Skin-subcutaneous tissue-broadest muscle of the back-erector spinal muscle.

(2) **Innervation and vasculature:** In the superficial layer, there are the lateral cutaneous branches of the posterior branches of the 7th and 8th thoracic nerves and the accompanying artery and vein. In the deep layer, there are the phretic nerve, the dorsal scapulocostal nerve, the muscular branches of the posterior branches of the 7th and 8th thoracic nerves and the branches of the thoracodorsal artery.

[Indications] Vomiting, belching, difficulty in swallowing, constriction in the chest, regidity and pain of the lower back.

[Operation] Puncture obliquely 0.5-0.8 *cun*.

35. BL 47 (*hún mén*)

[Location] On the back, below the spinous process of the 9th thoracic vertebra, 3 *cun* lateral to the posterior midline.

[Anatomy]

(1) Layer of needling: Skin-subcutaneous tissue-broadest muscle of the back-erector spinal muscle.

(2) Innervation and vasculature: In the superficial layer, there are the lateral cutaneous branches of the posterior branches of the 9th and 10th thoracic nerves and the accompanying artery and vein. In the deep layer, there are the muscular branches of the posterior branches of the 9th and 10th thoracic nerves and the branches of the thoracodorsal artery.

[Indications] Pain in the chest and hypochondriac region, vomiting, back pain.

[Operation] Puncture obliquely 0.5-0.8 *cun*.

36. BL 52 (*zhì shì*)

[Location] On the lower back, below the spinous process of the 2nd lumbar vertebra, 3 *cun* lateral to the posterior midline.

[Anatomy]

(1) Layer of needling: Skin-subcutaneous tissue-broadest muscle of the back-erector spinal muscle.

(2) Innervation and vasculature: In the superficial layer, there are the lateral cutaneous branches of the posterior branches of the 1st and 2nd lumbar nerves and the accompany artery and vein. In the deep layer, there are the muscular branches of the posterior branches of the thoracodorsal nerve and the 1st and 2nd lumbar nerves and the branches of the 1st lumbodorsal artery.

[Indications] Seminal emission, impotence, vaginal pain, dysuresia, edema, stiffness and pain in the lower back.

[Operation] Puncture perpendicularly 0.5~1 *cun*.

37. BL 54 (*zhì biān*)

[Location] On the buttock, on the level of the 4th posterior sacral foramen, 3 *cun* lateral to the median sacral crest.

[Anatomy]

(1) Layer of needling: Skin-subcutaneous tissue-greatest gluteal muscle-lower border of the piniform muscle.

(2) **Innervation and vasculature:** In the superficial layer, there are the middle and inferior clunial nerves. In the deep layer, there are the branches of the inferior gluteal nerve and artery, and the posterior cutaneous nerve of the thigh and the sciatic nerve.

[Indications] Pain in the lower back and leg, numbness and motor impairment of the lower limbs, pain in the penis, hemorrhoids.

[Operation] Puncture perpendicularly 1.5~3 *cun*.

38. BL 57 (*chéng shān*)

[Location] On the posterior midline of the leg, between BL 4 (*wěi zhōng*) and BL 60 (*kūn lún*), in the pointed depression directly below the belly of the gastrcnemius muscle when the leg is stretched or the heel is lifted.

[Anatomy]

(1) **Layer of needling:** Skin-subcutaneous tissue-gastrocnemius muscle-soleus muscle.

(2) **Innervation and vasculature:** In the superficial layer, there are the branches of the medial cutaneous nerve of the calf. In the deep layer, there are the tibial nerve and branches of the posterior tibial artery, medial nerve trunk of the calf, the small saphenous vein, the tibial nerve trunk and the trunk of the posterior tibial artery.

[Indications] Lower back and back pain, spasm of the lower leg, hemorrhoids, constipation, abdominal pain, hernia.

[Operation] Puncture perpendicularly 1~2 *cun*.

39. BL 59 (*fū yáng*) Point of the Yang Heel Vessel; *Xi*-Cleft Point

[Location] On the posterior side of the leg, posterior to the lateral malleolus, 3 *cun* directly above BL 60 (*kūn lún*).

[Anatomy]

(1) **Layer of needling:** Skin-subcutaneous tissue-short peroneal muscle-long flexor muscle of the great toe.

(2) **Innervation and vasculature:** In the superficial layer, there are the branches of the cutaneous nerve of the calf and the small saphenous vein. In the deep layer, there are the branches of the superifical peroneal nerve, tibial nerve and the peroneal artery.

[Indications] Headache, heaviness sensation of the head, pain in the lower back and leg, paralysis of the lower limbs, red swollen external malleolus.

[Operation] Puncture perpendicularly 0.8~1.2 *cun*.

40. BL 60 (*kūn lún*) *Jing*-River Point

[Location] Posterior to the lateral malleolus, in the depression between the tip of the external malleolus and Achilles tendon.

[Anatomy]

(1) Layer of needling: Skin-subcutaneous tissue-between the short peroneal muscle and the achilles tendon.

(2) Innervation and vasculature: In the superficial layer, there are the branches of the cutaneous nerve of the calf and the small saphenous vein, the sural nerve trunk and the small saphenous vein. In the deep layer, there are the branches or of the posterior artery of the external malleolus (from the peroneal artery).

[Indications] Headache, neck rigidity, blurred vision, epistaxis, malaria, pain and stiffness in the shoulder and back, pain in the heel, epilepsy, difficult labor.

[Operation] Puncture perpendicularly 0.5~0.8 *cun*.

41. BL 62 (*shēn mài*) Confluence Point that links the Yang Heel Vessel

[Location] On the lateral side of the foot, in the depression directly below the external malleolus.

[Anatomy]

(1) Layer of needling: Skin-subcutaneous tissue-crucial ligament of the foot-short extensor muscle of the toe.

(2) Innervation and vasculature: There are the branches of the lateral dorsal cutaneous nerve of the foot and the small saphenous vein. In the deeper layer, there are the muscular branches of the deep peroneal nerve and the lateral branches of the peroneal artery.

[Indications] Epilepsy, mania, headache, insomnia, dizziness, lower back pain, red painful eyes, neck rigidity.

[Operation] Puncture perpendicularly 0.3~0.5 *cun*.

42. BL 66 (*zú tōng gŭ*) *Ying*-Spring Point

[Location] On the lateral side of the foot, in the depression anterior to the 5th metatarsophalangeal joint, at the junction of the red and white skin.

[Anatomy]

(1) Layer of needling: Skin-subcutaneous tissue.

(2) Innervation and vasculature: There are the branches of the lateral dorsal cutaneous nerve and artery of the foot, the proper digital plantar nerve and artery.

[Indications] Headache, neck rigidity, blurred version, epistaxis, mania.

[Operation] Puncture perpendicularly 0.2~0.3 *cun*.

43. BL 67 (*zhì yīn*) *Jing*-Well Point

[Location] On the lateral side of the distal segment of the little toe, 0.1 *cun* posterior to the corner of the toenail.

[Anatomy]

(1) Layer of needling: Skin-subcutaneous tissue.

(2) Innervation and vasculature: There are the branches of the dorsal digital nerve and artery.

[Indications] Headache, stuffy nose, epistaxis, eye pain, retention of placenta, malposition of fetus, difficult labor.

[Operation] Puncture 0.1 *cun*.

Section 8 The Kidney Channel of Foot *Shaoyin*

1. KI 1 (*yǒng quán*) *Jing*-Well Point

[Location] On the sole, in the depression appearing when the foot is curled up, at the junction of the anterior third and posterior two-thirds of the line that links the heel and the toe web between the 2nd and the 3rd toes.

[Anatomy]

(1) Layer of needling: Skin-subcutaneous tissue-plantar aponeurosis-short flexor muscle of the toe-2nd lumbrical muscle.

(2) Innervation and vasculature: In the superficial layer, there are the cutaneous branches of the lateral medial nerve of the sole. In the deep layer, there are the muscular branches of the lateral nerve and medial artery of the sole and the 2nd common digital nerve of the sole and the 2nd plantar metatarsal arterial trunk.

[Indications] Headache, dizziness, dysuresia, constipation, infantile convulsion, feverish sensation in the soles, loss of consciousness.

[Operation] Puncture perpendicularly 0.5~1 *cun*.

2. KI 2 (*rán gŭ*) *Ying*-Spring Point

[Location] On the medial border of the foot, below the tuberosity of the navicular bone, at the junction of the red and white skin.

[Anatomy]

(1) Layer of needling: Skin-subcutaneous tissue-abductor muscle of the great toe.

(2) Innervation and vasculature: In the superficial layer, there are the branches of the saphenous nerve and vein. In the deep layer, there are the branches of the medial nerve and artery of the sole.

[Indications] Menstrual irregularity, morbid leucorrhea, seminal emission, dysuresia, diarrhea, pain and fullness in the chest and hypochondriac region, hemoptysis, neonatal tetanus, lockjaw, jaundice, pain, numbness and motor impairment of the lower limbs, painful instep.

[Operation] Puncture perpendicularly 0.5~0.8 *cun*.

3. KI 3 (*tài xī*) *Shu*-Stream Point; *Yuan*-Source Point

[Location] On the medial side of the foot, posterior to the medial malleolus, in the depression between the tip of the medial malleolus and the Achilles tendon.

[Anatomy]

(1) Layer of needling: Skin-subcutaneous tissue-long flexor muscle of the toe.

(2) Innervation and vasculature: In the superficial layer, there are the branches of the saphenous nerve and the great great saphenous vein. In the deep layer, there are the branches of the tibial nerve and the posterior tibial artery.

[Indications] Headache, blurred vision, sore throat, toothache, deafness, tinnitus, asthma, chest pain, spitting of blood, wasting and thirst disorder, menstrual irregularity, insomnia, poor memory, seminal emission, impotence, frequency of micturition, pain in the lower back, cold lower limbs, painful swollen medial malleolus.

[Operation] Puncture perpendicularly 0.5~1 *cun*.

4. KI 5 (*shuĭ quán*) *Xi*-Cleft Point

[Location] On the medial side of the foot, posterior and inferior to the medial malleolus, 1 *cun* directly below KI 3 (*tài xī*), in the depression anterior to the medial side of the tuberosity of the calcaneum.

[Anatomy]

(1) Layer of needling: Skin-subcutaneous tissue-calcaneal bone.

(2) Innervation and vasculature: In the superficial layer, there are the branches of the saphenous nerve and the great saphenous vein. In the deep layer, there are the tibial artery trunk and the posterior tibial artery trunk.

[Indications] Menstrual irregularity, dysmenorrhea, dysuresia, abdominal pain, blurred vision.

[Operation] Puncture perpendicularly 0.3~0.5 *cun*.

5. KI 6 (*zhào hăi*) Confluence Point that links the Yin Heal Vessel

[Location] On the medial side of the foot, in the depression below the tip of the medial malleolus.

[Anatomy]

(1) Layer of needling: Skin-subcutaneous tissue-tendon of posterior tibial muscle.

(2) Innervation and vasculature: In the superficial layer, there are the branches of the saphenous nerve and the great saphenous vein. In the deep layer, there are the muscular branches of the medial nerve of the medial heel and the branches of the posterior tibial artery.

[Indications] Epilepsy, insomnia, dysuresia, frequency of micturition, dry throat, sore throat, red painful swollen eye, menstrual irregularity, dysmenorrhea, morbid leucorrhea.

[Operation] Puncture perpendicularly 0.5~1 *cun*.

6. KI 7 (*fù liū*) *Jing*-River Point

[Location] On the medial side of the foot, 2 *cun* directly above KI 3 (*tài xī*), anterior to the Achilles tendon.

[Anatomy]

(1) Layer of needling: Skin-subcutaneous tissue-long flexor muscle of the great toe.

(2) Innervation and vasculature: In the superficial layer, there are the branches of the saphenous nerve, the medial cutaneous nerve of the leg and the great saphenous vein. In the deep layer, there are the muscular branches of the tibial nerve and the branches of the posterior tibial artery.

[Indications] Diarrhea, borboryguma, edema, abdominal distension, swollen leg, muscular atrophy of the foot, night sweating, febrile disease without sweating, lower back pain and rigidity.

[Operation] Puncture perpendicularly 0.5~1 *cun*.

7. KI 8 (*jiāo xìn*) Point of Yin Heel Vessel; *Xi*-Cleft Point

[Location] On the medial side of the leg, 2 *cun* directly above KI 3 (*tài xī*), 0.5 *cun* anterior to KI 7 (*fù liū*), posterior to the medial border of the tibia.

[Anatomy]

(1) Layer of needling: Skin-subcutaneous tissue-long flexor muscle of the great toe.

(2) Innervation and vasculature: In the superficial layer, there are the branches of the saphenous nerve and the great saphenous vein. In the deep layer, there are the muscular branches of the tibial nerve and the branches of the posterior tibial artery and vein.

[Indications] Menstrual irregularity, metrorrhagia or metrostaxis, prolapse of the uterus, diarrhea, constipation, painful swollen testis, stranguria, hernia, vaginal itching, passing bloody purulent stools, pain in the knees and medial side of the thigh.

[Operation] Puncture perpendicularly 0.6~1.2 *cun*.

8. KI 10 (*yīn gǔ*) *He*-Sea Point

[Location] On the medial side of the popliteal fossa, with the knee flexed, between the tendons of the semitendinous and semimembranous muscles.

[Anatomy]

(1) Layer of needling: Skin-subcutaneous tissue-between the tendons of semimemnranous. Muscle and semitendinous muscle-medial head of the gastrocnemius muscle.

(2) Innervation and vasculature: In the superficial layer, there are the saphenous nerve and the great saphenous vein. In the deep layer, there are the muscular branches of the tibial nerve and artery, and the branches of the medial superior genicular artery.

[Indications] Impotence, hernia, menstrual irregularity, metrorrhagia or metrostaxis, dysuresia, vaginal pain, mania, pain in the knees and medial side of the thigh.

[Operation] Puncture perpendicularly 1~1.5 *cun*.

9. KI 12 (*dà hè*)

[Location] On the lower abdomen, 4 *cun* below the centre of the umbilicus, 0.5 *cun* lateral to the anterior midline.

[Anatomy]

(1) Layer of needling: Skin-subcutaneous tissue-anterior sheath of the rectus muscle of the abdomen-rectus muscle of the abdomen.

(2) Innervation and vasculature: In the superficial layer, there are the cutaneous branches of the iliohypogastric nerve and the branches of the superficial epigastric artery. In the deep layer, there are the muscular branches of the subcostal nerve and the branches of the inferior epigastric artery.

[Indications] Prolapse of the uterus, seminal emission, morbid leucorrhea, menstrual irregularity, dysmenorrhea, diarrhea.

[Operation] Puncture perpendicularly 1~1.5 *cun*.

10. KI 13 (*qì xué*)

[Location] On the lower abdomen, 3 *cun* below the centre of the umbilicus, 0.5 *cun* lateral to the anterior midline.

[Anatomy]

(1) Layer of needling: Skin-subcutaneous tissue-anterior sheath of the rectus muscle of the abdomen-rectus muscle of the abdomen.

(2) Innervation and vasculature: In the superficial layer, there are the cutaneous subcostal nerve and the branches of the superficial epigastric artery. In the deep layer, there are the muscular branches of the subcostal nerve and the branches of the inferior epigastric artery.

[Indications] Menstrual irregularity, morbid leucorrhea, dysuresia, diarrhea.

[Operation] Puncture perpendicularly 1~1.5 *cun*.

11. KI 16 (*huāng shù*)

[Location] On the lower abdomen, 0.5 *cun* lateral to the anterior midline.

[Anatomy]

(1) Layer of needling: Skin-subcutaneous tissue-anterior sheath of the rectus muscle of the abdomen-rectus muscle of the abdomen.

(2) Innervation and vasculature: In the superficial layer, there are the anterior cutaneous branches of the 10th intercostal nerve and the periumbilical venous network. In the deep layer, there are the muscular branches of the 10th intercostal nerve and the branches of the superior-inferior epigastric arteries.

[Indications] Abdominal distending pain, vomiting, constipation, diarrhea.

[Operation] Puncture perpendicularly 1~1.5 *cun*.

Section 9 The Pericardium Channel of Hand *Jueyin*

1. PC 3 (*qǔ zé*) *He*-Sea Point

[Location] In the middle of the transverse cubital crease, at the ulnar side of the biceps muscle of the arm.

[Anatomy]

(1) Layer of needling: Skin-subcutaneous tissue-round pronator muscle-branchial muscle.

(2) Innervation and vasculature: In the superficial layer, there are the medial cutaneous nerve of the forearm, medial cubital vein and cutaneous vein. In the deep layer, there are the median nerve and the brachial artery.

[Indications] Heart pain, palpitation, stomachache, vomiting, diarrhea, febrile disease, contracture and pain in the elbow and arm.

[Operation] Puncture perpendicularly 0.8~1 *cun* or prick to bleed.

2. PC 4 (*xì mén*) *Xi*-Cleft Point

[Location] On the palmar side of the forearm and on the line that connects PC 3 (*qǔ zé*) and PC 7 (*dà líng*), 5 *cun* above the transverse crease of the wrist.

[Anatomy]

(1) Layer of needling: Skin-subcutaneous tissue-superficial flexor muscle of the fingers-deep flexor muscle of the fingers.

(2) Innervation and vasculature: In the superficial layer, there are the medial and lateral cutaneous nerves of the forearm and the median veins of the forearm. In the deep layer, there are the median nerve trunk and the accompanying median nerve, and the anterior interosseous artery.

[Indications] Heart pain, pain in the chest, hematemesis, hemoptysis, epilepsy.

[Operation] Puncture perpendicularly 0.5~1 *cun*.

3. PC 5 (*jiān shǐ*) *Jing*-River Point

[Location] On the palmar side of the forearm and on the line that links PC 3 (*qū zé*) and PC 7 (*dà líng*), 3 *cun* above the crease of the wrist, between the long palmar muscle and radial flexor muscle of the wrist.

[Anatomy]

(1) Layer of needling: Skin-subcutaneous tissue-superficial flexor muscle of the fingers-deep flexor muscle of the fingers-quadrate pronator muscle.

(2) Innervation and vasculature: In the superficial layer, there are the lateral and medial cutaneous nerves and the median vein of the forearm. In the deep layer, there are the median nerve and the accompanying artery and vein and the anterior interosseous nerve and artery.

[Indications] Heart pain, palpitation, stomachache, vomiting, febrile disease, malaria, mania and epilepsy, pain in the arm.

[Operation] Puncture perpendicularly 0.5~1 *cun*.

4. PC 6 (*nèi guān*) *Luo*-Connecting Point; Confluence Point that links the Yin Link Vessel

[Location] On the palmar side of the forearm and on the line that connects PC 3 (*qū zé*) and PC 7 (*dà líng*), 2 *cun* above the crease of the wrist, between the long palmar muscle and the radial flexor muscle of the wrist.

[Anatomy]

(1) Layer of needling: Skin-subcutaneous tissue-between the long palmar muscle and the radial flexor muscle of the wrist-quadrate pronate muscle.

(2) Innervation and vasculature: In the superficial layer, there are the branches of the medial and lateral cutaneous nerves and the median vein of the forearm. In the deep layer, there are the median nerve trunk and the accompanying median artery, the anterior interosseous nerve and artery.

[Indications] Heart pain, palpitation, chest distress, pain in the chest, stomachache, vomiting, hiccups, epilepsy, febrile disease, impediment and pain of the arm, insomnia, dizziness, migraine.

[Operation] Puncture perpendicularly 0.5~1 *cun*.

5. PC 7 (*dà líng*) *Shu*-Stream Point; *Yuan*-Source Point

[Location] At the midpoint of the transverse crease of the wrist, between the long palmar muscle and the radial flexor muscle of the wrist.

[Anatomy]

(1) Layer of needling: Skin-subcutaneous tissue-annular ligament (transverse carpal ligament).

(2) **Innervation and vasculature:** In the superficial layer, there are the lateral superficial carpometacarpal venous network and the branches of the median nerve. In the deep layer, there are median nerve and the lateral carpometacarpal artrerial network.

[Indications] Heart pain, palpitation, stomachache, vomiting, mania, pain in the chest and costal region, pain in the wrist joint.

[Operation] Puncture perpendicularly 0.3~0.5 *cun*.

6. PC 8 (*láo gōng*) *Ying*-Spring Point

[Location] In the centre of the palm, between the 2nd and the 3rd metacarpal bones, adjacent to the latter, and in the part where the middle finger tip touches when a fist is made.

[Anatomy]

(1) **Layer of needling:** Skin-subcutaneous tissue-palmar aponeurosis-superficial and deep flexor muscle of the fingers.

(2) **Innervation and vasculature:** In the superficial layer, there are the cutaneous branches of the median nerve of the palmar side. In the deep layer, there are the branches of the digital nerve of the median nerve, the deep palmar branch of the ulnar nerve, the superficial palmar arch and its branches, and the common palmar digital artery and its branches, and the metacarpal arteries.

[Indications] Heart pain, vomiting, mania, aphtha, foul breath.

[Operation] Puncture perpendicularly 0.3~0.5 *cun*.

Section 10 The *Sanjiao* Channel of Hand *Shaoyang*

1. SJ 2 (*yè mén*) *Ying*-Spring Point

[Location] On the dorsum of the hand, between the 4th and the 5th fingers, at the junction of the red and white skin, posterior to the web.

[Anatomy]

(1) **Layer of needling:** Skin-subcutaneous tissue.

(2) **Innervation and vasculature:** There are the dorsal digital nerve (branches of the nerve) and the dorsal arterial network of the hand.

[Indications] Headache, red eyes, deafness, tinnitus, sore throat, malaria, pain in the arm.

[Operation] Puncture perpendicularly 0.3~0.5 *cun*.

2. SJ 3 (*zhōng zhǔ*) *Shu*-Stream Point

[Location] On the dorsum of the hand, posterior to the 4th metacarpophalangeal joint, in the depression between the 4th and the 5th metacarpal bones.

[Anatomy]

(1) Layer of needling: Skin-subcutaneous tissue-dorsal interosseous muscle.

(2) Innervation and vasculature: In the superficial layer, there are the dorsal venous network of the hand, the cutaneous branches of the ulnar nerve. In the deep layer, there are the muscular branches of the ulnar nerve and the dorsal metacarpal artery.

[Indications] Headache, red eyes, deafness, tinnitus, sore throat, febrile disease, motor impairment of fingers.

[Operation] Puncture perpendicularly 0.3~0.5 *cun*.

3. SJ 4 (*yáng chí*) *Yuan*-Source Point

[Location] At the midpoint of the dorsal crease of the wrist, in the depression on the ulnar side of the extensor muscle of fingers.

[Anatomy]

(1) Layer of needling: Skin-subcutaneous tissue-annular ligament of the wrist.

(2) Innervation and vasculature: In the superficial layer, there are the dorsal branches of the ulnar nerve. In the deep layer, there are the dorsal carpal ulnar artery.

[Indications] Red swollen painful eyes, deafness, sore throat, malaria, wasting and thirst disorder, pain in the wrist.

[Operation] Puncture perpendicularly 0.3~0.5 *cun*.

4. SJ 5 (*wài guān*) *Luo*-Connecting Point; Confluence Point that links the Yang Link Vessel

[Location] On the dorsal side of the forearm, on the line that links SJ 4 (*yáng chí*) and the tip of the olecranon, 2 *cun* above the transverse crease of the wrist, between the radius and ulna.

[Anatomy]

(1) Layer of needling: Skin-subcutaneous tissue-extensor muscle of the little finger-long extensor muscle of the thumb-extensor muscle of the index finger.

(2) Innervation and vasculature: In the superficial layer, there are the posterior cutaneous nerve of the forearm. In the deep layer, there are the posterior interosseous nerve and artery.

[Indications] Febrile disease, headache, painful cheeks, red swollen painful eyes, tinnitus, deafness, scrofula, pain in the hypochondriac region, pain and impediment of the upper limbs.

[Operation] Puncture perpendicularly 0.5~1 *cun*.

5. SJ 6 (*zhī gōu*) *Jing*-River Point

[Location] On the dorsal side of the forearm, on the line that links SJ 4 (*yáng*

chí) and the tip of the olecranon, 3 *cun* above the transverse crease of the wrist, between the radius and ulna.

[Anatomy]

(1) Layer of needling: Skin-subcutaneous tissue-long extensor muscle of the little finger-long extensor muscle of the thumb.

(2) Innervation and vasculature: In the superficial layer, there are the posterior cutaneous nerve of the forearm. In the deep layer, there are the posterior interosseous nerve and artery.

[Indications] Tinnitus, deafness, sudden aphonia, scrofula, pain in the hypochondriac region, constipation, febrile disease.

[Operation] Puncture perpendicularly 0.5~1 *cun*.

6. SJ 10 (*tiān jǐng*) *He*-Sea Point

[Location] On the lateral side of the upper arm, in the depression 1 *cun* above the tip of the olecranon when the elbow is flexed.

[Anatomy]

(1) Layer of needling: Skin-subcutaneous tissue-brachial triceps muscle.

(2) Innervation and vasculature: In the superficial layer, there is the posterior brachial cutaneous nerve. In the deep layer, there are the the muscular branches of the radial nerve and the arterial network of the elbow joint.

[Indications] Migraine, deafness, scrofula, pain in the hypochondriac region, epilepsy.

[Operation] Puncture perpendicularly 0.5~1 *cun*.

7. SJ 13 (*nào huì*)

[Location] On the lateral side of the upper arm, on the line that links the tip of the olecranon and SJ 14 (*jiān liáo*), 3 *cun* below SJ 14 (*jiān liáo*), on the posterior border of the deltoid muscle.

[Anatomy]

(1) Layer of needling: Skin-subcutaneous tissue-brachial triceps muscle.

(2) Innervation and vasculature: In the superficial layer, there is the posterior brachial cutaneous nerve. In the deep layer, there are the muscular branches of the radial nerve and the deep brachial artery.

[Indications] Goiter, scrofula, pain and impediment of the upper limbs.

[Operation] Puncture perpendicularly 0.5~1 *cun*.

8. SJ 14 (*jiān liáo*)

[Location] On the posterior shoulder, in the depression posterior and inferior to the acromion when the arm is abducted.

[Anatomy]

(1) Layer of needling: Skin-subcutaneous tissue-deltoid muscle-infraspinous muscle.

(2) Innervation and vasculature: In the superficial layer, there is the lateral supraclavicular nerve. In the deep layer, there are the axillary nerve and the posterior circumflex humeral artery.

[Indications] Arm pain, heaviness sensation and motor impairment of the shoulder.

[Operation] Puncture perpendicularly 0.5~1 *cun* towards the articulation of the shoulder.

9. SJ 17 (*yì fēng*)

[Location] Posterior to the ear lobe, in the depression between the mandibular angle and mastoid process.

[Anatomy]

(1) Layer of needling: Skin-subcutaneous tissue-parotid gland.

(2) Innervation and vasculature: In the superficial layer, there are the great auricular nerve, the auricular branches of the facial nerve and the posterior auricular vein. In the deep layer, there are the facial nerve trunk, the parotid branch of the glossopharyngeal nerve, the posterior auricular artery and the pterygoid venous plexus.

[Indications] Tinnitus, deafness, deviation of the eye and mouth, lockjaw, toothache, swollen cheeks, scrofula.

[Operation] Puncture perpendicularly 0.8~1.2 *cun*.

10. SJ 20 (*jiăo sūn*)

[Location] On the head, with the ear flexed forward, directly above the ear apex, within the hairline.

[Anatomy]

(1) Layer of needling: Skin-subcutaneous tissue-superior auricular muscle-temporal muscle.

(2) Innervation and vasculature: There are the cutaneous branches of the auriculotemporal nerve. In the deep layer, there are the muscular branches of the auriculotemporal nerve and the superficial temporal artery.

[Indications] Swollen cheeks, parotitis, toothache, neck rigidity.

[Operation] Puncture horizontally 0.3-0.5 *cun*.

11. SJ 21 (*ěr mén*)

[Location] On the face, anterior to the supratragic notch, at the posterior border of the condyloid process of the mandible, in the depression with the mouth open.

[Anatomy]

(1) Layer of needling: Skin-subcutaneous tissue-parotid gland.

(2) Innervation and vasculature: In the superficial layer, there are the auriculotemporal nerve, the superficial temporal arterial nerve trunk. In the deep layer, there are the branches of the parotid branch of the glossopharyngeal nerve.

[Indications] Tinnitus, deafness, ear pain, toothache.

[Operation] Puncture perpendicularly 0.5~1 *cun* when the mouth is open.

12. SJ 23 (*sī zhú kōng*)

[Location] On the face, in the depression of the lateral end of the eyebrow.

[Anatomy]

(1) Layer of needling: Skin-subcutaneous tissue-orbicular muscle of the eye.

(2) Innervation and vasculature: In the superficial layer, there are the zygomaticotemporal branches of the mandibular nerve and the superficial temporal artery. In the deep layer, there are the temporal branches of the facial nerve and the muscular branches of the superficial temporal artery.

[Indications] Headache, red swollen painful eyes, twitching of eyelid, toothache, mania and epilepsy.

[Operation] Puncture horizontally 0.5-1 *cun*.

Section 11 The Gallbladder Channel of Foot *Shaoyang*

1. GB 1 (*tóng zǐ liáo*)

[Location] On the face, lateral to the outer canthus, on the lateral border of the orbit.

[Anatomy]

(1) Layer of needling: Skin-subcutaneous tissue-orbicular muscle of the eye-temporal muscle.

(2) Innervation and vasculature: In the superficial layer, there are the phthalmic nerve of the trigeminal nerve and the superior maxillary nerve. In the deep layer, there are the temporal and zygomatic branches of the facial nerve, and the superficial temporal artery.

[Indications] Headache, red swollen painful eyes, cloudy cornea, optic atrophy.

[Operation] Puncture horizontally 0.3~0.5 *cun* or prick to bleed.

2. GB 2 (*tīng huì*)

[Location] On the face, anterior to the intertragic notch, on the posterior border of the condyloid process of the mandible, in the depression with the mouth open.

[Anatomy]

(1) Layer of needling: Skin-subcutaneous tissue-messeteric fascia-parotid gland.

(2) Innervation and vasculature: In the superficial layer, there are the auriculotemporal nerve, the great auricular nerve and the superficial temporal artery. In the deep layer, there are the branches of the facial nerve plexus, the muscular branches of the mandibular nerve, and the branches of the glossopharyngeal nerve.

[Indications] Tinnitus, deafness, ear pain, painful cheeks, toothache, deviation of the mouth.

[Operation] Puncture perpendicularly 0.5~1 *cun* when the mouth is open.

3. GB 4 (*hán yàn*)

[Location] Within the hairline of the temporal region, at the junction of the upper 1/4 and lower 3/4 of the curved line that links ST 8 (*tóu wéi*) and GB 7 (*qū bìn*).

[Anatomy]

(1) Layer of needling: Skin-subcutaneous tissue-temporal muscle.

(2) Innervation and vasculature: There are the 2nd branch of the trigeminal nerve, the temporal branch of the facial nerve and the superficial temporal artery.

[Indications] Migraine, blurred vision, tinnitus, toothache, epilepsy.

[Operation] Puncture horizontally 0.3~0.5 *cun*.

4. GB 6 (*xuán lí*)

[Location] Within the hairline of the temporal region, at the junction of the upper 3/4 and lower 1/4 of the curved line that links ST 8 (*tóu wéi*) and GB 7 (*qū bìn*).

[Anatomy] Same as GB 4 (*hàn yàn*).

[Indications] Migraine, red swollen painful eyes, tinnitus.

[Operation] Puncture horizontally 0.5-0.8 *cun*.

5. GB 7 (*qū bìn*)

[Location] On the head, at the crossing point of the vertical posterior border of the temple and the horizontal line through the ear apex.

[Anatomy]

(1) Layer of needling: Skin-subcutaneous tissue-superior auricular muscle-temporal muscle.

(2) Innervation and vasculature: In the superficial layer, there are the auriculotemporal nerve and the superficial temporal artery. In the deep layer, there are the branches of the posterior auricular nerve and facial nerve, and the muscular branches of the mandibular nerve.

[Indications] Headache, toothache, lockjaw, sudden aphonia.

[Operation] Puncture horizontally 0.5-0.8 *cun*.

6. GB 8 (*shuài gŭ*)

[Location] On the head, superior to the ear apex, 1.5 *cun* above the hairline, directly above SJ 20 (*jiăo sūn*).

[Anatomy]

(1) Layer of needling: Skin-subcutaneous tissue-temporal muscle.

(2) Innervation and vasculature: In the superficial layer there are the auriculotemporal nerve, the greater occipital nerve, and the superficial temporal artery. In the deep layer there are the muscular branches of the mandibular nerve.

[Indications] Migraine, vertigo, infantile acute and chronic convulsion.

[Operation] Puncture horizontally 0.5-1 *cun*.

7. GB 12 (*wán gŭ*)

[Location] On the head, in the depression posterior and inferior to the mastoid process.

[Anatomy]

(1) Layer of needling: Skin-subcutaneous tissue-sternocleidomastoid muscle.

(2) Innervation and vasculature: In the superficial layer, there are the lesser occipital nerve and the posterior auricular artery. In the deep layer, there are the accessory nerve, the cervical nerve plexus and the occipital artery.

[Indications] Headache, pain and regidity of the neck, deviation of the mouth, malaria, epilepsy.

[Operation] Puncture obliquely 0.5-0.8 *cun*.

8. GB 14 (*yáng bái*)

[Location] On the forehead, directly above the pupil, 1 *cun* above the eyebrow.

[Anatomy]

(1) Layer of needling: Skin-subcutaneous tissue-frontal belly of the occipitofrontal muscle.

(2) Innervation and vasculature: There are the supraorbital artery and verin, the supraorbital nerve, and the frontal branches of the superficial temporal artery and vein in this area.

[Indications] Headache, giddiness, eye pain, blurred vision, twitching of eyelids.

[Operation] Puncture horizontally 0.5-0.8 *cun*.

9. GB 17 (*zhèng yíng*)

[Location] On the head, 2.5 *cun* above the hairline, 2.25 *cun* lateral to the front midline of the head.

[Anatomy]

(1) Layer of needling: Skin-subcutaneous tissue-epicranial aponeurosis.

(2) Innervation and vasculature: There are the greater occipital nerve, auriculotemporal nerve, supraorbital nerve and superficial temporal artery.

[Indications] Headache, blurred vision, lockjaw, toothache.

[Operation] Puncture horizontally 0.5-0.8 *cun*.

10. GB 18 (*chéng líng*)

[Location] On the head, 4 *cun* above the hairline, 2.25 *cun* lateral to the front midline of the head.

[Anatomy]

(1) Layer of needling: Skin-subcutaneous tissue-epicranial aponeurosis.

(2) Innervation and vasculature: There are the greater and lesser occipital nerves, the occipital artery and posterior auricular artery.

[Indications] Headache, aversion to wind and cold, stuffy nose, epistaxis, asthma.

[Operation] Puncture horizontally 0.5-0.8 *cun*.

11. GB 20 (*fēng chí*)

[Location] On the nape, inferior to the occipital bone, in the depression between the upper portion of the sternocleidomastoid muscle and the upper border of the trapezius muscle.

[Anatomy]

(1) Layer of needling: Skin-subcutaneous tissue-splenius muscle of the head-semispinal muscle of the head.

(2) Innervation and vasculature: In the superficial layer, there are the lesser occipital nerve. In the deep layer, there is the suboccipital nerve.

[Indications] Headache, blurred vision, red swollen painful eyes, nasal obstruction, epistaxis, tinnitus, deafness, pain and regidity of the neck, common cold, epilepsy, stroke, febrile disease, malaria, goiter.

[Operation] Puncture obliquely 0.8-1.3 *cun* towards the tip of the nose horizontally as medulla is in the deep part. It is essential to control the needling angle and depth, or puncture horizontally to go through DU 16 (*fēng fŭ*).

12. GB 21 (*jiān jĭng*)

[Location] On the shoulder, directly above the nipple, at the midpoint of the line that links DU 14 (*dà zhuī*) and the acromion.

[Anatomy]

(1) Layer of needling: Skin-subcutaneous tissue-trapezius muscle-levator muscle of the scapula.

(2) Innervation and vasculature: In the superficial layer, there are the medial branches of the supraclavicular nerve. In the deep layer, there are the accessory nerve, the dorsal scapular nerve, the transverse cervical artery, and deeper, the cervical pleura.

[Indications] Pain and regidity of the neck, shoulder and back pain, motor impairment of the arm, difficult labor, galactostasis, scrofula.

[Operation] Puncture perpendicularly 0.5~0.8 *cun*. The apex of the lung is located here, so deep insertion of the needle is forbidden. Never administer acupuncture to this point in pregnant women.

13. GB 24 (*rì yuè*) Front-*Mu* Point of the Gallbladder Channel

[Location] On the upper abdomen, directly below the nipple, in the 7th intercostal space, 4 *cun* lateral to the anterior midline.

[Anatomy]

(1) Layer of needling: Skin-subcutaneous tissue-external oblique muscle of the abdomen-intercostal muscle.

(2) Innervation and vasculature: In the superficial layer, there are the lateral cutaneous branches of the 7th intercostal nerve. In the deep layer, there are the 7th intercostal nerve and artery.

[Indications] Vomiting, acid regurgitation, pain in the hypochondriac region, hiccups, jaundice.

[Operation] Puncture obliquely 0.5~0.8 *cun* or horizontally 0.5~0.8 *cun*. Never puncture deeply to prevent injury to the lung.

14. GB 25 (*jīng mén*) Front-*Mu* Point of the Kidney Channel

[Location] On the lateral lower back, 1.8 *cun* posterior to LV 13 (*zhāng mén*), below the free end of the 12th rib.

[Anatomy]

(1) Layer of needling: Skin-subcutaneous tissue-external oblique muscle of the abdomen-internal oblique muscle of the abdomen-transverse muscle of the abdomen.

(2) Innervation and vasculature: In the superficial layer, there are the anterior cutaneous branches of the 11th and 12th thoracic nerves. In the deep layer, there are the 11th and 12th thoracic nerves.

[Indications] Dysuresia, edema, lower back pain, abdominal distension, diarrhea.

[Operation] Puncture perpendicularly 0.3~0.5 *cun*. Never puncture deeply to prevent injury to the lung.

15. GB 26 (*dài mài*)

[Location] On the lateral side of the abdomen, 1.8 *cun* posterior to LV 13 (*zhāng mén*), at the crossing point of a vertical line through the free end of the 11th rib and a horizontal line through the centre of the umbilicus.

[Anatomy]

(1) Layer of needling: Skin-subcutaneous tissue-external oblique muscle of the abdomen-internal oblique muscle of the abdomen-transverse muscle of the abdomen.

(2) Innervation and vasculature: In the superficial layer, there are the lateral cutaneous branches of the 10th thoracic nerve. In the deep layer, there are the subcostal nerve and artery.

[Indications] Amenorrhea, menstrual irregularity, morbid leucorrhea, abdominal pain, hernia, pain in the lower back and the hypochondriac region.

[Operation] Puncture perpendicularly 1~1.5 *cun*.

16. GB 28 (*wéi dào*)

[Location] On the lateral side of the abdomen, anterior and inferior to the anteriosuperior iliac spine, 0.5 *cun* anterior and inferior to GB 27 (*wǔ shū*).

[Anatomy]

(1) Layer of needling: Skin-subcutaneous tissue-external oblique muscle of the abdomen-transverse muscle of the abdomen.

(2) Innervation and vasculature: In the superficial layer, there are the lateral cutaneous branches of the anterior branches of the 11th and 12th thoracic and 1st lumbar nerves and accompanying arteries and veins. In the deep layer, there are the deep circumflex iliac artery and vein, the muscular branches of the anterior branches of the 11th and 12th thoracic and the 1st lumbar nerves and the related arteries and veins.

[Indications] Abdominal pain, hernia, morbid leucorrhea, prolapse of the uterus.

[Operation] Puncture perpendicularly 1~1.5 *cun*,or puncture obliquely and anteroinferiorly.

17. GB 29 (*jù liáo*)

[Location] On the hip, at the midpoint of the line that links the anteriosuperior iliac spine and the prominence of the great trochanter.

[Anatomy]

(1) Layer of needling: Skin-subcutaneous tissue-fascia lata-tensor muscle of the facia lata.

(2) Innervation and vasculature: In the superficial layer, there are the cutaneous nerve of the thigh. In the deep layer,there are the superior gluteal nerve and the ascending branches of the lateral femoral circumflex artery.

[Indications] Lower back pain, muscular atrophy of the lower limbs, paralysis, hernia.

[Operation] Puncture perpendicularly 1~1.5 *cun*.

18. GB 30 (*huán tiào*)

[Location] On the lateral side of the thigh, at the junction of the lateral third and medial third of the line that links the great prominence of the trochanter and the sacral hiatus of the sacrum when the patient is in a lateral recumbent position with the thigh flexed.

[Anatomy]

(1) Layer of needling: Skin-subcutaneous tissue-greatest gluteal muscle.

(2) Innervation and vasculature: In the superficial layer, there is the inferior cutaneous gluteal nerve. In the deep layer, there are the sciatic nerve trunk, the inferior gluteal nerve and artery.

[Indications] Pain in the lumbar region and thigh, hemiplegia, muscular atrophy of the lower limbs.

[Operation] Puncture perpendicularly 1~1.5 *cun*.

19. GB 31 (*fēng shì*)

[Location] On the lateral midline of the thigh, 7 *cun* above the transverse popliteal crease or at the place where the middle finger touches when the patient stands straightly with the arms hanging down freely.

[Anatomy]

(1) Layer of needling: Skin-subcutaneous tissue-iliotibial tract-lateral muscle of the thigh-intermediate vastus muscle of the thigh.

(2) Innervation and vasculature: In the superficial layer, there is the lateral cutaneous nerve of the thigh. In the deep layer,there are the muscular branches of the gluteal nerve and the branches of the lateral circumflex femoral artery.

[Indications] Hemiplegia, muscular atrophy of the lower limbs, general pruritus, beriberi.

[Operation] Puncture perpendicularly 1~2 *cun*.

20. GB 33 (*xī yáng guān*)

[Location] On the lateral side of the knee, 3 *cun* above GB 34 (*yáng líng quán*), in the depression above the external epicondyle of the femur.

[Anatomy]

(1) Layer of needling: Skin-subcutaneous tissue-biceps muscle of the arm-lateral head of the gastrocnemius muscle.

(2) Innervation and vasculature: In the superficial layer, there is the lateral cutaneous nerve of the thigh. In the deep layer, there are the sciatic nerve and the lateral superior genicular artery.

[Indications] Painful swollen and rigid knee, numbness of the lower leg.

[Operation] Puncture perpendicularly 0.8~1 *cun*.

21. GB 34 (*yáng líng quán*) *He*-Sea Point; Lower *He*-Sea Point of the Gallbladder Channel; Influential Point of the Tendon

[Location] On the lateral side of the leg, in the depression anterior and inferior to the head of the fibula.

[Anatomy]

(1) Layer of needling: Skin-subcutaneous tissue-long peroneal muscle-long extensor muscle of the toe.

(2) Innervation and vasculature: In the superficial layer, there is the lateral sural cutaneous nerve. In the deep layer,there are the superficial, deep peroneal nerve, anterior tibial artery and the lateral inferior genicular artery.

[Indications] Pain in the hypochondriac region, bitter taste in the mouth, vomiting, hemiplegia, muscular atrophy of the lower limbs, beriberi, jaundice, infantile convulsion.

[Operation] Puncture perpendicularly 1~1.5 *cun*.

22. GB 37 (*guāng míng*) *Luo*-Connecting Point

[Location] On the lateral side of the leg, 5 *cun* directly above the tip of the external malleolus, on the anterior border of the fibula.

[Anatomy]

(1) Layer of needling: Skin-subcutaneous tissue-short peroneal muscle-long extensor muscle of the toe-long extensor muscle of the great toe.

(2) Innervation and vasculature: In the superficial layer, there are the lateral cutaneous nerve of the calf, and the superficial peroneal nerve. In the deep layer, there are the superficial and deep peroneal nerves and the anterior tibial artery, deeper, there are the deep peroneal nerve trunk and the anterior tibial artery.

[Indications] Eye pain, night blindness, muscular atrophy of the lower limbs, distending pain in the breasts.

[Operation] Puncture perpendicularly 1~1.5 *cun*.

23. GB 39 (*xuán zhōng*) Influential Point of the Marrow

[Location] On the lateral side of the leg, 3 *cun* above the tip of the external malleolus, on the anterior border of the fibula.

[Anatomy]

(1) Layer of needling: Skin-subcutaneous tissue-long extensor muscle of the toe.

(2) Innervation and vasculature: In the superficial layer, there is the lateral cutaneous peroneal nerve. In the deep layer, there are the branches of the deep peroneal nerve and artery, deeper, the deep peroneal nerve trunk and the anterior tibial artery and vein.

[Indications] Neck rigidity, distending pain in the chest and hypochondriac region, muscular atrophy of the lower limbs, sore throat, beriberi, hemiplegia, hemorrhoids.

[Operation] Puncture perpendicularly 0.8~1 *cun*.

24. GB 40 (*qiū xū*) *Yuan*-Source Point

[Location] Anterior and inferior to the external malleolus, in the depression lateral to the tendon of the long extensor muscle of the toes.

[Anatomy]

(1) Layer of needling: Skin-subcutaneous tissue-cruciate ligament of the leg (anterior extensor retinaculum)-short extensor muscle of the toe.

(2) Innervation and vasculature: In the superficiallayer, there are the dorsal cutaneous nerve of the foot (branches of the sural nerve), and the superficial cutaneous peroneal nerve. In the deep layer, there are the muscular branches of the peroneal nerve and the anterior lateral malleolar artery.

[Indications] Neck pain, distending pain in the chest and hypochondriac region, muscular atrophy of the lower limbs, malaria.

[Operation] Puncture perpendicularly 0.5~0.8 *cun*.

25. GB 41 (*zú lín qì*) *Shu*-Stream Point; Confluence Point that links the Belt Vessel

[Location] On the lateral side of the instep, posterior to the 4th metatarsophalangeal joint, in the depression lateral to the extensor muscle of the little toe.

[Anatomy]

(1) Layer of needling: Skin-subcutaneous tissue-4th dorsal interosseous muscle and the 3rd plantar interosseous muscle.

(2) Innervation and vasculature: There are the intermediate dorsal cutaneous nerve of the foot (branches of the superficial peroneal nerve) and the dorsal venous network of the foot. In the deep layer, there are the muscular branches of the lateral plantar nerve and the 4th dorsal metatarsal artery (starting from the dorsal artery of the foot).

[Indications] Red swollen painful eyes, pain in the hypochondriac region, menstrual irregularity, enuresis, acute mastitis, malaria, pain in the dorsum of the foot.

[Operation] Puncture perpendicularly 0.3~0.5 *cun*.

26. GB 43 (*xiá xī*) *Ying*-Spring Point

[Location] On the lateral side of the instep, between the 4th and 5th toes, at the junction of the red and white skin, proximal to the margin of the web.

[Anatomy]

(1) Layer of needling: Skin-subcutaneous tissue.

(2) Innervation and vasculature: In the superficial layer, there are the intermediate dorsal cutaneous nerve of the foot and the dorsal venous network. In the deep layer, there are the 4th dorsal digital artery and vein of the foot.

[Indications] Headache, blurred vision, tinnitus, deafness, red swollen painful eyes, febrile disease, pain in the hypochondriac region, acute mastitis.

[Operation] Puncture perpendicularly 0.3~0.5 *cun*.

Section 12 The Liver Channel of Foot *Jueyin*

1. LV 1 (*dà dūn*) *Jing*-Well Point

[Location] On the lateral side of the distal segment of the great toe, 0.1 *cun* from the corner of the toenail.

[Anatomy]

(1) Layer of needling: Skin-subcutaneous tissue.

(2) Innervation and vasculature: There are the dorsal digital nerve of the foot (cutaneous branches of the peroneal nerve) and the dorsal digital artery of the foot.

[Indications] Hernia, enuresis, menstrual irregularity, amenorrhea, metrorrhagia or metrostaxis, prolapse of the uterus, epilepsy.

[Operation] Puncture obliquely 0.1-0.2 *cun*.

2. LV 2 (*xíng jiān*) *Ying*-Spring Point

[Location] On the instep, between the 1st and 2nd toes, at the junction of the red and white skin, proximal to the margin of the web.

[Anatomy]

(1) Layer of needling: Skin-subcutaneous tissue.

(2) Innervation and vasculature: There are the dorsal digital nerve and the artery of the foot.

[Indications] Headache, blurred vision, redswollen painful eyes, bluish blindness, deviation of the mouth, pain in the hypochondriac region, hernia, dysuresia, metrorrhagia or metrostaxis, epilepsy, menstrual irregularity, dysmenorrhea, morbid leucorrhea, stroke.

[Operation] Puncture perpendicularly 0.5~0.8 *cun*.

3. LV 3 (*tài chōng*) *Shu*-Stream Point; *Yuan*-Source Point

[Location] On the instep, in the depression of the posterior end of the 1st interosseous metatarsal space.

[Anatomy]

(1) Layer of needling: Skin-subcutaneous tissue-1st lateral dorsal intermetatarsal muscle-oblique head of the adductor pollicis.

(2) Innervation and vasculature: In the superficial layer, there are the dorsal digital nerve and venous network of the foot. In the deep layer, there are the lateral plantar nerve and the 1st dorsal metatarsal artery.

[Indications] Headache, blurred vision, red swollen painful eyes, pain in the hypochondriac region, enuresis, hernia, metrorrhagia or metrostaxis, menstrual irregularity, epilepsy, vomiting, infantile convulsion, muscular atrophy of the lower limbs.

[Operation] Puncture perpendicularly 0.5~0.8 *cun*.

4. LV 4 (*zhōng fēng*) *Jing*-River Point

[Location] On the instep, anterior to the medial malleolus, on the line that links SP 5 (*shāng qiū*) and ST 41 (*jiě xī*), in the depression medial to the anterior tibial muscle.

[Anatomy]

(1) Layer of needling: Skin-subcutaneous tissue-inferior extensor retinaculum (the cruciate ligament of the leg)-anterior tibial muscle.

(2) Innervation and vasculature: In the superficial layer, there are the cutaneous saphenous nerve, the dorsal cutaneous nerve of the foot and the great sephenous vein. In the deep layer, there are peroneal nerve and the dorsal artery of the foot.

[Indications] Hernia, seminal emission, dysuresia, abdominal pain, painful swollen medial malleolus.

[Operation] Puncture perpendicularly 0.5~0.8 *cun*.

5. LV 5 (*lí gōu*) *Luo*-Connecting Point

[Location] On the medial side of the leg, 5 *cun* above the medial malleolus, in the centre of the medial side of the tibia.

[Anatomy]

(1) Layer of needling: Skin-subcutaneous tissue-long flexor muscle of the toe-posterior tibial muscle.

(2) Innervation and vasculature: There are the great saphenous nerve and the saphenous nerve. In the deep layer, there are the tibial nerve and the posterior tibial artery.

[Indications] Dysuresia, enuresis, menstrual irregularity, morbid leucorrhea, muscular atrophy of the lower limbs.

[Operation] Puncture horizontally 0.5-0.8 *cun*.

6. LV 6 (*zhōng dū*) *Xi*-Cleft Point

[Location] On the medial side of the leg, 7 *cun* above the medial malleolus, in the centre of the medial side of the fibula.

[Anatomy] Same as LV 5 (*lí gōu*).

[Indications] Hernia, metrorrhagia or metrostaxis, diarrhea, lochiorrhea.

[Operation] Puncture horizontally 0.5-0.8 *cun*.

7. LV 7 (*xī guān*)

[Location] On the medial side of the leg, posterior and inferior to the medial epicondyle of the tibia, 1 *cun* posterior to SP 9 (*yín líng quán*), in the upper portion of the medial head of the gastrocnemius muscle.

[Anatomy]

(1) Layer of needling: Skin-subcutaneous tissue-medial head of the gastrocnemius muscle.

(2) Innervation and vasculature: In the superficial layer, there are the saphenous nerve and the great saphenous vein. In the deep layer, there are the muscular branches of the tibial nerve and the medial inferior genicular artery.

[Indications] Painful swollen knees, muscular atrophy of the lower limbs.

[Operation] Puncture perpendicularly 0.5~0.8 *cun*.

8. LV 8 (*qŭ quán*) *He*-Sea Point

[Location] On the medial side of the knee, with the knee flexed, at the medial end of the transverse popliteal crease, posterior to the medial epicondyle of the thigh, in the depression of the anterior border of the insertions of the semimembranous and semitendinous muscles.

[Anatomy]

(1) Layer of needling: Skin-subcutaneous tissue-sartorius muscle-gracilis muscle-semimembranous muscle-medial head of the gastrocnemius muscle.

(2) Innervation and vasculature: In the superficial layer, there are the saphenous nerve and the great saphenous vein. In the deep layer, there are the muscular branches of the femoral nerve and the obturator nerve, the branches of the tibial nerve and the medial superior genicular artery, deeper, the tibial nerve trunk,artery and vein.

[Indications] Abdominal pain, dysuresia, seminal emission, pruritus vulvae, painful knees, menstrual irregularity, dysmenorrhea, morbid leucorrhea.

[Operation] Puncture perpendicularly 1~1.5 *cun*.

9. LV 10 (*zú wŭ lĭ*)

[Location] On the medial side of the thigh, 3 *cun* directly below ST 30 (*qì chōng*), at the proximal end of the thigh, inferior to the pubic tubercle, on the lateral border of the long abductor muscle.

[Anatomy]

(1) Layer of needling: Skin-subcutaneous tissue-long adductor muscle-short adductor muscle-great adductor muscle.

(2) Innervation and vasculature: In the superficial layer, there are the anterior cutaneous branches of the femoral nerve and the obtrurator nerve, the branches of the ilioinguinal nerve and the great saphenous vein. In the deep layer, there are the obtrurator artery.

[Indications] Lower abdominal pain, incontinence of urine, prolapse of the uterus, painful swollen testis, somnolence, scrofula.

[Operation] Puncture perpendicularly 1~1.5 *cun*.

10. LV 12 (*jí mài*)

[Location] Lateral to the pubic tubercle, lateral and inferior to ST 30 (*qì chōng*) in the inguinal groove where the pulsation of the femoral artery is palpable, 2.5 *cun* to the front midline.

[Anatomy]

(1) Layer of needling: Skin-subcutaneous tissue-pectineal muscle-lateral obturator muscle.

(2) Innervation and vasculature: In the superficial layer, there are the anterior cutaneous branches of the femoral nerve, ilioinguinal nerve and the superficial epigastric vein. In the deep layer, there are the muscular branches of the femoral nerve and the obturator nerve, the external pudendal artery and the obturator artery, and inferiorly, the obturator nerve trunk and the inferoposterior femoral artery and vein.

[Indications] Hernia, lower abdominal pain, prolapse of the uterus.

[Operation] Puncture perpendicularly 0.5~0.8 *cun*. Avoid the artery.

11. LV 13 (*zhāng mén*) Front-*Mu* Point Point of the Spleen Channel; Influential Point of the Zang Organs

[Location] On the lateral side of the abdomen, below the free end of the 11th floating rib.

[Anatomy]

(1) Layer of needling: Skin-subcutaneous tissue-external oblique muscle of the abdomen-internal oblique muscle of the abdomen-transverse muscle of the abdomen.

(2) Innervation and vasculature: In the superficial layer, there are the lateral cutaneous branches of the 10th and 11th thoracic nerves and the superficial thoracoepigastric vein. In the deep layer, there are the 10th and 11th thoracic nerves and the intercostal artery.

[Indications] Abdominal distending pain, diarrhea, pain in the hypochondriac region, abdominal mass.

[Operation] Puncture obliquely 0.5-0.8 *cun*.

12. LV 14 (*qī mén*) Front-*Mu* Point of the Liver Channel

[Location] On the chest, directly below the nipple, in the 6th intercostal space, 4 *cun* lateral to the anterior midline.

[Anatomy]

(1) Layer of needling: Skin-subcutaneous tissue-external oblique muscle of the abdomen-external intercostal muscle-internal intercostal muscle.

(2) Innervation and vasculature: In the superficial layer, there are the lateral cutaneous branches of the 6th intercostal nerve. In the deep layer, there are the 6th intercostal nerve and artery.

[Indications] Distending pain in the hypochondriac region, abdominal distension, vomiting, acute mastitis.

[Operation] Puncture obliquely 0.5-0.8 *cun* or horizontally 0.5-0.8 *cun*.

Section 13 The *Du* Vessel

1. DU 1 (*cháng qiáng*) *Luo*-Connecting Point

[Location] Below the tip of the coccyx, at the midpoint of the line that links the tip of the coccyx and anus.

[Anatomy]

(1) Layer of needling: Skin-subcutaneous tissue-anococcygeal ligament-deep external sphincter muscle of the anus-levator ani muscle.

(2) Innervation and vasculature: In the superficial layer, there are the cutaneous branches of the anal nerve (branch of the pudendal nerve). In the deep layer, there are the muscular branches of the anal nerve and the anal artery (internal branch of the pudendal artery).

[Indications] Diarrhea, passing bloody stools, constipation, hemorrhoids, mania, epilepsy, pain in the lower back, coccygeal and sacral region.

[Operation] Puncture 0.5~1 *cun* obliquely with the needle tip towards upward and on the level of the sacral bone. Never puncure through the rectum to avoid infection.

2. DU 2 (*yāo shù*)

[Location] On the sacrum, on the posterior midline, just at the sacral hiatus.

[Anatomy]

(1) Layer of needling: Skin-subcutaneous tissue-sacral bone.

(2) Innervation and vasculature: In the superficial layer, there are the middle clunial nerve. In the deep layer, there are the posterior branches of the median sacral artery and the inferior gluteal artery.

[Indications] Menstrual irregularity, hemorrhoids, pain and regidity of the lower back, muscular atrophy of the lower limbs, epilepsy.

[Operation] Puncture superiorly and obliquely 0.5-1 *cun*.

3. DU 3 (*yāo yáng guān*)

[Location] On the lower back, on the posterior midline, in the depression below the spinous process of the 4th lumbar vertebra.

[Anatomy]

(1) Layer of needling: Skin-subcutaneous tissue-supraspinal ligament-interspinal ligament.

(2) Innervation and vasculature: In the superficial layer, there are the posterior branches of the lumbar nerve. In the deep layer, there are the posterior branches of the lumbar nerve and the lumbar artery.

[Indications] Menstrual irregularity, seminal emission, impotence, pain in the lower back, muscular atrophy of the lower limbs.

[Operation] Puncture superiorly and obliquely 0.5-1 *cun*.

4. DU 4 (*mìng mén*)

[Location] On the lower back, on the posterior midline, in the depression below the spinous process of the 2nd lumbar vertebra.

[Anatomy] Same as DU 3 (*yāo yáng guān*).

[Indications] Impotence, seminal emission, morbid leucorrhea, enuresis, frequency of micturition, menstrual irregularity, diarrhea, pain in the lower back, cold sensation of the limbs.

[Operation] Puncture superiorly and obliquely 0.5-1 *cun*.

5. DU 10 (*líng tái*)

[Location] On the back, on the posterior midline, in the depression below the spinous process of the 6th thoracic vertebra.

[Anatomy]

(1) Layer of needling: Skin-subcutaneous tissue-supraspinal ligament-interspinal ligament.

(2) Innervation and vasculature: In the superficial layer, there are the medial cutaneous branches of the posterior branches of the 11th thorocic nerve and the accompanying artery and vein. In the deep layer, there are the external (posterior) vertical venous plexus between the adjacent spinous processes, the branches of the posterior branches of the 11th thoracic nerve and the branches or tributaries of the dorsal branches of the 11th posterior intercostal artery and vein.

[Indications] Cough, shortness of breath, furuncle, pain and rigidity of the back.

[Operation] Puncture superiorly and obliquely 0.5~1 *cun*.

6. DU 12 (*shēn zhù*)

[Location] On the back, on the posterior midline, in the depression below the spinous process of the 3rd thoracic vertebra.

[Anatomy] Same as DU 10 (*líng tái*).

[Indications] Cough, shortness of breath, epilepsy, pain and rigidity of the back.

[Operation] Puncture superiorly and obliquely 0.5~1 *cun*.

7. DU 13 (*táo dào*)

[Location] On the back, on the posterior midline, in the depression below the spinous process of the 1st thoracic vertebra.

[Anatomy] Same as DU 10 (*líng tái*).

[Indications] Headache, malaria, febrile disease, regidity of the back.

[Operation] Puncture superiorly and obliquely 0.5~1 *cun*.

8. DU 14 (*dà zhuī*)

[Location] On the posterior midline, in the depression below the 7th cervical vertebra.

[Anatomy]

(1) Layer of needling: Skin-subcutaneous tissue-supraspinal ligament-interspinal ligament.

(2) Innervation and vasculature: In the superficial layer, there are the cutaneous branches of the posterior branches of the 8th cervical nerve. In the deep layer, there are the posterior branches of the 8th cervical nerve and the transverse cervical artery.

[Indications] Febrile disease, malaria, cough, shortness of breath, steaming bone disorder, night sweating, epilepsy, headache, stiff neck, pain in the shoulder and back, pain and regidity of the lower back, rubella.

[Operation] Puncture perpendicularly 0.5~1 *cun*.

9. DU 16 (*fēng fǔ*)

[Location] On the nape, 1 *cun* directly above the midpoint of the posterior hairline, directly below the external occipital protuberance, in the depression between the trapezius muscle on both sides.

[Anatomy]

(1) Layer of needling: Skin-subcutaneous tissue-between left and right trapezius muscle-nuchal ligament (between left and right splenius muscles of the head)-between left and riht semispinal muscles of the head.

(2) Innervation and vasculature: In the superficial layer, there are the 3rd occipital nerve and the subcutaneous vein. In the deep layer, there are the branches of the posterior branches of the 2nd and 3rd cervical nerves, the external (posterior) vertebral venous plexus and the branches or tributaries of the occipital artery and vein.

[Indications] Headache, stiff neck, dizziness, vertigo, sore throat, aphonia, mania, apoplexy.

[Operation] Puncture perpendicularly 0.5~1 *cun*. It is forbidden to puncture deeply to avoid injury to the medulla.

10. DU 17 (*nǎo hù*)

[Location] On the head, 2.5 *cun* directly above the midpoint of the posterior hairline, 1.5 *cun* above DU 16 (*fēng fǔ*), in the depression of the superior border of the external occipital protuberance.

[Anatomy]

(1) Layer of needling: Skin-subcutaneous tissue-occipital belly of the occipitofrontal muscle.

(2) Innervation and vasculature: There are the branches of the greater occipital nerve. In the deep layer, there are the posterior auricular branches of the facial nerve and the occipital artery.

[Indications] Headache, dizziness, vertigo, stiff neck, aphonia, epilepsy.

[Operation] Puncture horizontally 0.5-0.8 *cun*.

11. DU 20 (*bǎi huì*)

[Location] On the head, 5 *cun* directly above the midpoint of the posterior hairline, or at the midpoint of the line that links the apexes of both ears.

[Anatomy]

(1) Layer of needling: Skin-subcutaneous tissue-epicranial aponeurosis.

(2) Innervation and vasculature: There are the supratrochlear nerve and the superficial temporal artery.

[Indications] Headache, dizziness, vertigo, apoplexy, aphonia, mania, prolapse of the rectum and uterus, diarrhea, poor memory, insomnia.

[Operation] Puncture horizontally 0.5-0.8 *cun*.

12. DU 23 (*shàng xīng*)

[Location] On the head, 1 *cun* directly above the midpoint of the anterior hairline.

[Anatomy]

(1) Layer of needling: Skin-subcutaneous tissue-epicranial aponeurosis.

(2) Innervation and vasculature: In the superficial layer, there are the supratrochlear nerve. In the deep layer, there are the temporal branches of the facial nerve and the supraorbital artery.

[Indications] Headache, eye pain, nasosinusitis, epistaxis, mania, malaria, febrile disease.

[Operation] Puncture horizontally 0.5~1 *cun*.

13. DU 24 (*shén tíng*)

[Location] On the head, 0.5 *cun* directly above the midpoint of the anterior hairline.

[Anatomy] Same as DU 23 (*shàng xīng*).

[Indications] Headache, dizziness, vertigo, insomnia, nasosinusitis, epilepsy.

[Operation] Puncture horizontally 0.5-0.8 *cun*.

14. DU 26 (*shuǐ gōu*)

[Location] On the face, at the junction of the upper third and the middle third of the philtrum.

[Anatomy]

(1) Layer of needling: Skin-subcutaneous tissue-orbicular muscle of mouth.

(2) Innervation and vasculature: In the superficial layer, there are the infraorbital nerve. In the deep layer, there are the buccal branches of the facial nerve and the superior labial artery (branch of the facial artery).

[Indications] Coma, syncope, mania, epilepsy, deviation of the mouth, pain and regidity of the lower back.

[Operation] Puncture superiorly and obliquely 0.3-0.5 *cun*.

Section 14 The *Ren* Vessel

1. RN 2 (*qū gǔ*)

[Location] On the lower abdomen and on the anterior midline, at the midpoint of the upper border of the public symphysis.

[Anatomy]

(1) **Layer of needling:** Skin-subcutaneous tissue-linea alba or the straight muscle of the abdomen-transverse fascia.

(2) **Innervation and vasculature:** In the superficial layer, there are the inferior cutaneous branches of the iliohypogastric nerve and the superficial abdominal artery. In the deep layer, there are the abdominal branches of the iliohypogastric nerve and the inferior epigastric artery, deeper, the urinary bladder.

[Indications] Dysuresia, enuresis, seminal emission, impotence, menstrual irregularity, morbid leucorrhea.

[Operation] Puncture perpendicularly 0.5~1 *cun*. Acupuncture is applied after passing of urine as internally there is the urinary bladder. Be cautious with pregnant women.

2. RN 3 (*zhōng jí*) Front-*Mu* Point of the Bladder Channel

[Location] On the lower abdomen and on the anterior midline, 4 *cun* below the centre of the umbilicus.

[Anatomy]

(1) **Layer of needling:** Skin-subcutaneous tissue-linea alba-transverse fascia.

(2) **Innervation and vasculature:** In the superficial layer, there are the inferior cutaneous branches of the iliohypogastric nerve and the branches of the superficial epigastric artery. In the deep layer, there are the iliohypogastric nerve and the inferior epigastic artery.

[Indications] Dysuresia, enuresis, hernia, seminal emission, impotence, menstrual irregularity, metrorrhagia or metrostaxis, morbid leucorrhea, prolapse of the uterus, infertility.

[Operation] Puncture perpendicularly 0.5~1 *cun*. Be cautious with pregnant women.

3. RN 4 (*guān yuán*) Front-*Mu* Point of the Small Intestine Channel

[Location] On the lower abdomen and on the anterior midline, 3 *cun* below the centre of the umbilicus.

[Anatomy]

(1) **Layer of needling:** Skin-subcutaneous tissue-linea alba-transverse fascia.

(2) **Innervation and vasculature:** In the superficial layer, there are the anterior cutaneous branches of the subcostal nerve and the superficial epigastic artery. In the deep layer, there are the subcostal nerve and the inferior epigastic artery, deeper, the abdominal cavity.

[Indications] Enuresis, frequency of micturition, retention of urine, diarrhea, abdominal pain, seminal emission, impotence, hernia, menstrual irregularity, morbid leucorrhea, infertility, apoplexy, consumptive disease.

[Operation] Puncture perpendicularly 1~2 *cun*. Be cautious with pregnant women.

4. RN 5 (*shí mén*) Front-*Mu* Point of the *Sanjiao* Channel

[Location] On the lower abdomen and on the anterior midline, 2 *cun* below the centre of the umbilicus.

[Anatomy]

(1) Layer of needling: Skin-subcutaneous tissue-linea alba-transverse fascia.

(2) Innervation and vasculature: In the superficial layer, there are the anterior cutaneous branches of the intercostal nerve and the epigastic artery. In the deep layer, there are the intercostal nerve and the inferior epigastic artery.

[Indications] Abdominal pain, edema, hernia, dysuresia, diarrhea, amenorrhea, morbid leucorrhea, metrorrhagia or metrostaxis.

[Operation] Puncture perpendicularly 1~2 *cun*. Be cautious with pregnant women.

5. RN 6 (*qì hăi*)

[Location] On the lower abdomen and on the anterior midline, 1.5 *cun* below the centre of the umbilicus.

[Anatomy] Same as RN 5 (*shí mén*).

[Indications] Abdominal pain, diarrhea, constipation, enuresis, hernia, seminal emission, impotence, menstrual irregularity, amenorrhea, metrorrhagia or metrostaxis, collapse, consumptive disease.

[Operation] Puncture perpendicularly 1~2 *cun*. Be cautious with pregnant women.

6. RN 11 (*jiàn lǐ*)

[Location] On the upper abdomen and on the anterior midline, 3 *cun* above the centre of the umbilicus.

[Anatomy]

(1) Layer of needling: Skin-subcutaneous tissue-linea alba-transverse fascia-extraperitoneal fat tissue-parietal peritoneum.

(2) Innervation and vasculature: In the superficial layer, there are the anterior cutaneous branches of the anterior branch of the 9th thoracic nerve or the tributaries of the superficial epigastric vein. In the deep layer, there are the branches of the anterior branch of the 9th thoracic nerve.

[Indications] Stomachache, vomiting, poor appetite, abdominal distension, edema.

[Operation] Puncture perpendicularly 1~2 *cun*.

7. RN 12 (*zhōng wǎn*) Front-*Mu* Point of the Stomach Channel; Influential Point of the *Fu* Organ

[Location] On the upper abdomen and on the anterior midline, 4 *cun* above the centre of the umbilicus.

[Anatomy] Same as RN 11 (*jiàn lǐ*).

[Indications] Stomachache, vomiting, hiccups, abdominal distension, diarrhea, jaundice, mania.

[Operation] Puncture perpendicularly 1~1.5 *cun*.

8. RN 13 (*shàng wǎn*)

[Location] On the upper abdomen and on the anterior midline, 5 *cun* above the centre of the umbilicus.

[Anatomy] Same as RN 11 (*jiàn lǐ*).

[Indications] Stomachache, vomiting, hiccups, abdominal distension, epilepsy.

[Operation] Puncture perpendicularly 1~1.5 *cun*.

9. RN 14 (*jù quē*) Front-*Mu* Point of the Heart Channel

[Location] On the upper abdomen and on the anterior midline, 6 *cun* above the centre of the umbilicus.

[Anatomy] Same as RN 11 (*jiàn lǐ*).

[Indications] Pain in the chest and the cardiac region, palpitation, abdominal distension, mania and epilepsy.

[Operation] Puncture superiorly and obliquely 0.5-1 *cun*. Never puncture deeply to prevent injury to the lung.

10. RN 15 (*jiū wěi*) *Luo*-Connecting Point

[Location] On the upper abdomen and on the anterior midline, 3 *cun* above the centre of the umbilicus, 1 *cun* below the xiphisternal synchondrosis.

[Anatomy] Same as RN 11 (*jiàn lǐ*).

[Indications] Pain in the chest, hiccups, mania and epilepsy.

[Operation] Puncture superiorly and obliquely 0.5-1 *cun*.

11. RN 17 (*dàn zhōng*) Front-*Mu* Point of the Pericardium Channel; Influential Point of Qi

[Location] On the chest and on the anterior midline, on the level of the 4th intercostal space, at the midpoint of the line that links both nipples.

[Anatomy]

(1) Layer of needling: Skin-subcutaneous tissue-breast bone.

(2) Innervation and vasculature: There are the anterior cutaneous branches of the 4th intercostal nerve. In the deep layer, there are the 4th intercostal nerve and the perforating branches of the internal thoracic artery.

[Indications] Cough, shortness of breath, pain in the chest, palpitation, insufficient lactation, vomiting, dysphagia.

[Operation] Puncture horizontally 0.3-0.5 *cun*.

12. RN 22 (*tiān tū*)

[Location] On the neck, in the centre of the suprasternal fossa.

[Anatomy]

(1) Layer of needling: Skin-subcutaneous tissue-between the left and right sterna and the hyoid bones, and the sternocleidomastoid muscles-superior mediastinum areolar tissue-anterior space of the trachea.

(2) Innervation and vasculature: In the superficial layer, there are the transverse cervical nerve, the branches of the cervical venous arch. In the deep layer, there are the descending branch of the hypoglossal nerve and the inferior thyroid artery, deeper, the trachea. When it goes further down the needle may touch the posterior manubrium of the sternum, the thymus gland, the left anonymous vein and the aortic arch.

[Indications] Cough, shortness of breath, pain in the chest, sore throat, sudden aphonia, goiter, globus hystericus, dysphagia.

[Operation] First puncture perpendicularly 0.2 *cun*, then direct the needle inferiorly and insert into the place along the posterior sternum 1~1.5 *cun*.

13. RN 23 (*lián quán*)

[Location] On the neck and on the anterior midline, above the laryngeal protuberance, in the depression above the upper border of the hyoid bone.

[Anatomy]

(1) Layer of needling: Skin-subcutaneous tissue-mylohyoid muscle.

(2) Innervation and vasculature: In the superficial layer, there are the branches of the transverse cervical nerve, hypoglossal nerve, lingual artery and the superior artery of the thyroid.

[Indications] Sublingual swelling and pain, salivation, aphasia, stiffness of the tongue, sudden aphonia, laryngalgia, difficulty in swallowing.

[Operation] Puncture towards the root of the tongue 0.5~0.8 *cun*.

14. RN 24 (*chéng jiāng*)

[Location] On the face, in the central depression of the mentolabial groove.

[Anatomy]

(1) Layer of needling: Skin-subcutaneous tissue-orbicular muscle of the mouth.

(2) Innervation and vasculature: In the superficial layer, there is the mental nerve. In the deep layer, there are the manibular branch of the facial nerve and the inferior labial artery.

[Indications] Painful swollen mouth and gums, salivation, sudden aphonia, mania.

[Operation] Puncture obliquely 0.3-0.5 *cun*.

Chapter 5

Commonly Used Extra Points

1. EX-HN1 (*sì shén cōng*)

[Location] On the vertex of the head, 1 *cun* posterior, anterior, and lateral to DU 20 (*bǎi huì*), a group of 4 points.

[Anatomy] Greater occipital nerve,supratrochlear nerve,auriculotemporal nerve.

[Indications] Headache, dizziness, insomnia, poor memory, mania, epilepsy, eye disease, stroke.

[Operation] Puncture horizontally 0.5-0.8 *cun*.

2. EX-HN4 (*yú yāo*)

[Location] On the forehead, directly above the pupil, in the midpoint of the eyebrow.

[Anatomy] In the orbicular muscle of the eye, in the superficial layer there is the supraorbital nerve. In the deep layer, there are the temporal branches of the facial nerve.

[Indications] Pain in the supraorbital region, twitching of the eyelids, ptosis, red swollen painful eyes, cloudy cornea, deviation of the mouth and eye.

[Operation] Puncture horizontally 0.3-0.5 *cun*.

3. EX-HN3 (*yìn táng*)

[Location] On the forehead, at the midpoint between the eyebrows.

[Anatomy] In the superficial layer, there is the supratrochlear nerve. In the deep layer, there are the temporal branches of the facial nerve and the branches of the inner canthus artery.

[Indications] Mental disorders: dementia,epilepsy, insomnia, poor memory, depressive psychosis, headache, dizziness, epistaxis, nasosinusitis.

[Operation] Puncture horizontally 0.3-0.5 *cun* or prick to bleed.

4. EX-HN5 (*tài yáng*)

[Location] At the temporal part of the head, between the lateral end of the eyebrow and the outer canthus, in the depression about 1 finger breadth behind them.

[Anatomy] In the temporal fascia and the temporal muscle, in the superficial layer, there are the temporal branches of the maxillary nerve and the superficial temporal artery. In the deep layer, there are the muscular branches of the mandibular nerve.

[Indications] Eye disease, headache, dizziness, deviation of the eye and mouth.

[Operation] Puncture perpendicularly or obliquely 0.3~0.5 *cun*, or prick to bleed.

5. EX-HN6 (*ěr jiān*)

[Location] Above the auricle, at the tip of the auricle when the ear is folded forward.

[Anatomy] In the deep layer, there are the auricular branches of the facial nerve and the posterior branches of the occipital nerve.

[Indications] Eye disease, headache, sore throat.

[Operation] Puncture perpendicularly 0.1~0.2 *cun* or prick to bleed.

6. EX-HN7 (*qiú hòu*)

[Location] On the face, at the junction of the lateral 1/4 and the medial 3/4 of the infraorbital margin.

[Anatomy] In the orbicular muscle of the eye, deeper, the eye muscle; In the superficial layer, there are the zygomatic branches of the maxillar nerve and the inferoorbital nerve. In the deep layer, there are the zygomatic branches of the facial nerve. When it is inserted into the orbit, the needle may touch the inferoorbital nerve trunk, the inferior retus muscle, the inferior oblique muscle and the adpose body of the orbit, the ophthalmic nerve and the oculomoter nerve.

[Indications] Eye diseases.

[Operation] Push the eyeball gently upward. Puncture slowly and perpendicularly along the lower border of the orbit 0.5~1.5 *cun*.

7. EX-HN8 (*shàng yíng xiāng*)

[Location] On the face, at the junction of the alar cartilage and the nasal concha, near the upper end of the nasolabial groove.

[Anatomy] In the nasal muscle and cartilage of the wing of the nose. In the superficial layer, there are the infraorbital nerve and the trochlear nerve. In the deep layer, there are the buccal branches of the facial nerve.

[Indications] Nasal sinusitis, boils of the nose, nasal disease.

[Operation] Puncture horizontally, interiorly and superiorly 0.3~0.5 *cun*.

8. EX-HN14 (*yì míng*)

[Location] On the nape, 1 *cun* posterior to SJ 17 (*yì fēng*).

[Anatomy] On the sternocleidomastoid muscle; In the superficial layer, there are the great auricular nerve and less occipital nerve. In the deep layer, there are the accessory nerve and the posterior branches of cervical nerve, deeper, the vagus nerve trunk, accessory nerve trunk and cervical artery and vein.

[Indications] Headache, dizziness, insomnia, eye disease, tinnitus.

[Operation] Puncture perpendicularly 0.5~1 *cun*. Moxibustion is applicable.

9. *Ān mián*

[Location] On the nape, at the midpoint between SJ 17 (*yì fēng*) and DU 20 (*fēng chí*).

[Anatomy] Same as EX-HN14 (*yì míng*).

[Indications] Insomnia, vertigo, dizziness, headache, palpitation, mania.

[Operation] Puncture perpendicularly 0.8~1.2 *cun*.

10. EX-CA1 (*zǐ gōng*)

[Location] On the lower abdomen, 4 *cun* below the centre of the umbilicus, 3 *cun* lateral to RN 3 (*zhōng jí*).

[Anatomy] In the oblique muscle of the abdomen; In the deep layer, there are the muscular branches of the iliohypogastric nerve and the inferior epigastric artery.

[Indications] Prolapse of the uterus, menstrual irregularity, metrorrhagia or metrostaxis, infertility, and other gynecological diseases.

[Operation] Puncture perpendicularly 0.8~1.2 *cun*.

11. EX-B1 (*dìng chuǎn*)

[Location] Below the spinous process of the 7th cervical vertebra, 0.5 *cun* lateral to the posterior midline.

[Anatomy]

In the trapezius muscle, rhomboid muscle,superior posterior serratus muscle and plenius muscle of the neck; In the superficial layer, there are the cutaneous branches of the posterior branches of the cervical nerve. In the deep layer, there are muscular branches of the posterior branches of the cervical nerve, accessory nerve, the transverse cervical artery and the deep cervical artery.

[Indications] Asthma, cough, headache, stiff neck.

[Operation] Puncture perpendicularly 0.5~0.8 *cun*.

12. EX-B2 (*jiá jǐ*)

[Location] On the back and lower back, below the spinous processes from the 1st thoracic to the 5th lumbar vertebrae, 0.5 *cun* lateral to the posterior midline, 17 points on each side, all together 34 points.

[Anatomy] In the superficial muscles of the back, there are the trapezius muscle, rhomboid muscle, thoracolumbar fascia, posterior serratus muscle. In the deep muscles of the back, there are the erector spinal muscle. In the superficial layer, there are the cutaneous branches of the posterior branches of the thoracia or the lumbar nerves. In the deep layer, there are the posterior branches of the thoracic or lumbar nerves, posterior intercostal artery and lumbar arteries.

[Indications] Diseases in the upper limbs: C1~C3; diseases in the lower limbs: L1~L5; diseases in the chest: T1~T8; diseases in the abdominal region: T6~L5.

[Operation] Puncture perpendicularly 0.3~0.5 *cun*. The plum-blossom needle therapy is also applied.

Notes: EX-B2 (*jiá jǐ*) (from C2~C7): In the nape, on both sides of the correpondent posterior spinous processes of the cervical vertebra, 0.5 *cun* to the posterior midline.

13. EX-B3 (*wèi guǎn xià shù*)

[Location] On the back, below the spinous process of the 8th thoracic vertebra, 1.5 *cun* lateral to the posterior midline.

[Anatomy] In the trapezius muscle and in the broadest muscle of the back, in the superficial layer, there are the cutaneous branches of the posterior branch of the 8th thoracic nerve. In the deep layer, there are the muscular branches of the posterior branch of the 8th thoracic nerve and the posterior intercostal artery.

[Indications] Diabetes, stomachache, abdominal pain, pain in the chest and the hypochondriac region.

[Operation] Puncture obliquely 0.3-0.5 *cun*.

14. EX-B7 (*yāo yǎn*)

[Location] On the lower back, in the depression below the spinous process of the 4th lumbar vertebra, 3.5 *cun* lateral to the posterior midline.

[Anatomy] In the broadest muscle of the back, in the quadrate muscle of the loins; In the superficial layer, there are the cutaneous branches of the posterior branch of the 4th lumbar nerve.In the deep layer, there are the muscular branches of the posterior branch of the 4th lumbar nerve and the lumbar artery.

[Indications] Lower back pain, menstrual irregularity, morbid leucorrhea, consumptive disease.

[Operation] Puncture perpendicularly 1~1.5 *cun*.

15. *Jiān qián* (*jiān nèi líng*)

[Location] Sitting straight while relaxing the shoulders, on the midpoint between the end of the anterior axillary fold and LI 15 (*jiān yú*).

[Anatomy] In the deltoid muscle; In the superficial layer, there are the lateral branches of the supraclavicular nerve. In the deep layer, there are the axillar nerve, musculocutaneous nerve and the thoracoacromial artery.

[Indications] Pain in the shoulder and arm, failure of the arm to raise, paralysis of the upper limbs.

[Operation] Puncture perpendicularly 1~1.5 *cun*.

16. EX-UE2 (*èr bái*)

[Location] On the palmar side of the forearm, 4 *cun* above the transverse crease of the wrist, on each side of the radial flexor muscle of the wrist, two points on each side.

[Anatomy] In the superficial digital flexor muscle, the long flexor muscle of the thumb and the deep flexor muscle of the finger (ulnar side); In the superficial layer, there are the lateral cutaneous nerve of the forearm. In the deep layer, there are the radial arterial trunk, the superficial branches of the radial nerve (ulnar side), and the median nerve (ulnar side).

[Indications] Hemorrhoids, prolapse of the rectum, pain in the forearm, chest and hypochondriac region.

[Operation] Puncture perpendicularly 0.5~0.8 *cun*.

17. EX-UE4 (*zhōng kuí*)

[Location] On the midpoint of the proximal interphalangeal joint of the middle finger at the dorsal side when a fise is made.

[Anatomy] The radial and ulnar nerves and the dorsal digital artery.

[Indications] Vomiting, hiccups, difficulty in swallowing, poor appetite, stomach and spleen disorders.

[Operation] Puncture perpendicularly 0.2~0.3 *cun*.

18. EX-UE7 (*yāo tòng diǎn*)

[Location] On the dorsum of the hand, between the 2nd and 3rd metacarpal bones and between the 4th and 5th metacarpal bones, at the midpoint between the dorsal crease of the wrist and metacarpophalangeal joint, two points on one hand.

[Anatomy] On the ulnar short extensor muscle (ulnar side) and the extensor muscle of the little finger (ulnar side).

[Indications] Acute lumbar sprain.

[Operation] Puncture obliquely 0.5~0.8 *cun* from both sides of the palm towards the centre.

19. EX-UE8 (*lào zhěn*) (*wài láo gōng*)

[Location] On the dorsum of the hand, between the 2nd and 3rd metacarpal bones, about 0.5 *cun* posterior to the metacarpophalangeal joint.

[Anatomy]

In the 2nd dorsal lateral intersseous muscle and the superficial dorsal digital nerve.

[Indications] Stiff neck, painful swollen hand and arm, neonatal tetanus.

[Operation] Puncture perpendicularly 0.5~0.8 *cun*.

20. EX-UE9 (*bā xié*)

[Location] On the dorsum of the hand when a loose fist is made, at the junction of the white and red skin proximal to the margin between the five fingers, altogether eight points.

[Anatomy] In the adductor muscle of the thumb (*bā xié* 1) and the intersseous muscle (*bā xié* 2, 3, 4), in the superficial layer, there are the superficial branches of the dorsal branch of the radial nerve, and the dorsal branches of the ulnar nerve. In the deep layer, there are the muscular branches of the ulnar nerve and the dorsal metacarpal arterial network.

[Indications] Painful swollen back of the hand, numbness of the fingers, intense heat, eye pain, bite by poisonous insects.

[Operation] Puncture obliquely 0.5-0.8 *cun* or prick to bleed.

21. EX-UE11 (*shí xuān*)

[Location] On the tips of the ten fingers, 0.1 *cun* from the free margin of the nails.

[Anatomy] Proper palmar digital nerve (starting from the median nerve of the three half fingers in the radial side, and from the ulnar nerve of one and half fingers in the ulnar side).

[Indications] Coma, epilepsy, high fever, sore throat, numbness of the fingers.

[Operation] Puncture 0.1-0.2 *cun* or prick to bleed.

22. EX-UE6 (*xiǎo gǔ kōng*)

[Location] On the dorsal side of the little finger, at the tip of the proximal interphalangeal joint.

[Anatomy] The ulnar nerve and the dorsal digital nerve.

[Indications] Pain of the fingers, eye pain.

[Operation] Puncture perpendicularly 0.2~0.3*cun*. Moxibustion is applicable.

23. EX-LE3 (*bǎi chóng wō*)

[Location] On the medial side of the thigh, 3 *cun* above the medial superior corner of the patella with the knee flexed, ie 1 *cun* above SP 10 (*xuè hǎi*).

[Anatomy] In the medial intermuscle of the thigh; In the superficial layer, there are the muscular branches of the femoral nerve and the femoral artery.

[Indications] Malnutrition due to parasitic infestation, eczema, rubella, abscess of the pudendum.

[Operation] Puncture perpendicularly 1.5~2 *cun*.

24. EX-LE6 (*dăn náng*)

[Location] In the depression anterior and inferior to the head of the fibula, 2 *cun* directly below GB 34 (*yáng líng quán*).

[Anatomy] In the long peroneal muscle; In the superficial layer, there is the lateral sural cutaneous nerve. In the deep layer, there are the deep peroneal nerve, the anterior tibial artery and vein and the muscular branches of the peroneal nerve.

[Indications] Acute and chronic cholecystitis, cholelithiasis, biliary ascariasis and other biliary diseases, muscular atrophy and numbness of the lower limbs.

[Operation] Puncture perpendicularly 1~2 *cun*.

25. EX-LE7 (*lán wĕi*)

[Location] 5 *cun* below ST 35 (*dú bí*), 2 *cun* below ST 36 (*zú sān lĭ*), one finger breadth lateral to the anterior crest of the tibia.

[Anatomy] In the anterior tibial muscle, the interosseous membrane of the leg and the posterior tibial muscle,. in the superficial layer, there are the lateral sural cutaneous nerve. In the deep layer, there are the deep peroneal nerve trunk, the anterior tibial artery and vein, the muscular branches of the deep peroneal nerve and the tibial nerve.

[Indications] Acute and chronic appendicitis, indigestion, atrophy and numbness of the lower limbs.

[Operation] Puncture perpendicularly 1.5~2 *cun*.

Part 2 The Clinical Practice

Chapter 1

Introduction

Section 1 Highlights of Syndrome Differentiation and Treatment

Differential diagnosis of syndromes is the basis of treatment in traditional Chinese medicine. The dermal needling therapy is guided by the theory of channels and collaterals, and its differentiation of syndromes and treatment is based on the four examinations and eight principles.

1. Eight-Principle Syndrome Differentiation

The eight principles are the general guiding rule in the differentiation of syndromes. They are yin and yang, exterior and interior, cold and heat, and deficiency and excess, to collectively categorize complicated manifestations of diseases, indicating the site of a disease, its nature and contrast of the power between pathogenic factors and healthy qi.

Yin and yang are the key principle in the differentiation of syndromes. Only when the yin or yang syndrome is determined, can the correct treating principle be designed. The exterior, heat and excess syndromes fall into the category of *yang,* while the interior, cold and deficiency syndromes are in the category of yin. In treatment of the former the reducing method with strong tapping is performed, while of the latter the reinforcing method with gentle tapping is performed.

Differentiation of the exterior and interior syndromes is an approach to know the prognosis and progression of a disease. Generally, disorders in the skin, muscular fibers, channels and collaterals attribute to an exterior syndrome, while that in the *zang-fu* organs, qi and blood and bone marrow belong to an interior syndrome.

Differentiation of the cold and heat syndromes is an approach to determine the nature of a disease.The former is due to exposure to exogenous pathogenic cold or insufficient yang qi, while the latter is due to exposure to pathogenic heat or excessive yang qi.

Differentiation of deficiency and excess syndromes is an approach to distinguish the condition of pathogenic factors and healthy qi. A deficiency syndrome indicates insufficiency of healthy qi, while an excess syndrome abundance of pathogenic factors.

2. *Zang-Fu* Organ Syndrome Differentiation

To distinguish the type of syndrome, one must analyze the physiological characteristics of the *zang-fu* organs, the site of a disease, the nature and condition of the pathogenic factors and healthy qi.

(1) The Lung

(i) The Lung Restrained by Wind-Cold

Main manifestations: Aversion to cold, fever, headache and stuffy nose with watery discharge or expectoration of thin sputum, thin and white fur, floating and tense pulse.

Treatment: Select points of the Lung Channel of Hand *Taiyin* and the Large Intestine Channel of Hand *Yangming*.

(ii) Accumulation of Heat in the Lung

Main manifestations: Cough, thick and yellow sputum, or expectoration of bloody pus, chest constriction and pain in the chest, fever, thirst, epistaxis, swollen sore throat, red tongue with yellow fur, rapid pulse.

Treatment: Select points of the Lung Channel of Hand *Taiyin*, and the Large Intestine Channel of Hand *Yangming*.

(iii) The Lung Obstructed by Sputum

Main manifestations: Cough and dyspnea, wheezing, excessive thick sputum, fullness in the chest and hypochondrium, white and greasy fur, slippery or slippery and rapid pulse.

Treatment: Select points of the Lung Channel of Hand *Taiyin*, Spleen Channel of Foot *Taiyin* and the Stomach Channel of Foot *Yangming*.

(iv) Body Fluids Impaired by Lung Heat

Main manifestations: Dry cough, hemoptysis, dry throat and mouth, tidal fever and night sweating, red tongue with scanty fur, thready and rapid pulse.

Treatment: Select points of the Lung Channel of Hand *Taiyin*, Spleen Channel of Foot *Taiyin* and the Kidney Channel of Foot *Shaoyin*.

(v) Lung Qi Deficiency

Main manifestations: Cough, shortness of breath, thin sputum, fatigue and disinclination to talk, pale complexion, spontaneous perspiration, pale tongue with white fur, deficient pulse.

Treatment: Select points of the Lung Channel of Hand *Taiyin*, Spleen Channel of Foot *Taiyin* and the relevant Back-*Shu* points.

(2) The Large Intestine

(i) Deficiency and Cold in the Large Intestine

Main manifestations: Abdominal pain alleviated by pressure, diarrhea with borborygmus, prolapse of rectum, pale tongue with white slippery fur, deep and slow pulse.

Treatment: Select points of the Large Intestine Channel of Hand *Yangming*, the Stomach Channel of Foot *Yangming* and *Ren* Vessel.

(ii) Excessive Heat in the Large Intestine

Main manifestations: Constipation or dysentery with foul smell, or stools with bright blood, heat sensation and pain in the anus, red tongue with yellow fur, deep and forceful or slippery and rapid pulse.

Treatment: Select points of the Large Intestine Channel of Hand *Yangming*, the Stomach Channel of Foot *Yangming*, Front-*Mu* and lower *He*-Sea points of the Large Intestine Channel.

(3) Spleen

(i) Spleen Yang Deficiency

Main manifestations: Abdominal pain alleviated by warmth, less intake of food, abdominal bloating, loose stools or stools with large volume of undigested food, thin and clear leucorrhea, cold limbs and preference for warmth, pale tongue with slippery fur, deep and slow pulse.

Treatment: Select points of the Spleen Channel of Foot *Taiyin*, the Stomach Channel of Foot *Yangming*, the *Shu*-Stream and Front-*Mu* points of the Spleen Channel.

(ii) Spleen Qi Deficiency

Main manifestations: Abdominal bloating, loose stools, lusterless complexion, disinclination to talk due to deficiency of qi, lassitude, or menorrhagia, metrorrhagia or metrostaxis, pale tongue with tooth mark on its edge and white fur, soggy and moderate pulse.

Treatment: Select points of the Spleen Channel of Foot *Taiyin*, the Stomach Channel of Foot *Yang ming* and the Back-*Shu* points of the Spleen Channel.

(iii) Sinking of Spleen Qi

Main manifestations: Dizziness, feeble voice and breathing, sense of droopingand bloating in the stomach and abdomen, or prolapse of the rectum or uterus.

Treatment: Select points of the *Ren* Vessel, the Stomach Channel of Foot

Yangming and the Back-*Shu* points of the Spleen Channel.

(iv) Dampness Disturbance of the Spleen

Main manifestations: Fullness in the stomach and abdomen or abdominal pain, nausea, anorexia, sticky sensation in the mouth, absence of thirst, heaviness sensation of the head and body or edema, unsurfaced fever, sallow complexion, yellow eyes, loose stools, concentrated urine, white or yellow greasy fur, soggy, moderate or moderate rapid pulse.

Treatment: Select points of the Spleen Channel of Foot *Taiyin*, the Stomach Channel of Foot *Yang-ming* and the Front-*Mu* points of the Spleen Channel.

(4) The Stomach

(i) Stomach Qi Deficiency

Main manifestations: Anorexia, nausea and hiccups, fullness in the stomach, pale red tongue with white and thin fur, thready and weak pulse.

Treatment: Select points of the Stomach Channel of Foot *Yangming*, the Back-*Shu* and Front-*Mu* points of the Stomach Channel.

(ii) Stomach Yang Deficiency

Main manifestations: Cold pain in the stomach,alleviated by heat and pressure, vomiting with clear water, or vomiting after meals, borborygmus aggravated by cold, pale tongue with white and slippery fur, deep or slow pulse.

Treatment: Select points of the Stomach Channel of Foot *Yangming*, the Spleen Channel of Foot *Taiyin,* and the Back-*Shu* and Front-*Mu* points of the Stomach Channel.

(iii) Intense Stomach Fire

Main manifestations: Fever, thirst and preference for cold drinks, foul breath, or toothache and swollen gums, epigastric burning pain, acid regurgitation and gastric upset, abnormal increased appetite with frequent hunger, constipation, or delirium, red tongue with yellow dry fur, slippery, rapid, surging and large pulse.

Treatment: Select points of the Large Intestine Channel of Hand *Yangming*, the Stomach Channel of Foot *Yangming*, and the Front-*Mu* points of the Stomach Channel.

(5) The Heart

(i) Heart Yang Deficiency

Main manifestations: Oppression and pain in the chest, palpitations and shortness of breath worse when active, aversion to cold, cold limbs, pallor, pale or purplish enlarged tongue with white fur, thready, weak or knotted and intermittent pulse.

Treatment: Select points of the Heart Channel of Hand *Shaoyin*, the Pericardium Channel of Hand *Jueyin*, and the Back-*Shu* and Front-*Mu* points of the Heart Channel.

(ii) Heart Yin Deficiency

Main manifestations: Palpitations and restlessness, amnesia, dream-disturbed sleep, or tidal fever, flushed cheeks, night sweating, nocturnal emission, red dry tongue with scanty coating, thready and rapid pulse.

Treatment: Select points of the Pericardium Channel of Hand *Jueyin*, the Kidney Channel of Foot *Shaoyin*, and the Back-*Shu* points of the Heart Channel.

(iii) The Heart Agitated by Phlegm-Fire

Main manifestations: Insomnia, dream-disturbed sleep, restlessness, or incoherent speech, weeping and laughing with no reasons, mania and violent action or epilepsy, red tongue with yellow greasy fur, slippery and rapid pulse.

Treatment: Select points of the Heart Channel of Hand *Shaoyin*, the Pericardium Channel of Hand *Jueyin*, the Stomach Channel of Foot *Yangming* and the *Du* Vessel.

(iv) Blazing of Heart Fire

Main manifestations: Restlessness, insomnia, flushed face, thirst, ulcers in the mouth and tongue, red tongue with yellow fur, rapid pulse.

Treatment: Select points of the Heart Channel of Hand *Shaoyin*, the Pericardium Channel of Hand *Jueyin*.

(v) Heart Vessel Obstruction

Main manifestations: Palpitations, oppression or stabbing pain in the chest with the shoulder, back and the medial aspect of the arm involved sometimes, purplish tongue with petechia or ecchymosis, thready choppy or knotted and intermittent pulse.

Treatment: Select points of the Pericardium Channel of Hand *Jueyin*, the Heart Channel of Hand *Shaoyin*, the Back-*Shu* and Front-*Mu* points of the Heart Channel.

(6) The Small Intestine

(i) Deficiency-Cold in the Small Intestine

Main manifestations: Constant abdominal pain alleviated by heat and pressure, borborygmus and diarrhea, pale tongue with white fur, thready and slow pulse.

Treatment: Select the Back-*Shu*, Front-*Mu* and lower *He*-Sea points of the Small Intestine Channel.

(ii) Excessive Heat in the Small Intestine

Main manifestations: Restlessness, insomnia, ulcerous mouth and tongue, brown urine and painful urination, pain in the penis, red tongue with yellow fur, slippery and rapid pulse.

Treatment: Select points of the Small Intestine Channel of Hand *Taiyang*, the Heart Channel of Hand *Shaoyin*, the Front-*Mu* and lower *He*-Sea points of the Small Intestine Channel.

(7) The Kidney

(i) Kidney Yang Deficiency

Main manifestations: Aching pain and cold in the lower back and knees, dizziness, aversion to cold and cold limbs, night polyuria, impotence, premature ejaculation, infertility, persistent diarrhea or edema, pale thick and delicate tongue with white and slippery fur, deep and slow pulse.

Treatment: Select points of the Kidney Channel of Foot *Shaoyin*, the Spleen Channel of Foot *Taiyin*, the *Ren* Vessel, the *Du* Vessel, and the Back-*Shu* points of the Kidney Channel.

(ii) Failure of the Kidney to grasp Qi

Main manifestations: Shortness of breath and panting,worse when active, spontaneous sweating, disinclination to talk, feeble voice, puffy face and pale complexion, pale tongue with thin fur, thready and weak pulse.

Treatment: Select points of the Kidney Channel of Foot *Shaoyin*, the *Ren* Vessel and the Back-*Shu* points of the Kidney Channel.

(iii) Kidney Yin Deficiency

Main manifestations: Dizziness, tinnitus, insomnia and amnesia, aching pain and weakness in the lower back and knees, tidal fever and night sweating, feverish sensation in the chest, palms and soles, flushed cheeks, dry throat, seminal emission, hypomenorrhea or amenorrhea, red tongue with scanty fur, thready and rapid pulse.

Treatment: Select points of the Heart Channel of Hand *Shaoyin*, the Kidney Channel of Foot *Shaoyin*, the Spleen Channel of Foot *Taiyin* and the Back-*Shu* points of the Kidney Channel.

(8) The Urinary Bladder

(i) Deficiency in the Bladder

Main manifestations: Frequent urination or enuresis, cold pain in the lower abdomen, pale tongue with white and slippery fur, deep and thready pulse.

Treatment: Select the Front-*Mu* points and points of the Bladder Channel of Foot *Taiyang*, the Kidney Channel of Foot *Shaoyin*.

(ii) Heat Retention in the Bladder

Main manifestations: Frequency and urgency of urination, difficult urination, brown urine or anuria or hematuria, or urolithic stranguria, red tongue with yellow or yellow greasy fur, slippery and rapid pulse.

Treatment: Select points of the *Ren* Vessel, the Bladder Channel of Foot *Taiyang* and the Front-*Mu* points of the Bladder Channel.

(9) The Pericardium

Concerning the main manifestations and treatment, consult the section of "The Heart".

(10) The *Sanjiao*

(i) Deficiency-Cold in the *Sanjiao*

Main manifestations: General edema, fullness in the abdomen with cold sensation, reversed flow of qi, or enuresis, incontinence of urine, pale tongue with white and slippery fur, deep and thready pulse.

Treatment: Select the Back-*Shu* and Front-*Mu* points of the *Sanjiao* Channel and the points of the Kidney Channel of Foot *Shaoyin* and the *Ren* Vessel.

(ii) Heat Accumulation in the *Sanjiao*

Main manifestations: Fever, reversed flow of qi, general edema, dysuresia, distending pain in the lower abdomen, red tongue with yellow fur and rapid pulse.

Treatment: Select the Front-*Mu* points and lower *He*-Sea points of the *Sanjiao* Channel and the points of the Kidney Channel of Foot *Shaoyin*.

(11) The Liver

(i) Stagnation of Liver Qi

Main manifestations: Depression, distending pain in the hypochondriac regions or breasts, constriction in the chest, sighing, irritability, poor appetite, dysmenorrhea, menstrual irregularity or foreign body sensation in the throat, or scrofula, goiter, acid regurgitation, white fur and wiry pulse.

Treatment: Select points of the Liver Channel of Foot *Jueyin*, the Gallbladder Channel of Foot *Shaoyang* and the Stomach Channel of Foot *Yangming*.

(ii) Blazing of Liver Fire

Main manifestations: Dizziness, distending sensation in eyes, tinnitus, red swollen eyes, bitter taste and dryness in the mouth, irritability, restlessness, insomnia or dream-disturbed sleep, red tongue with yellow dry fur, wiry and rapid pulse.

Treatment: Select points of the Liver Channel of Foot *Jueyin* and the Gallbladder Channel of Foot *Shaoyang*.

(iii) Stirring of Liver Wind

Main manifestations: Sudden loss of consciousness, stiff tongue, aphasia, hemiplegia, deviation of the mouth and tongue, or convulsion, opisthotonus, white thick or yellow greasy fur, and wiry rapid pulse.

Treatment: Select points of the Liver Channel of Foot *Jueyin*, the *Du* Vessel and *Ren* Vessel.

(12) The Gallbladder

(i) Hyperactivity of Gallbladder Fire

Main manifestations: Vertigo, tinnitus, headache and distending sensation in eyes, bitter taste and dryness in the mouth, hypochondriac pain, red tongue with yellow fur, wiry slippery or rapid pulse.

Treatment: Select points of the Gallbladder Channel of Foot *Shaoyang* and the front-*mu* points of the Gallbladder Channel.

(ii) Gallbladder Qi Deficiency with Timidity

Main manifestations: Being in a state of apprehension, timidity, palpitation, dream-disturbed sleep, blurred vision, thin white fur, wiry and thready pulse.

Treatment: Select the back-*shu* points and points of the Gallbladder Channel of Foot *Shaoyang*, the Pericardium Channel of Hand *Jueyin* and the Liver Channel of Foot *Jueyin*.

3. Differentiation of Syndromes according to the Theory of Channels and Collaterals

When acupuncture is used in treatment, it is essential to know the symptoms and signs and pathological changes of a given *zang-fu* organ or channel. To clarify, treat a disease with the affected channels and *zang-fu* organs, to make an accurate diagnosis, which is the basis for treatment. This is called differentiation of syndromes according to the theory of channels.

(1) Syndromes and Treatment of Disorders of the Lung Channel of Hand *Taiyin*

(i) Invasion by Wind-Heat

Main manifestations: Aching pain in the anterior medial aspect of the arm, muscular atrophy, numbness and pain in shoulder and arm.

Treatment: Select points and *Luo*-Connection points of the Lung Channel.

(ii) Upward Attack by Pathogenic Heat

Main manifestations: Epistaxis, sore throat, pain in the supraclavicular fossa.

Treatment: Select points of the Lung Channel and the Large Intestine Channel.

(2) Syndromes and Treatment of Disorders of the Large Intestine Channel of Hand *Yangming*

(i) Obstruction by Wind-Cold

Main manifestations: Aching pain in the anterior, lateral aspect of the upper limb, muscular atrophy, numbness, difficulty of raising the painful shoulder.

Treatment: Select points of the Large Intestine Channel.

(ii) Upward Attack by Pathogenic Heat

Main manifestations: Headache, yellow sclera, toothache, swollen cheeks, twitching of lips, epistaxis, deviation of the mouth, sore throat, foul breath.

Treatment: Select points of the Large Intestine and Stomach Channels.

(3) Syndromes and Treatment of Disorders of the Stomach Channel of Foot *Yangming*

(i) Invasion by Pathogenic Wind-Cold-Dampness

Main manifestations: Swollen, painful knee joints, aching pain, heaviness sensation or numbness of the anterior aspect of the lower limbs.

Treatment: Select points of the Stomach Channel.

(ii) Upward Attack by Stomach Fire

Main manifestations: Ulcerous mouth and lips, foul breath, toothache, swollen neck, sore throat, or epistaxis, thick and sticky nasal discharge and pain in the breasts.

Treatment: Select points of the Large Intestine Channel and the Stomach Channel.

(4) Syndromes and Treatment of Disorders of the Spleen Channel of Foot *Taiyin*.

(i) Invasion by Pathogenic Wind-Cold-Dampness

Main manifestations: Pain in the medial aspect of the thigh and knee, swollen painful instep, difficult flexion of limbs and muscular atrophy.

Treatment: Select points of the Spleen Channel.

(ii) Upward Disturbance by Pathogenic Heat

Main manifestations: Stiff tongue, aphasia, or stiff painful tongue, sluggishness, jaundice, belching and abdominal distension.

Treatment: Select points of the Spleen Channel and the Stomach Channel.

(5) Syndromes and Treatment of Disorders of the Heart Channel of Foot *Shaoyin*.

(i) Invasion by Pathogenic Wind-Cold-Dampness

Main manifestations: Pain in the chest, cold pain and numbness in the shoulder blade and medial aspect of the upper arm.

Treatment: Select points of the Heart Channel and the Small Intestine Channel.

(ii) Blazing of Heart Fire

Main manifestations: Dry mouth, yellow sclera, ulcerous mouth and tongue, epistaxis, red tongue and rapid pulse.

Treatment: Select points of the Heart Channel.

(6) Syndromes and Treatment of Disorders of the Small Intestine Channel of Hand *Taiyang*

(i) Obstruction by Exogenous Pathogenic Factors

Main manifestations: Stiff and painful nape, lower abdominal pain, pain numbness or muscular atrophy of the shoulder, arm and the lateral aspect of the elbow.

Treatment: Select points of the Small Intestine Channel.

(ii) Upward Disturbance by Pathogenic Heat

Main manifestations: Swollen jaw, yellow sclera, deafness and tinnitus.

Treatment: Select points and the lower *He*-Sea points of the Small Intestine Channel.

(7) Syndromes and Treatment of Disorders of the Urinary Bladder Channel of Foot *Taiyang*

(i) Collaterals Attacked by Wind-Cold

Main manifestations: Aching pain, numbness or spasm in the nape, lower back, buttocks and the posterior aspect of the lower limbs.

Treatment: Select points of the Bladder Channel.

(ii) Accumulation of Pathogenic Heat

Main manifestations: Epistaxis, headache, red swollen painful eyes.

Treatment: Select points of the Bladder Channel.

(8) Syndromes and Treatment of Disorders of the Kidney Channel of Foot *Shaoyin*

Invasion of the Channel by Pathogenic Factors

Main manifestations: Aching pain, heaviness numbness or flaccidity of the posterior-medial aspect of the lower limbs, cold feet, difficult to stand.

Treatment: Select points of the Kidney Channel.

(9) Syndromes and Treatment of Disorders of the Pericardium Channel of Hand *Jueyin*

(i) Invasion by Pathogenic Wind-Cold-Dampness

Main manifestations: Pain in the chest and axilla, pain and numbness of the medial aspect of the upper arm.

Treatment: Select points of the Pericardium Channel.

(ii) Accumulation of Heat in the Channel

Main manifestations: Palpitations, restlessness, depressive manic psychosis, feverish sensation in palms.

Treatment: Select points of the Pericardium Channel and the Liver Channel.

(10) Syndromes and Treatment of Disorders of the *Sanjiao* Channel of Hand *Shaoyang*

(i) Invasion by Pathogenic Wind-Cold-Dampness

Main manifestations: Aching distending pain and numbness of the shoulder, lateral aspect of the arm, elbow and little finger.

Treatment: Select points of the *Sanjiao* Channel.

(ii) Upward Disturbance by Pathogenic Heat

Main manifestations: Dizziness, tinnitus, sudden deafness, eye pain, swollen cheeks, sore throat and scrofula.

Treatment: Select points of *Sanjiao* Channel and the Gallbladder Channel.

(11) Syndromes and Treatment of Disorders of the Gallbladder Channel of Foot *Shaoyang*

(i) Obstruction by Wind-Cold-Dampness

Main manifestations: Pain and numbness along the lateral aspect of the chest, hypochondrium, thigh and knees, and motor impairment of the little toe.

Treatment: Select points of the Gallbladder Channel.

(ii) Upward Disturbance by Pathogenic Heat

Main manifestations: Bitter taste in the mouth, vertigo, deafness, tinnitus, pain in the hypochondrium and swollen axilla.

Treatment: Select points of the Gallbladder Channel and the Liver Channel.

(12) Syndromes and Treatment of Disorders of the Liver Channel of Foot *Jueyin*

(i) Invasion of the Collaterals by Pathogenic Cold

Main manifestations: Cold pain in the lower abdomen, hernia, pain and hanging down of the testes, aversion to cold, alleviated by heat, or pain and numbness in the medial aspect of the lower limbs, or calf muscular cramp.

Treatment: Select points of the Liver Channel.

(ii) Upward Disturbance by Wind-Heat

Main manifestations: Dizziness and vertigo, muscular twitching of eyelids and face, red swollen painful eyes.

Treatment: Select points of the Liver Channel and the Pericardium Channel.

Section 2 Principles of Treatment

Principles of treatment are worked out under the guidance of the holistic concept and differentiation of syndromes and treatment, which has significance in design of the strategies of treatment and point combination.

1. The Tip, Root, Acute and Chronic

The "tip" and "root" are relative concepts which have multiple meanings, indicating the primary and secondary aspects in a disease course. In terms of healthy qi and pathogenic factors, the former is the root, and the latter is the tip, and in terms of the cause of a disease and symptoms, the former is the root while the latter the tip. In terms of the site of a lesion, the internal organs are the root, whereas the body surface is at the tip. In terms of an old illness and a recent illness, the former is primary and the latter secondary.

(1) Treating the Root

With differentiation of syndromes, we can see through the appearance to grasp the essence and find out the fundamental cause of a disease, then to make out the corresponding method to treat the disease from the root.

(2) Treating the Acute Symptoms in Emergency Cases

Generally, treating the primary aspect of a disease is the basic approach, however, under some circumstances, the symptoms are more acute than the root cause, and if they are neglected, symptoms may deteriorate and a critical condition occurs. That is why we first relieve the symptoms, and then treat the root cause. In this way, the condition is alleviated and there is a favorable background in the treatment of the root cause, the purpose of which is to treat the disease from the root.

(3) Treating the Root in Chronic Cases

When the condition is stable, or when an old illness may not bring about other lesions, and no critical condition occurs, or acute symptoms are relieved after treatment, stress is put on treatment of the root.

(4) Treating the Primary and Secondary Aspects of a Disease Simultaneously

When the symptoms and the root are both in the state of being relieved or acute, the principle of "treating both the symptoms and the root simultaneously" is applicable.

2. Reinforcing the Healthy Qi and Eliminating the Pathogenic Factors

The healthy qi refers to man's ability to resist diseases. A course of disease is one in which there is a combat between the healthy qi and the pathogenic factors. If the former overcomes the latter, disease retreats but, if the pathogenic factors win the battle, the condition deteriorates. Reinforcing the healthy qi is used for a deficiency syndrome while eliminating the pathogenic factors is for an excess syndrome. If it is a deficiency-excess complex syndrome, the above two methods are used in combination.

Section 3 Point Combination and Selection of Points

Point combination of the dermal needling therapy is based on the guiding principle of "syndrome differentiation and treatment," in which appropriate selection of points and tapping manipulations are integrated. Selection of points is closely related to the therapeutic effect, so it is important to select the right points. This section focuses on the principle of point selection and the method of point combination.

1. Principle of Point Selection

Selection of points is guided by the theory of channels and collaterals. Different points are selected for different cases. Selection of the adjacent and distal points, and selection of points according to symptoms are the usual practice.

(1) Selection of the Adjacent Points

It is based on the universal law that needling applied to all points can treat the local or nearby disorders, which reflect on the local or nearby surface of the body. For example, LV 14 (*qī mén*) and RN 12 (*zhōng wǎn*) are selected respectively for liver disease and stomach disease. BL 1 (*jīng míng*), SI 12 (*bǐng fēng*) and SI 9 (*jiān zhēn*) are selected for eye problem and shoulder pain respectively.

(2) Selection of the Distant Points

It is an approach to select points on the body surface away from the diseased area based on the theory of traditional Chinese medicine and the indications of the fourteen channels. In practice, it has two methods: selection of points on the affected channel and on the related channel.

- **Selection of points on the affected channel:** It means to select points on the diseased channel. For instance, ST 36 (*zú sān lǐ*) is selected for stomachache, HT 6 (*yīn xì*) for cardiac pain and DU 26 (*shuǐ gōu*) for acute lower back pain.
- **Selection of points from the related channel:** It refers to a selection of points on the channel that is interiorly-exteriorly related to the diseased channel, or from other related channels. For example, SP 4 (*gōng sūn*) and SP 5 (*shāng qiū*) are selected for stomachache, as the Stomach Channel and the Spleen Channel are interiorly-exteriorly related. For cough caused by failure of the kidney to grasp qi, LU 5 (*chǐ zé*), LU 7 (*liè quē*), KI 3 (*tài xī*), BL 13 (*fèi shù*) and BL 23 (*shèn shù*) are selected. For painful stiff nape, LU 7 (*liè quē*) is selected.

(3) Selection of points according to symptoms

It is based on the theory of traditional Chinese medicine and specific therapeutic effect of some points, used for general symptoms. For instance, DU 14 (*dà zhuī*) and LI 11 (*qū chí*) are selected to treat fever and DU 26 (*shuǐ gōu*) and EX-UE11 (*shí xuān*) for loss of consciousness.

2. Point Combination

Point combination is based on the principles of point selection and the indications of the fourteen channels.

Point combination starts from the whole in light of the condition, and points are selected on differentiation of syndromes. Only with this can the synergetic effect of points play its full role.

(1) Combination of the Same Channel Points

It means that when a particular *zang-fu* organ or channel gets blocked or disharmonized, the points of the channel are selected in a prescription. For example, for fullness in the stomach with indigestion and abdomen, the adjacent point ST 21 (*liáng mén*) and the distal point ST 36 (*zú sān lǐ*) are selected. For posterior headache, the adjacent point BL 10 (*tiān zhù*) and the distal point BL 66 (*zú tōng gǔ*) are selected.

(2) Point Combination of the Interiorly-Exteriorly Related Channels

When a particular *zang-fu* organ or channel is diseased, points of the interiorly-exteriorly related channels are selected. This method is based on the yin-yang and interiorly-exterior relation between the *zang-fu* organs and channels. For example, for fever, cough, sore throat due to fettering of the lung by wind-cold, the points selected are LU 5 (*chǐ zé*), LU 7 (*liè quē*), LI 11 (*qǔ chí*) and LI 4 (*hé gǔ*), which have an interior-exterior relation with the Lung Channel, as the Lung Channel and Large Intestine Channel are interiorly-exteriorly related. The *yuan*-source and *luo*-connecting point combination is also in this category.

(3) Superior-Inferior Point Combination

It is a method of point combination in which points above the lower back are paired with points on the lower limbs. In practice, superior and inferior points can be used separately. For parietal pain, disorder of the Liver Channel, LV 3 (*tài chōng*) is selected, or DU 20 (*bǎi huì*) is selected for rectal prolapse, or they are selected together. For sore throat, LU 7 (*liè quē*), KI 6 (*zhào hǎi*) and the confluent points of the eight extraordinary vessels are selected.

(4) Anterior-Posterior Point Combination

It is also named "abdomen-back yin-yang point combination". The anterior refers to the chest and abdomen, attributable to yin while the posterior refers to the back and lower back, attributable to yang. *The Treatise on Needle in Formal Use in Miraculous Pivot* names it "paired needling". For example, RN 12 (*zhōng wǎn*) and ST 21 (*liáng mén*) are combined with BL 50 (*wèi cāng*) in the posterior to treat stomachache. The combination of the back-*shu* points and the front-*mu* points is of this category. For instance, RN 14 (*jù quē*) in the anterior and BL 15 (*xīn shù*) in the posterior are selected for constriction in the chest and heart pain.

(5) Left-Right Point Combination

It is a method of point combination in which bilateral points of a given channel are selected. It is called "contralateral needling" and "contralateral collateral needling" in *The Inner Classic*. It is characterized by needling the points of the right side when the left side is diseased, or vice versa. For example, for ptosis of the left angle of the mouth, right LI 4 (*hé gŭ*) is selected. Left corresponding points or points on both sides are selected when hemiplegia is seen on the right side.

Chapter 2

Treatment

Section 1 Internal Diseases

1. Common Cold

[Overview]

It is a disease from external pathogenic wind or epidemic pathogens, leading to dysfunction of the lung in the line of defense, manifested by stuffy and running nose, sneezing, cough, headache, aversion to cold, fever and general malaise.

Among diseases from external contraction, common cold is a most commonly seen illness. It may occur all year round but mostly in winter and spring. It is not only closely related to the outbreak and progress of acute bronchitis and acute attack of chronic bronchitis, but it is also related to the progression and deterioration of angina pectoris, edema and impediment diseases. It endangers the life of children, the aged and debilitated. Influenza must be actively prevented and treated as it always outbreaks and spreads fast with critical conditions and possible death.

In this section, common cold and influenza are discussed, with emphasis on prevention and treatment of the former. This section can be referred to when the diseases according to Western diagnosis of common cold, influenza and acute upper respiratory tract infection are treated.

[Cause and Mechanism of Disease]

Pathogenic wind and epidemic pathogens attack the human body through two pathways, either from the nose and mouth, or the skin and hair. Invasion of the lung by pathogenic factors via the nose and mouth, results in a series of symptoms of the lung. The hair and skin are the barriers of the human body against pathogenic factors. When these barriers are warmed, moistened and nourished by the defensive qi and fluids, they may resist the pathogenic factors to protect the exterior. When they attack the body and the defensive function of the hair and skin weakens, pathogenic factors may invade the lung via the skin and hair and cause a series of symptoms related to the lung.

The lesion is usually in the lung, which is related to skin and hair. The ventilating function of the lung warms and moistens them. Thus, when they are affected, dysfunction of the lung occurs. Diseased hair and skin leads to dysfunction of the lung. The window of the lung is the nose so when the lung qi fails to disperse freely, common cold occurs, which is marked by stuffy and running nose, cough, sore throat, aversion to cold, fever, headache and general pain.

Due to the changes in seasons, weather, and health condition, there are different syndromes of this condition, such as diseases from wind-cold, wind-heat and summer-dampness. In the course of diseases due to cold and heat, the symptoms may transform or coincide each other.

In traditional Chinese medicine, it is also called "wind affection." The term "influenza" is shared by Western medicine and traditional Chinse medicine.

[Types of Syndromes]

Main manifestations: Fever or aversion to cold, stuffy and running nose, headache and general pain.

(1) Severe wind-cold: Severe aversion to cold and mild fever, general aching pain, headache, absence of sweating, stuffy nose, low muffled voice, running nose with thin nasal discharge, sneezing, thin and white fur, and floating tight pulse.

(2) Wind-heat: Fever, aversion to wind, headache, slight sweating, running nose with yellow and sticky discharge, cough, sore throat, thirst with a desire for drinks, thin and yellow fur, and floating rapid pulse.

(3) Summer-dampness: Low grade fever, sweating without relief, slight aversion to cold, heaviness in the head, sluggishness, heaviness and aching pain of limbs, cough with sticky sputum, running nose with thick nasal discharge, irritability, thirst without a desire for drinks, short and brown urine, yellow and greasy fur, and soggy rapid pulse.

[Syndrome Differentiation and Treatment]

Treatment: To disperse cold, clear heat, disseminate lung qi to relieve coughing

Point combination 1:

Main points:

GB 20 (*fēng chí*)	BL 12 (*fēng mén*)	BL 13 (*fèi shù*)

Secondary points:

Wind-cold: SJ 5 (*wài guān*), LI 4 (*hé gŭ*)

Wind-heat: DU 14 (*dà zhuī*), LI 11 (*qŭ chí*)

Summer-dampness: SP 9 (*yīn líng quán*), ST 36 (*zú sān lĭ*)

Stuffy and running nose: LI 20 (*yíng xiāng*)
Cough: RN 22 (*tiān tū*), LU 10 (*yú jì*)
Sore throat: LU 11 (*shào shāng*), LU 7 (*liè quē*)
Point combination 2 (for common cold due to wind-heat):
Main points:

DU 14 (*dà zhuī*)	LI 11 (*qǔ chí*)	LI 4 (*hé gǔ*)

Secondary points:
Headache: GB 20 (*fēng chí*), EX-HN5 (*tài yáng*), LU 7 (*liè quē*)
Cough: RN 22 (*tiān tū*), LU 5 (*chǐ zé*), LU 9 (*tài yuān*)
Stuffy and running nose: LI 20 (*yíng xiāng*)
Point combination 3:
Ear points: Ear Apex (HX 6.7i), Lung (CO 14) on the back auricle
Secondary points:
Forehead pain: Forehead (AT 1)
Pain in the back of the head: Occiput (AT 3)
Migraine: Temple (AT 2)
Point combination 4: The Lung Channel, the Large Intestine Channel, the *Du* Vessel, the first line 1.5 *cun* lateral to the posterior midline on the back of the Bladder Channel.

Operation: After routine sterilization, moderate tapping is used for wind-cold syndrome until light red skin appears, while for wind-heat syndrome a little bleeding appears. Strictly sterilize the ear if ear acupuncture treatment is applied. Treatment is given once a day and five treatments make a course.

[Differential Diagnosis]

(1) The clinical manifestations of allergic rhinitis is similar to that of common cold, but it has an acute onset, frequent sneezing with thin nasal discharge. After a few minutes, the symptoms disappear. It is usually accompanied by other allergic disease.

(2) Many acute infectious diseases have symptoms of common cold, for example, epidemic cerebrospinal meningitis, measles, typhoid, paratyphoid and typhus. In epidemic areas and seasons, it should be intimately observed and make differential diagnosis.

[Nursing and Prevention]

(1) Keep warm and indoor air fresh. Avoid wind-cold. When one contracts it, have light meals, and quit smoking and alcohol dependence.

(2) Do not go to public places as much as possible during the influenza period to avoid infection.

(3) Tapping or moxibustion is applied to ST 36 (*zú sān lǐ*) daily to prevent influenza.

2. Acute Bronchitis

[Overview]

It is due to invasion of the lung by the six external pathogenic factors, or to dysfunction of the *zang-fu* organs which injures the lung and disables lung qi to disperse. Coughing and spitting phlegm are the main manifestations. Acute bronchitis is a most commonly seen condition with high incidence, especially in the cold areas.

When acute coughing is the chief symptom of conditions such as upper respiratory infection, bronchodilation and pneumonia, consult this section for treatment, along with referral to treat other disorders complicated by acute coughing.

[Cause and Mechanism of Disease]

It is usually due to invasion of the lung by six external pathogenic factors, or dysfunction of other *zang-fu* organs, which disturbs the dispersion of lung qi, and forces qi to go upward, resulting in coughing.

(1) External pathogenic factors attacking lung: It is due to six external pathogenic factors which invade the lung via either the nose or mouth, or the skin and hair. As a result, lung qi is fettered and the lung loses the function of dispersion.

(2) Internal pathogenic factors attacking lung: It is also caused by dysfunction of the lung due to an attack by internal pathogenic factors. There are two possibilities, one is lesion of other *zang-fu* organs, and the other is lesion of the lung itself. In the former condition, emotional stress affects smooth flow of liver qi, and stagnant qi turns into fire, which flames and invades the lung. In the latter condition, improper diet, smoking, alcohol consumption, or preference for spicy food all assist fire, which scorches the lung and stomach, resulting in phlegm; likewise, overeating greasy food leads to impeded transportation of the spleen, resulting in production of phlegm, which blocks the lung airway, making rise of lung qi, and finally causing coughing.

Coughing due to external contraction attributes to the excess syndrome. It is caused by invasion of the lung by external pathogenic factors and obstruction of lung qi. If they are not expelled in time, wind-cold may transform into heat, or wind-heat into dryness, or phlegm produced from lung heat.

Coughing due to internal injury mostly attributes to the excess with deficiency complication. The main pathogenic factors are phlegm and fire. Retained phlegm may turn into fire, and fire may scorch body fluids into phlegm. For example, when liver fire attacks the lung, lung fluid is impaired and phlegm produces. When phlegm-dampness attacks the lung, the spleen fails in transportation and the refined essence of drinks and food do not go upward to nourish the lung. They accumulate and form phlegm and store in the lung. As a result, lung qi accumulates and goes up to induce coughing. If it retains in the lung, accompanied by external contraction, phlegm-dampness may generate heat, marked by phlegm-heat and coughing. If it causes cold formation, cold-phlegm and cough are found.

[Types of Syndromes]

Main manifestations: Coughing, spitting thin phlegm

(1) Wind-cold: Heavy cough, itching of the throat, shortness of breath, thin white phlegm, aversion to cold, absence of sweating, thin, white fur and floating tight pulse.

(2) Wind-heat: Coughing with spitting thick and yellow phlegm, sore throat, yellow nasal discharge, fever, sweating, thirst with a desire for drinks, thin yellow fur, and floating rapid pulse.

[Syndrome Differentiation and Treatment]

Treatment: To disperse cold, clear heat, disseminate lung qi to relieve coughing.

Point combination 1:

Main pionts:

BL 13 (*fèi shù*)	LU 7 (*liè quē*)	LI 4 (*hé gŭ*)
LU 9 (*tài yuān*)	LU 5 (*chĭ zé*)	

Secondary points:

Wind cold: BL 12 (*fēng mén*), SJ 5 (*wài guān*)

Wind heat: LI 11 (*qū chí*), DU 14 (*dà zhūi*)

Sore throat: LU 11 (*shào shāng*)

Much phlegm: ST 40 (*fēng lóng*), SP 9 (*yīn líng quán*)

Point combination 2 (for wind-cold coughing):

BL 13 (*fèi shù*)	LU 7 (*liè quē*)	LU 5 (*chĭ zé*)
LI 4 (*hé gŭ*)		

Point combination 3 (for wind-heat coughing):

BL 13 (*fèi shù*)	LU 5 (*chĭ zé*)	GB 20 (*fēng chí*)
DU 14 (*dà zhuī*)		

Point combination 4: The Lung Channel, the *Du* Vessel, the first line lateral to the Bladder Channel.

Operation: After routine sterilization, moderate tapping is applied to the above points until the skin becomes flushed, while for wind-heat coughing, tap the skin until a little bleeding occurs. Treatment is given once a day or once every other day and five treatments make a course.

[Nursing and Prevention]

(1) Put on or take off clothes with weather change. Ventilate the room to keep air fresh. Avoid exposure to oily smell and dust.

(2) Quit smoking and alcohol dependence. Don't eat spicy and greasy foods.

3. Chronic Bronchitis

[Overview]

It usually develops from persistent acute bronchitis. It has a long disease course and repeated attacks. Coughing and expectoration of phlegm are the main manifestations.

Chronic bronchitis is the most commonly seen condition with high incidence. In China, the incidence is about 3%~5%. Among people over 50, the incidence is 10%~15% and there is a high incidence in cold regions of China. In the treatment of disease involving coughing as its chief complaint, refer to this section. Acute onset of chronic bronchitis marked by acute coughing is treated according to the method mentioned in the previous section.

[Cause and Mechanism of Disease]

It is due to the lung affected by diseased zang-fu organ. Then lung qi fails in dispersion, and instead, it rises, resulting in this condition.

(1) Liver fire invading lung: It is due to emotional stress. When it fails to flow smoothly, the stagnant liver qi turns into fire and inflames up along the channels to attack the lung, causing failure of lung qi to disperse, consequently inducing cough.

(2) Turbid phlegm obstructing lung: It is due to improper diet, smoking, alcohol dependence, or preference for spicy foods, which scorches the lung and stomach to trigger production of phlegm. Overeating greasy food impedes normal transportation of the spleen and results in production of phlegm, which goes upward to the lung and blocks the airway. Finally, adverse rising of lung qi leads to coughing.

(3) Lung yin deficiency: It is usually caused by persistent lung disorders, which results in debility of the lung and consumption of yin when it fails to govern qi. The lung is not able to bring qi down, and instead, qi goes up, leading to coughing.

Coughing in chronic bronchitis usually attributes to excess and deficiency complication. Phlegm and fire are the chief pathogenic factors. Retained phlegm may turn into fire and fire may scorch body fluids into phlegm. Excessive pathogenic factors and diminished healthy qi often affect some organs as well as the lung. For example, when liver fire attacks the lung, fluids of the lung are impaired, and phlegm produces. Failure of the spleen in transportation is often seen in the case of invasion of the lung by phlegm-dampness. The nutrients from food and drinks cannot transform into refined substances to nourish the lung. They retain in the lung and generate phlegm, which then goes upward and resides in the lung. When lung qi goes up, coughing occurs. In a chronic disease, deficiency in the lung and kidney impedes qi to transform into fluid. Phlegm is easily produced. This is why we say "the spleen is the source of phlegm, and the lung is the depositor of phlegm." If the kidney is involved, coughing may develop into asthma. If phlegm-dampness retains in the lung with external contraction, it may turn into heat, and phlegm-heat coughing occurs. If it turns to cold, phlegm-cold coughing occurs. If coughing is due to lung problems, a deficiency syndrome may turn to an excess syndrome.

Insufficiency of lung yin usually leads to hyperactivity of fire, which scorches body fluids and produces phlegm. When the lung is not moistened, adverse rising of lung qi results in coughing, or lung qi fails to disperse and can't transform into body fluids, which accumulates and forms phlegm. As a result, lung qi adversely rises and coughing occurs.

[Types of Syndromes]

Main manifestations: Recurrent unhealed coughing

(1) Liver fire invading lung: Coughing with chest pain involving the hypochondrium, scanty sticky phlegm, difficult to expectorate, flushed cheeks, irritability, bitter taste in the mouth, dry throat, thin yellow fur, and wiry rapid pulse.

(2) Turbid phlegm obstructing lung: Recurrent heavy coughing, fullness and constriction in the chest, profuse sticky phlegm or in mass, anorexia, loose stools, white greasy fur, soggy or slippery pulse.

(3) Lung yin deficiency: Slow onset, short faint coughing, dry cough with scanty phlegm or without phlegm, dry mouth, tidal fever, flushed cheeks, night sweating, wearing away, emaciation, red tongue with scanty coating, and thin rapid pulse.

[Syndrome Differentiation and Treatment]

Treatment: To replenish yin, clear the lung, invigorate the spleen, resolve phlegm, purge fire, relieve coughing.

Point combination 1:

Main pionts:

BL 13 (*fèi shù*)	LU 9 (*tài yuān*)	LU 5 (*chĭ zé*)

Secondary points:

Liver fire invading lung: LV 2 (*xíng jiān*), LU 10 (*yú jì*)

Turbid phlegm obstructing lung:

BL 20 (*pí shù*)	RN 12 (*zhōng wăn*)	ST 40 (*fēng lóng*)
ST 36 (*zú sān lĭ*)		

Lung yin deficiency: BL 43 (*gāo huāng*), LU 1 (*zhōng fŭ*), KI 7 (*fù liū*).

Point Combination 2: The Lung Channel and the Stomach Channel

Operation: After routine sterilization, moderate or strong tapping is applied to the above points or along the corresponding channels for the excess syndrome until the skin becomes flushed or slightly bleeding, while for the deficiency syndrome light tapping is applied until the skin becomes flushed. Treatment is given once every two to three days and ten treatments make a course.

[Nursing and Prevention]

(1) Keep warm and avoid exposure to wind-cold in weather change. Try to refrain from going to public places to prevent infection.

(2) Do physical exercises to build up health, or take part in outdoor activities to enhance cold-resistant capability.

(3) Take care of environmental sanitation. Keep air fresh in the room. Do not expose to oily smoke and dust.

(4) Take light meals and avoid spicy greasy food.

4. Bronchial Asthma

[Overview]

It is a commonly seen recurrent condition. According to traditional Chinese medicine, it is divided into two types: wheezing and panting. Although both of them are in the category of dyspnea, their manifestations are different. Wheezing is characterized by a whistling type of continuous sound, while panting is a labored or difficult breathing. In severe cases patients may gasp and raise shoulders.

It occurs all year round, especially during the cold season and sudden weather change. In the treatment of asthmatic bronchitis, lung infection, pneumonia, emphysema, cardiac asthma, pulmonary tuberculosis, pneumosilicosis and hysteria accompanied by asthma, this section can be consulted.

[Cause and Mechanism of Disease]

Bronchial asthma is caused by external contraction or internal injury. When it is triggered by external contraction, food, emotional factor, tiredness, phlegm may obstruct the air passage, followed by failure of lung qi to disperse, causing air passage contracture.

(1) Wind-cold fettering lung: When the lung is fettered by wind-cold or wind-heat, which is not driven out of the body in time and retains in the lung, lung qi fails to flow smoothly and disperse, followed by its adverse rising, causing asthma.

(2) Phlegm-heat obstructing lung: It is also caused by phlegm-heat obstructing the lung in acute or chronic conditions. When lung qi is restricted, normal distribution of qi and body fluids are impeded, coagulation of fluids generates phlegm. This may be caused by dysfunction of the spleen in transportation, where phlegm is produced and transforms into fire, which disturbs the lung and obstructs the air passage. Failure of lung qi to disperse leads to asthma.

(3) Liver fire invading lung: Asthma occurs when there are emotional problems that make qi stagnate. Asthma may also occur if liver qi fails to flow freely, or when liver qi is impaired by fury, leading to stagnation of liver qi, which transforms into fire, followed by invasion of the lung by liver fire and adverse rise of lung qi.

(4) Poor health and chronic disease: It is caused diminished function of the lung in a chronic disease, in which lung qi is impaired by persistent coughing. When the lung fails to govern qi, asthma occurs. The condition deteriorates in cases of insuffcient lung qi and impeded flow of blood, resulting in deficiency of qi and stagnation of blood. In a chronic case, the spleen is involved. Dysfunction of the spleen leads to accumulation of dampness which turns to phlegm. Overstrain or excessive sexual activities damage the kidney and kidney essence. If lung qi fails to nourish the kidney, the latter is deficient. In turn, the kidney cannot aid the lung to grasp qi. When the lung inhales less and exhales more, asthma occurs. Further more, when kidney yang is deficient and the kidney fails to dominate water, water floods and disturbs the lung and and heart, leading to insufficiency of heart yang, and consequently, asthma occurs. This is a syndrome of deficiency complicated by excess.

[Types of Syndromes]

Main manifestations: Recurrent attack, shortness of breath, dyspnea, wheezing.

(1) Asthma of the excess syndrome: Sudden onset, difficult hoarse breathing, gasping and raising shoulders, fullness and constriction in the chest, relief with breathing out.

(i) Wind-cold fettering lung: Coughing, shortness of breath, expectoration of thin white phlegm, complicated by aversion to cold and fever, headache, absence of sweating, thin white fur, and floating tight pulse.

(ii) Phlegm-heat obstructing lung: Shortness of breath, hoarse breathing, fever, thirst, restlessness, difficult expectoration of thick yellow phlegm, yellow thick or greasy fur, and slippery rapid pulse.

(iii) Liver fire invading lung: Shortness of breath, adverse rising of qi, coughing, bloated pains in the chest and hypochondrium, restlessness, irritability, scanty and sticky phlegm difficult to expectorate, thin yellow dry fur, and wiry rapid pulse.

(2) Asthma of the deficiency syndrome: Slow onset, long disease course, shortness of breath with low sound, aggravated when active, spontaneous sweating, less qi in the chest, relieved by deep breath.

(i) Lung deficiency: Shortness of breath, aggravated when active, weak coughing, aversion to cold, thin phlegm, thin white fur, and thready weak pulse.

(ii) Spleen deficiency: Shortness of breath, low asthmatic sound, thin phlegm, lassitude, pale enlarged tongue, and soggy moderate pulse.

(iii) Kidney deficiency: Chronic asthma, aggravated when active, breathing out more than breathing in, aversion to cold, cold limbs, or general edema, pale tongue with white fur, and deep thready pulse.

[Syndrome Differentiation and Treatment]

(1) Excess Syndrome

Treatment: To disseminate lung qi to relieve asthma.

Point combination 1:

Main points: EX-B1 (*dìng chuǎn*) (below the spinous process of the 7th cervical vertebra, 0.5 *cun* lateral to the posterior midline), RN 17 (*dàn zhōng*), RN 22 (*tiān tū*)

Secondary points:

Wind-cold fettering lung: BL 12 (*fēng mén*), LU 7 (*liè quē*)

Phlegm-heat obstructing lung:

LU 5 (*chǐ zé*)	LU 10 (*yú jì*)	ST 40 (*fēng lóng*)

Liver fire invading lung:

LV 2 (*xíng jiān*)	LV 14 (*qī mén*)	LU 10 (*yú jì*)

(2) Deficiency Syndrome

Treatment: To reinforce healthy qi to relieve asthma.

Point combination 2:

Main points:

EX-B1 (*dìng chuǎn*)	BL 13 (*fèi shù*)	BL 43 (*gāo huāng*)
RN 6 (*qì hǎi*)		

Secondary points:

Lung deficiency:

LU 9 (*tài yuān*)	LU 8 (*jīng qú*)	LU 1 (*zhōng fǔ*)

Spleen deficiency:

BL 20 (*pí shù*)	ST 36 (*zú sān lǐ*)	SP 3 (*tài bái*)

Kidney deficiency:

BL 23 (*shèn shù*)	KI 3 (*tài xī*)	RN 4 (*guān yuán*)

Point combination 3:

Main points: For deficiency syndrome

BL 13 (*fèi shù*)	BL 43 (*gāo huāng shù*)	BL 20 (*pí shù*)
BL 23 (*shèn shù*)		

Secondary points:

Profuse phlegm: ST 36 (*zú sān lǐ*), ST 40 (*fēng lóng*)

Shortness of breath:

RN 22 (*tiān tū*)	LU 1 (*zhōng fǔ*)	LU 6 (*kǒng zuì*)

Aversion to cold and cold limbs: RN 4 (*guān yuán*), DU 4 (*mìng mén*)

Point combination 4:

Main points:

EX-B1 (*dìng chuǎn*)	BL 13 (*fèi shù*)	BL 12 (*fēng mén*)
DU 14 (*dà zhuī*)	SI 15 (*jiān zhōng shù*)	

Secondary points:

GB 20 (*fēng chí*)	BL 11 (*dà zhù*)	BL 23 (*shèn shù*)
BL 20 (*pí shù*)	BL 25 (*dà cháng shù*)	

Operation: After routine sterilization, for the excess syndrome moderate or strong tapping is applied, while for the excess-heat syndrome light tapping is applied, followed by cupping. Do not cause much bleeding. For the deficiency syndrome light tapping is applied. Treatment is given once a day or every other day and ten treatments make a course.

[Nursing and Prevention]

(1) Put on or take off clothes when weather changes. Keep warm and avoid cold.

(2) Take physical exercises to build up health.

(3) Keep the indoor air fresh. Avoid exposure to allergic substances, like pollen, dust or paint.

(4) Quit smoking and alcohol dependence. Take light meals and avoid greasy, rich spicy food.

5. Cerebrovascular Accidents

[Overview]

In traditional Chinese medicine, cerebrovascular accident is in the category of "wind-stroke", "apoplexy", or is caused by disorder of blood and qi, which produces wind, fire, phlegm and obstruction resulting in blood stasis of the brain arteries and veins, or cerebral hemorrhage. The main manifestations are sudden falling, loss of consciousness, hemiplegia, accompanied by deviated mouth, slurred speech, or only by deviation of the mouth and eye, hemiplegia and motion difficulties but without loss of consciousness. According to different degrees of injury, it is classified into two types: *zang-fu* stroke and channel stroke, marked by different manifestations. It is usually seen in middle-aged people, and occurs all year round but mostly in winter and spring.

Consult this section in the treatment of cerebral infarction, cerebral hemorrhage, subarachnoid hemorrhage caused by high blood pressure, arteriosclerosis, aneurysm, or cerebral embolism triggered by rheumatic heart disease, atrial fibrillation and bacterial endocarditis.

[Cause and Mechanism of Disease]

(1) Apoplexy involving collaterals: It is due to insufficiency of healthy qi, accompanied by sudden weather change, resulting in stagnation of qi and blood.

(2) Internal stirring of liver fire: It is due to emotion problems and disturbed liver qi flow, leading to stagnation of qi and blood in the brain vessels, or it is due to fury that impairs the liver, as a result, there is hyperactivity of liver yang or heart fire. Mutual stirring-up of wind and fire brings qi upward, followed by rising of blood, which attacks the brain.

(3) Phlegm heat and *fu*-organ excess: It is due to phlegm-heat accompanied by overeating of greasy and sweet foods or by alcohol indulgence, which impairs the spleen and stomach and makes the spleen fail to transport. As a result, phlegm produces and turns to heat. Phlegm and heat go together and block the channel and cloud the orifices, or it is due to hyperactivity of liver fire and qi stagnation, which impairs the function of the spleen, resulting in production of phlegm, or it is due to stagnated liver qi, which transforms into fire and scorches body fluids into phlegm. Then phlegm and stagnated qi work together to disturb the channels.

Lesion is in the brain, closely related to the heart, kidney, liver and spleen. In conclusion, its mechanism includes deficiency (yin deficiency, qi deficiency), fire (liver fire, heart fire), wind (liver wind, external wind), phlegm (wind-phlegm, damp-phlegm), disorder of qi (reversed flow of qi) and blood (blood stasis). They interact under certain circumstances. Deficiency is in origin but it appears superficially as excess, and simultaneously, deficiency in the upper and excess in the lower are the common characteristics. The chief trigger is deficiency of liver-kidney yin, qi and blood, while in the superficial cause it is mutual stirring-up of wind and heat, profuse phlegm-dampness and blood stasis, and disturbance of qi and blood. The basic cause is reversed flow of qi and blood that attack the brain.

[Types of Syndromes]

Main manifestations: Sudden falling, loss of consciousness, hemiplegia, accompanied by deviated mouth and slurred speech.

(1) Channel Stroke

Main manifestations: Numbness of one side, hemiplegia, deviation of the mouth and tongue, stiff tongue, slurred speech or aphasia.

(i) Apoplexy involving collaterals: Numb skin, hands and feet, sudden deviation of the mouth and eye, slurred speech, or hemiplegia in severe cases, thin white fur and wiry pulse.

(ii) Internal stirring of liver fire: Dizziness and headache, tinnitus, vertigo, insomnia, dream-disturbed sleep, reddened face, irritability, sudden deviation of the mouth and eye, slurred speech, or even hemiplegia, bright red tongue, scanty or greasy fur and wiry thin or wiry slippery pulse.

(iii) Phlegm heat and *fu*-organ excess: Sudden hemiplegia, numbness of one side of the body, sudden deviation of the mouth and eye, stiff tongue, slurred speech, dry stools or constipation, dizziness, wheezing, loss of consciousness, somnolence, yellow thick fur and wiry slippery or rapid pulse.

(iv) Qi deficiency and blood stasis: Hemiplegia, deviation of the mouth and tongue, slurred speech, tarnished complexion, listlessness, lassitude, disinclination to talk, pale and dark tongue or with petechia and white fur, thready and rough or deep and slow pulse.

(2) *Zang-fu* Organs Stroke

Main manifestations: Sudden loss of consciousness, hemiplegia, deviation of the mouth and tongue, stiff tongue, slurred speech, numbness of one side of the body.

(i) Excess syndrome: Syncope, restlessness, clenched jaw, wheezing, closed fists, constipation, anuresis, limb contracture or convulsion, white greasy or yellow greasy fur, and wiry slippery pulse.

(ii) Depletion syndrome: Syncope, eye close, mouth open, snoring, feeble breathing, cold limbs, dripping with sweat, oily sweat, urine and fecal incontinence, flaccidity, curled tongue,and thready weak or feeble pulse.

[Syndrome Differentiation and Treatment]

(1) Channel Stroke

Treatment: To nourish the kidney and liver, activate blood circulation and reinforce qi, extinguish wind and unblock channels.

(i) Hemiplegia

Point combination 1:

Main points:

Upper limbs:

LI 15 (*jiān yú*)	SJ 14 (*jiān liáo*)	LI 14 (*bì nào*)
LI 11 (*qū chí*)	LI 10 (*shǒu sān lǐ*)	LI 4 (*hé gǔ*)

Lower limbs:

GB 30 (*huán tiào*)	ST 32 (*fú tù*)	GB 34 (*yáng líng quán*)
ST 36 (*zú sān lǐ*)	ST 41 (*jiě xī*)	GB 39 (*xuán zhōng*)
BL 60 (*kūn lún*)		

(ii) Slurred Speech

Point combination 2: RN 23 (*lián quán*), HT 5 (*tōng lǐ*)

(iii) Deviation of the Mouth

Point combination 3:

Main points:

SI 18 (*quán liáo*)	ST 4 (*dì cāng*)	ST 6 (*jiá chē*)
LI 19 (*kǒu hé liáo*)	RN 24 (*chéng jiāng*)	LI 4 (*hé gǔ*)
LV 3 (*tài chōng*)		

Secondary points:

Channel attacked by wind:

GB 20 (*fēng chí*)	BL 12 (*fēng mén*)	GB 31 (*fēng shì*)

Stirring-up of liver wind:

BL 18 (*gān shù*)	BL 23 (*shèn shù*)	KI 7 (*fù liū*)
SP 10 (*xuè hǎi*)		

Phlegm-heat disturbance:

RN 12 (*zhōng wǎn*)	ST 40 (*fēng lóng*)	ST 25 (*tiān shū*)
ST 37 (*shàng jù xū*)	ST 44 (*nèi tíng*)	

Qi deficiency and blood stasis:

RN 6 (*qì hǎi*)	RN 4 (*guān yuán*)	SP 6 (*sān yīn jiāo*)
ST 36 (*zú sān lǐ*)	BL 17 (*gé shù*)	

Operation: After routine sterilization, moderate tapping is applied. In the acute stage treatment is given once a day. In the convalescent or sequela period treatment is given once every two to three days and ten treatments make a course.

Point combination 4:

Upper limbs: EX-B2 (*jiá jǐ*) (C4~T3); Lower limbs: EX-B2 (*jiá jǐ*) (L1~L5), upper and lower limbs where the three yang channels pass.

Operation: After routine sterilization, tapping is applied until skin becomes flushed. Divide the traveling course of the channels into several parts and apply tapping to each part separately. Treatment is given once every two to three days and ten treatments make a course.

(2) *Zang-fu* Organs Stroke

(i) Block Syndrome

Treatment: To extinguish wind, resolve phlegm, induce resuscitation.

Point Combination 5:

Main points: Twelve *Jing*-Well points:

DU 26 (*shuǐ gōu*)	DU 16 (*fēng fǔ*)	ST 40 (*fēng lóng*)
PC 6 (*nèi guān*)	PC 8 (*láo gōng*)	KI 1 (*yǒng quán*)

Secondary points:

Locked jaws:

ST 7 (*xià guān*)	ST 6 (*jiá chē*)	LI 4 (*hé gǔ*)

Closed fists: LI 4 (*hé gǔ*), SI 3 (*hòu xī*)

(ii) Collapse Syndrome

Treatment: To restore yang to save one from collapse.

Point Combination 6:

Main points:

RN 6 (*qì hǎi*)	RN 4 (*guān yuán*)	DU 20 (*bǎi huì*)

Secondary points:

Dripping of sweat: HT 6 (*yīn xì*), KI 7 (*fù liū*)

Incontinence of urine and feces: RN 3 (*zhōng jí*), SP 6 (*sān yīn jiāo*)

Operation: After routine sterilization, moderate tapping is applied to the depletion syndrome and to the twelve *Jing*-Well points until bleeding appears. Treatment is given once a day. Gentle tapping is applied to the depletion syndrome once a day, and ten treatments make a course.

Point Combination 7:

Main points: Scalp Acupuncture

Hemiplegia: The anterior oblique line of vertex-temporal (MS 6), the upper 3/5, the lateral line 2 of vertex (MS 8)

Numbness of one side of the body: The posterior oblige line of vertex-temporal, the upper 3/5, the lateral line 1 (MS 8) and lateral line 2 of vertex (MS 9)

Deviation of the mouth and eye: The anterior oblige line of vertex-temperal (MS 6), the lower 2/5

Slurred speech: The anterior oblige line of vertex-temperal line (MS 10), the lower 2/5

Operation: After routine sterilization, moderate tapping is used, once every two to three days and ten treatments make a course. Since there are multiple blood vessels on the head, in case of bleeding or people prone to infection, it is forbidden to use.

[Nursing and Prevention]

(1) Take care of diet structure. Eat more fresh vegetables and fruits, and eat less greasy food. Keep bowels movement free and quit smoking and alcohol dependence.

(2) Maintain good emotions. Don't get angry or exciting easily.

(3) Regular check up on blood pressure, BS, BF and keep them in the normal range. Pay attention to functional exercises of the body and speech training.

(4) Give emergency treatment if necessary.

6. Headache

[Overview]

Headache, a commonly seen disorder and a subjective complaint is triggered by external contraction and internal injury, that blocks related channels or disturbs the upper orifices. It may occur in multiple acute or chronic diseases, such as hypertension, neurotic headache, migraine, etc. It sometimes is also a pre-symptom of deterioration of related diseases.

[Cause and Mechanism of Disease]

(1) External contraction: It is often caused by carelessness in lifestyle and exposure to wind accompanied by cold, heat and dampness. Wind is a yang pathogen. It is said that *"the upper orifices are attacked first when wind invades the body," and "only wind could reach the top"*. Wind is the leader of six excesses and the chief pathogenic factor. Cold is a yin pathogen that impairs yang, and when yang is blocked with cold, blood stagnation occurs, and the channels are undernourished. Headache occurs as the channels become spasmodic. It is also caused by a disturbance of qi and blood, and malnutrition of channels, when wind attacks upward with heat, obstructing the upper orifices, impairing essence and blood, or making the brain and channels undernourished. When wind attacks the head with dampness, and yang is blocked, or the spleen does not function well, it leads to production of phlegm which clouds the brain, causing headache.

(2) Internal damage: It is usually closely related to the liver, spleen and kidney. When there is insufficient liver yin or kidney yin, uncontrolled liver yang becomes hyperactive, and headaches occur. When the spleen fails to perform its function because of improper diet, imbalance between work and rest, and production of phlegm, this results in yang rising and yin descending. When yang is blocked, phlegm and stagnant qi are integrated, then the brain lacks yang, essence and blood, and the channels are not adequately nourished. Sometimes, headache occurs after a disease or childbirth because of the loss of blood and malnourishment of the brain and channels. The kidney may be a source of the problem as well. It is because of poor constitution, insufficiency of kidney essence, or of overstrain and indulgent sexual activities, which impairs essence or the flow of qi, or dysfunction of the liver and spleen, and insufficiency of qi and essence production, or stagnation of liver qi, impeding the production of qi and essence, and nourishment of the brain and channels. Besides trauma or falling, chronic diseases may result in poor circulation of qi and blood, and malnutrition of channels, causing the occurrence of headaches.

[Types of Syndromes]

(1) Headaches due to External Contraction

Main manifestations: Acute onset with severe pain, usually an excess syndrome.

(i) Wind-cold syndrome: Whole head pain with neck and back involved, aggravated by cold, alleviated by warmth, aversion to cold and wind, thin white fur and floating tight pulse.

(ii) Wind-heat syndrome: Distending sharp headache, fever, aversion to wind, flushed cheeks and red eyes, thirst, a desire for cold drinks, constipation, yellow urine, red tongue with thin yellow fur, and floating rapid pulse.

(iii) Wind-dampness syndrome: Heavy headache, sluggishness, tastelessness in the mouth, no desire to drink, aggravated in overcast, rainy or windy days, white and greasy fur,and floating slippery pulse.

(2) Headache due to Internal Damage

Main manifestations: Slow onset with mild headache, a deficiency syndrome or an excess syndrome.

(i) Upper orifices obstructed by phlegm-dampness: Headache, as if the head was bound, chest fullness and constriction, lassitude, vomiting of saliva, anorexia, loose stools, white greasy fur, and slippery pulse.

(ii) Prickly headache due to blood stasis: Unhealed fixed pain, purplish tongue with ecchymosis or petechia, and wiry rough pulse.

(iii) Headache due to liver yang hyperactivity: Dizziness, aggravated when angry, restlessness, irascibility, bitter taste in the mouth and dry throat, hypochondriac bloated pain, flushed cheeks and red eyes, insomnia, red tongue with yellow fur, and wiry or wiry rapid pulse.

(iv) Headache due to deficiency of qi and blood: Occasional headache, aggravated when tired, probably alleviated after rest, lassitude, pale complexion, palpitation, insomnia and dream-disturbed sleep, pale tongue with tooth marks on the edge, thin white fur, and thready weak pulse.

(v) Headache due to kidney deficiency: Dizziness, aching pain and weakness of the lower back and knees, seminal emission, morbid leucorrhea, tinnitus, deafness, insomnia, amnesia, red tongue with less coating, and thready or deep thready pulse.

[Syndrome Differentiation and Treatment]

(1) Headache due to External Contraction

Treatment: To disperse wind and cold, clear heat, resolve dampness, remove obstruction from the upper orifices, relieve pain.

Point combination 1:

Main points:

DU 20 (*bǎi huì*)	GB 20 (*fēng chí*)	ST 8 (*tóu wéi*)
LI 4 (*hé gǔ*)	EX-HN5 (*tài yáng*)	

Secondary points:

Wind-cold: BL 12 (*fēng mén*), LU 7 (*liè quē*)

Wind-heat: DU 14 (*dà zhuī*), LI 11 (*qū chí*)

Wind-dampness:

BL 12 (*fēng mén*)	ST 40 (*fēng lóng*)	SP 9 (*yīn líng quán*)

Point combination 2:

Main points:

GB 20 (*fēng chí*)	BL 12 (*fēng mén*)	BL 13 (*fèi shù*)
LI 4 (*hé gǔ*)		

Secondary points:

Forehead pain:

ST 8 (*tóu wéi*)	EX-HN3 (*yìn táng*)	ST 43 (*xiàn gǔ*)

Pain in the vertex of the head: EX-HN1 (*sì shén cōng*), LV 3 (*tài chōng*)

Pain in the back of the head: BL 10 (*tiān zhù*), BL 60 (*kūn lún*)

Migraine:

GB 8 (*shuài gŭ*)	GB 12 (*wán gŭ*)	GB 41 (*zú lín qì*)

Operation: After routine sterilization, it had better to give moderate tapping. For the heat syndrome add cupping after tapping. Treatment is given once a day and five treatments make a course.

(2) Headache due to internal injury

Treatment: To reinforce the liver and kidney, invigorate the spleen, resolve phlegm, activate blood circulation and remove obstruction from orifices.

Point combination 3:

Upper orifices obstructed by turbid phlegm

Main points:

GB 20 (*fēng chí*)	ST 40 (*fēng lóng*)	LI 4 (*hé gŭ*)
RN 12 (*zhōng wăn*)	BL 20 (*pí shù*)	BL 21 (*wèi shù*)

Operation: Gentle tapping is applied to

RN 12 (*zhōng wăn*)	BL 20 (*pí shù*)	BL 21 (*wèi shù*)

Moderate tapping is applied to other points. Treatment is given every other day and five treatments make a course.

Point combination 4:

Blood stasis

Main points:

Ashi points	BL 17 (*gé shù*)	SP 10 (*xuè hăi*)
SP 6 (*sān yīn jiāo*)	LI 4 (*hé gŭ*)	LV 3 (*tài chōng*)

Operation: After routine sterilization, moderate or strong tapping is used. Bloodletting and cupping are applied to BL 17 (*gé shù*) and SP 10 (*xiè hăi*). Treatment is given once every other day and five treatments make a course.

Point Combination 5:

Liver yang hyperactivity

Main points:

GB 20 (*fēng chí*)	DU 16 (*fēng fǔ*)	DU 20 (*bǎi huì*)
GB 43 (*xiá xī*)	LV 2 (*xíng jiān*)	KI 3 (*tài xī*)
KI 7 (*fù liū*)		

Operation: After routine sterilization, gentle tapping is applied to KI 3 (*tài xī*) and KI 7 (*fù liū*), while moderate tapping for other points. Treatment is given once every two to three days and five treatments make a course.

Point Combination 6:

Both qi and blood deficiency

Main points:

BL 20 (*pí shù*)	BL 23 (*shèn shù*)	BL 18 (*gān shù*)
RN 6 (*qì hǎi*)	ST 36 (*zú sān lǐ*)	SP 6 (*sān yīn jiāo*)

Point Combination 7:

Kidney deficiency

Main points:

DU 20 (*bǎi huì*)	DU 23 (*shàng xīng*)	BL 23 (*shèn shù*)
BL 18 (*gān shù*)	RN 4 (*guān yuán*)	GB 39 (*xuán zhōng*)
KI 3 (*tài xī*)	SP 6 (*sān yīn jiāo*)	

Operation: After routine sterilization, gentle tapping is used once every two to three days and ten treatments make a course.

Point Combination 8:

The head and the neck where the *DU* Vessel, Bladder Channel and Gallbladder Channel pass.

Operation: After routine sterilization, gentle tapping is used for the deficiency syndrome, while for the excess syndrome strong tapping is used. Treatment is given once every two to three days and ten treatments make a course.

[Nursing and Prevention]

(1) Lead a regular life. Avoid over-strain, stress and agitation. Quit smoking and alcohol dependence.

(2) Do physical exercises to improve health. Don't be exposed to wind and cold.

(3) The cause must be made clear for unhealed headache. Treat primary

disease so as not to cause deterioration.

7. Facial Paralysis

[Overview]

It is characterized by deviation of the mouth and eye, usually seen in peripheral and central facial palsy. In the treatment of these two conditions, though they are different in pathology, this section can be referred to.

[Cause and Mechanism of Disease]

It is mainly due to invasion of the channels by wind from diminished healthy qi and defensive qi, leading to stagnation of qi and blood, malnutrition of the Sanjiao Channel, Large Intestine Channel and Stomach Channel in the face, the condition occurs.

[Types of Syndromes]

Main manifestations: Deviation of the mouth and eye, superficial forehead wrinkles or no wrinkles, incomplete closure of eyes, tears running or dry eyes, ptosis at the corner of the mouth

(1) Wind-cold attacking exterior: Aversion to wind-cold and superficial forehead wrinkles, slobbering, indigestion, hyperacusis, postauricular aching pain or migraine, thin white fur, and floating tight pulse.

(2) Channel and vessel obstruction: Flaccid facial muscles, enlargement of the palpebral fissure, incomplete closure of the eye, tears running or tenderness in the face, fixed pain, dark tongue, and wiry rough pulse.

(3) Both qi and blood deficiency: Prolonged duration, functional impairment accompanied by facial muscle spasm, atrophy, deviation of the mouth, pale dark tongue with white fur, and deep thready pulse.

[Syndrome Differentiation and Treatment]

Treatment: To dispel wind and cold, replenish qi and blood

Point combination 1:

Main points:

GB 14 (*yáng bái*)	ST 2 (*sì bái*)	ST 4 (*dì cāng*)
ST 6 (*jiá chē*)	LI 20 (*yíng xiāng*)	RN 24 (*chéng jiāng*)
LI 4 (*hé gǔ*)	LV 3 (*tài chōng*)	

Secondary points:

Wind-cold attacking exterior: GB 20 (*fēng chí*), SJ 5 (*wài guān*)

Channel and vessel obstruction:

BL 17 (*gé shù*)	BL 18 (*gān shù*)	RN 17 (*dàn zhōng*)

Both qi and blood deficiency:

ST 36 (*zú sān lǐ*)	SP 6 (*sān yīn jiāo*)	RN 12 (*zhōng wǎn*)
BL 20 (*pí shù*)	BL 21 (*wèi shù*)	

Postauricular pain: SJ 17 (*yì fēng*), GB 12 (*wán gǔ*)
Migraine: GB 8 (*shuài gǔ*), GB 41 (*zú lín qì*)
Hyperacusis: SJ 21 (*ěr mén*), SJ 3 (*zhōng zhǔ*)
Off-centre philtrum: DU 26 (*shuǐ gōu*)
Difficulty of moving the nose: EX-HN8 (*shàng yíng xiāng*)

Operation: At the early stage, gentle tapping is used, while moderate tapping is applied to the distal points. In case of qi and blood stagnation in channels, moderate and strong tapping is applied to the local points and distal points respectively. For deficiency of qi and blood, the local points receive the moderate tapping whereas the distal points the strong tapping.

At the acute stage treatment is given once a day and five treatments make a course. With an interval of two days, next course of treatment starts. At the convalescent or sequela stage, treatment is given once every two to three days and ten treatments make a course. Patients with tenderness in the face, pricking to bleed then cupping are used.

Point combination 2:
Main points:

GB 14 (*yáng bái*)	BL 2 (*cuán zhú*)	EX-HN5 (*tài yáng*)
ST 7 (*xià guān*)	ST 4 (*dì cāng*)	ST 6 (*jiá chē*)
SI 18 (*quán liáo*)	GB 20 (*fēng chí*)	

Operation: After routine sterilization, moderate tapping is applied until slightly bleeding. Treatment is given every other day and ten treatments make a course.

[Differential Diagnosis]

(1) Inferior facial muscle paralysis is only found in the central facial palsy. The forehead wrinkles and eye closure function are normal, mostly accompanied by symptoms or signs of other impaired cranial nerves or pyramidal tracts, such as tongue muscle paralysis and contralateral paralysis of limbs. With the help of

Head CT or NMR examination, an accurate diagnosis can be made.

(2) Facial paralysis caused by lesion of the posterior cranial fossa, such as in cerebellopontine angle tumor and basilar meningitis, nasopharyngeal carcinoma intracranial metastasis is mostly accompanied by auditory handicap and special manifestation of a primary disease.

(3) Acute infectious polyradiculoneuritis is characterized by peripheral nerve paralysis, usually on both sides. The typical symptoms are history of premonitory infection, symmetric limb movement and sensory disorder, lower limb motor nerve paralysis and albuminocytolgoic dissociation in cerebrospinal fluid.

[Nursing and Prevention]

(1) Keep warm. Avoid wind and cold. Don't be exposed to cold and wind after sweating and during sleep, especially in summer.

(2) It is better to wear eye patch to protect the cornea. Use the eyes less to rest them. Apply massage or hot compress to the affected muscles by oneself.

8. Facial Tic

[Overview]

It is an involuntary, paroxysmal spasm. In severe cases, eyes are not able to open. In traditional Chinese medicine, it is called "muscular twitching and cramp".

[Cause and Mechanism of Disease]

It is caused by invasion of the body by liver yang hyperactivity, channels obstructed by wind-phlegm and deficiency of qi and blood.

(1) Ascendant hyperactivity of liver yang: It is caused by excessive yang of the patient, or by impairment of liver yin due to fire transformed from stagnated liver qi over a long period of time, or by depression or anger, or persistent kidney yin deficiency and malnutrition of the liver. All the above factors lead to insufficiency of liver yin, hyperactivity of liver yang and internal stirring of liver wind, hereby, causing facial tic.

(2) Wind-phlegm obstructing vessels: It is caused by deficiency in the lung, spleen and kidney. Deficiency in the lung fails it to transport fluids and regulate the water passages, with a production of phlegm. Spleen deficiency disturbs its function. As a result, the fluids stagnate and congeal into phlegm. Deficiency of kidney qi results in uncontrolled water metabolism with production of phlegm-dampness. Disturbance of wind-phlegm causes the condition.

(3) Both qi and blood deficiency: It is also caused by deficiency of both qi and blood with the problem in the spleen. Impaired spleen leads to insufficient middle-*jiao* qi and failure of the middle-*jiao* in transportation, resulting in a lack of supply of essence and blood, followed by deficiency of qi and blood, deficient yin and hyperactive yang. The liver is involved and liver yang becomes hyperactive. In addition, when heart qi is insufficient and heart fire fails to disperse with hyperactivity of yin, tendons and limbs lack nutrition and the condition occurs.

[Types of Syndromes]

Main manifestations: Involuntary paroxysmal spasm of the orbicular muscles at the early stage, gradually spreading to one side of the face in different directions, occurs in accordance with pacemaker use, aggravated by agitation, stress or over-strain. Tic vanishes in sleeping.

(1) Ascendant hyperactivity of liver yang: Accompanied by dizziness, tinnitus, flushed cheeks, hypochondriac pain, bitter taste in the mouth and dry throat, irascibility, yellow urine, red tongue with yellow fur, and wiry pulse.

(2) Wind-phlegm obstructing vessels: Accompanied by dizziness, headache as if the head was bound, chest constriction, anorexia, thick greasy fur, and wiry slippery pulse.

(3) Both qi and blood deficiency: Accompanied by anorexia, lassitude, pale complexion, bloated abdomen, loose stools, pale tongue with white fur, and thin weak pulse.

[Syndrome Differentiation and Treatment]

Treatment: To pacify the liver, subdue yang, resolve phlegm, extinguish wind, replenish qi and blood

Point combination 1:

Main points:

GB 20 (*fēng chí*)	LI 4 (*hé gŭ*)	LV 3 (*tài chōng*)
Ashi points (pacemakers)		

Secondary points:

Ascendant hyperactivity of liver yang:

LV 2 (*xíng jiān*)	GB 41 (*zú lín qì*)	LV 8 (*qŭ quán*)

Wind-phlegm obstructing vessels:

SP 9 (*yīn líng quán*)	ST 40 (*fēng lóng*)	PC 6 (*nèi guān*)

Both qi and blood deficiency:

ST 36 (*zú sān lǐ*)	BL 20 (*pí shù*)	BL 21 (*wèi shù*)

Point combination 2:

Main points:

DU 16 (*fēng fǔ*)	DU 14 (*dà zhuī*)	LV 3 (*tài chōng*)
LI 4 (*hé gǔ*)		

Secondary points:

Lesion at the upper eyelid: GB 14 (*yáng bái*), EX-HN4 (*yú yāo*)

Lesion at the cheek from the lower eyelid to the place above the horizontal line of the mouth corner:

LI 20 (*yíng xiāng*)	SI 18 (*quán liáo*)	GB 29 (*jù liáo*)

Lesion at the cheek below the horizontal line of the mouth:

ST 4 (*dì cāng*)	ST 6 (*jiá chē*)	RN 24 (*chéng jiāng*)

Operation: After routine sterilization, gentle tapping is applied to ST 36 (*zú sān lǐ*), BL 20 (*pí shù*), BL 21 (*wèi shù*) and for other points moderate tapping is used. Treatment is given once every two to three days and ten treatments make a course.

[Nursing and Prevention]

Keep a cheerful state of mind. Have enough sleep. Avoid stress and overstrain.

9. Trigeminal Neuralgia

[Overview]

It is a recurrent, transient, tense pain of the trigeminal nerve pathway, but without sensibility impairment and pathological abnormity. It mostly occurs among people over 40, especially in women. Clinically, the second and third branches of the trigeminal nerve often involve only one side of the face. It is either a primary or secondary condition. In traditional Chinese medicine, it is called "face aching", "supra-orbital bone pains", or "head-wind."

[Cause and Mechanism of Disease]

(1) Cold syndrome: Cold is often the trigger that impairs yang. Attacked by cold, yang is suppressed and cold congeals and blood stagnates. Undernourishment of channels leads to this condition.

(2) Heat syndrome: It is also caused by fire from stagnated liver qi. Flaming of fire disturbs the face, as well as overeating, where the retained food produces heat, so that stomach fire goes up to the face along the Stomach Channel.

(3) Deficiency syndrome: Yin deficiency of the body or impairment of essence due to excessive sexual activities is another reason. Yin deficiency and yang hyperactivity result in flaming of deficiency-fire, causing this condition.

[Types of Syndromes]

Main manifestations: Sudden onset, paroxysmal, stabbing burning pain, accompanied by lateral facial tic, lacrimation and slobbering. Pain usually relieves several seconds or minutes later, and recurrent attacks in several successive hours or days. There are no symptoms between episodes. There exists a "trigger point," evoked by exposure to wind, washing the face, speaking and chewing. It recurs in six to twelve months.

(1) Cold syndrome: Facial pain caused by exposure to cold, aggravated by cold, alleviated by warmth, thin nasal discharge, white fur and floating tight pulse.

(2) Heat syndrome: Burning pain, flushed cheeks, red eyes, dry mouth, sore throat, thirst, desire for cold drinks, dry stools, yellow urine, red tongue with yellow or thick greasy fur, and wiry rapid or slippery rapid pulse.

(3) Deficiency syndrome: Unresolved recurrent pain, facial tic, dark complexion, lack of strength, disinclination to talk, dark tongue or with petechia, thin thready pulse.

[Syndrome Differentiation and Treatment]

Treatment: To disperse wind, clear heat, resolve stasis, free the orifices

Point combination 1:

Ashi points	LI 4 (*hé gǔ*)	ST 43 (*xiàn gǔ*)

Point combination 2:

Frontal headache (1st branch): GB 14 (*yáng bái*), EX-HN5 (*tài yáng*)

Maxillary pain (2nd branch):

SI 18 (*quán liáo*)	ST 7 (*xià guān*)	ST 3 (*jù liáo*)

Mandibular pain (3rd branch):

ST 6 (*jiá chē*)	ST 4 (*dì cāng*)	RN 24 (*chéng jiāng*)

Secondary points:

Cold syndrome:

GB 20 (*fēng chí*)	SJ 6 (*zhī gōu*)	ST 41 (*jiě xī*)

Heat syndrome:

Hyperactivity of liver-gallbladder fire:

LV 2 (*xíng jiān*)	GB 43 (*xiá xī*)	GB 41 (*zú lín qì*)

Excess stomach heat:

LI 2 (*èr jiān*)	ST 44 (*nèi tíng*)	LI 4 (*hé gǔ*)

Yin deficiency with effulgent fire:

KI 3 (*tài xī*)	KI 7 (*fù liū*)	SP 6 (*sān yīn jiāo*)

Deficiency syndrome:

BL 20 (*pí shù*)	BL 17 (*gé shù*)	ST 36 (*zú sān lǐ*)

Operation: After routine sterilization, gentle tapping is applied to local points, while moderate and strong tapping to distal points for the excess syndrome. For the deficiency syndrome, except BL 17 (*gé shù*), other points should be tapped gently. Treatment is given once every two to three days and ten treatments make a course. For patients with severe pain treatment is given once a day and five treatments make a course.

[Differential Diagnosis]

(1) Continuous dull toothache indicates lesion in the gums.

(2) Migraine may not confine the trigeminal nerve area. Pain often lasts for over dozens of minutes.

(3) Nasopharyngeal carcinoma manifests itself as the symptoms like trigeminal neuralgia. Isotope scanning or basilar X-ray examination is needed to make an accurate diagnosis.

(4) Mandibular arthritis is characterized by circumscribed continuous pain. Tenderness and functional disturbance are found in the mandibular articulation.

(5) Glossopharyngeal neuralgia is in the lingual root, soft palate, tonsilla, pharyngeal portion and external auditory canal.

(6) Trigeminal neuralgia is the first symptom of some demyelinating diseases in patients with multiple sclerosis, so it is important to know if the patient who suffers from trigeminal neuralgia has symptoms and signs related to the multiple

sclerosis. If necessary, make related examinations as early as possible.

[Nursing and Prevention]

(1) Keep a positive mindset. Avoid stress.

(2) Have a regular lifestyle, enough rest and sleep.

(3) Don't touch the "trigger point" if possible. Keep away from wind to the face.

(4) Help the patient have confidence in cure of the disease.

10. Myasthenia Gravis

[Overview]

It is characterized by muscular atrophy or flaccidity with motor impairment due to weakness of the limb muscles and tendons for a long period. Usually the lower limbs are affected, so it is also called "atrophic crippling" in traditional Chinese medicine. In the treatment of infectious polyneuritis or motor neuron disease having the same symptoms this section can be inferred to.

[Cause and Mechanism of Disease]

(1) Damp-heat emmersion: It is caused by exposure to damp-heat or rain which impairs the channels, leading to impeded flow of qi and blood, disturbance of the nutritiven and defensive aspects. As a result, this condition occurs with the production of heat and further impairment of qi and blood circulation, and malnutrition of the muscles and tendons. It is also caused by improper diet, overeating of greasy, sweet, spicy foods or alcohol dependence that impairs the spleen. Mysthenia gravis occurs owing to the production of internal damp-heat, interrupting the transportation of the spleen, leading to malnutrition of muscles and tendons. It may deteriorate owing to damp-heat in the Stomach Channel, impairing the lung. Lesion is in the spleen and stomach, and the spleen is disturbed by damp-heat. The middle-*jiao* qi is impaired, which causes deficiency and damp-heat in the spleen, or kidney yin is impaired when qi goes down. This is a combination of the deficiency and excess syndromes.

(2) Spleen-stomach deficiency: It is caused by spleen-stomach deficiency failure of refined nutritious substances to transport, or spleen-stomach deficiency in a chronic disease, which impairs the middle-*jiao* qi and disturbs the receiving, transporting and transforming functions. Since there lacks the source of qi, blood and body fluids, the five *zang* organs suffer from malnutrition with unsmooth flow of qi and blood. As a result, the bones and muscles are not nourished and articulations are impaired, causing this condition. Long spleen deficiency and stomach deteriorates the condition.

(3) Liver-kidney depletion: Myasthenia gravis may be caused by deficiency in the liver and kidney, reduction in marrow and muscular atrophy, or persistent kidney deficiency, indulgent sexual activities, intercourse during intoxication, or over-strain, leading to yin consumption, kidney yin deficiency and excessive kidney fire and malnutrition of the muscles and tendons.

[Types of Syndromes]

Main manifestations: On onset one or two side's ptosis, deep and low sound, dysphagia, masseter muscle and facial muscular flaccidity, or with the muscles of the whole body involved to different degrees, relieved in the morning and aggravated at night or when active, temporarily relieved after rest or taking anticholinesterase drugs.

(1) Spleen deficiency with dampness-heat: Accompanied by anorexia, lassitude, difficult bowels movements, brown urine, pale tongue with yellow greasy fur, and slippery rapid pulse.

(2) Spleen qi deficiency: Accompanied by sallow complexion, anorexia, profuse phlegm and urinal discharge, lassitude, loose stools, enlarged pale tongue with white fur, and moderate pulse.

(3) Kidney yin deficiency: Accompanied by aching pain in the lower back and knees, dizziness, tinnitus, feverish sensation in the chest, palms and soles, yellow urine, constipation, red tongue with scanty fur, and thready rapid pulse.

[Syndrome Differentiation and Treatment]

Treatment: To invigorate the spleen, replenish qi, resolve dampness and clear heat

Point combination 1:

Main points:

BL 20 (*pí shù*)	BL 21 (*wèi shù*)	ST 36 (*zú sān lǐ*)
SP 6 (*sān yīn jiāo*)		

Secondary points:

Spleen deficiency with dampness-heat:

SP 9 (*yīn líng quán*)	DU 14 (*dà zhuī*)	LI 11 (*qū chí*)

Spleen qi deficiency: RN 6 (*qì hǎi*), DU 20 (*bǎi huì*)

Kidney yin deficiency:

BL 23 (*shèn shù*)	KI 3 (*tài xī*)	KI 2 (*rán gǔ*)

Ocular muscle flaccidity:

GB 14 (*yáng bái*)	BL 2 (*cuán zhú*)	SJ 23 (*sī zhú kōng*)
LI 4 (*hé gǔ*)	BL 62 (*shēn mài*)	

Laryngeal muscle flaccidity:

RN 23 (*lián quán*)	ST 9 (*rén yíng*)	LU 7 (*liè quē*)
KI 6 (*zhào hǎi*)		

Upper limbs flaccidity:

LI 15 (*jiān yú*)	LI 14 (*bì nào*)	LI 11 (*qǔ chí*)
LI 10 (*shǒu sān lǐ*)	LI 4 (*hé gǔ*)	

Lower limbs flaccidity:

GB 30 (*huán tiào*)	BL 36 (*chéng fú*)	ST 31 (*bì guān*)
ST 32 (*fú tù*)	SP 10 (*xuè hǎi*)	

Operation: After routine sterilization, gentle tapping is applied. Treatment is given once every two to three days and ten treatments make a course.

Point combination 2:

Along the traveling course of the Bladder Channel on the lower back and back, DU Vessel and three yang channels on the upper and lower limbs.

Upper limbs: EX-B2 (*jiá jǐ*) (C3~T3)

Lower limbs: EX-B2 (*jiá jǐ*) (L1~L5)

Chest: From EX-B2 (*jiá jǐ*) (T2~T8)

Abdomen: EX-B2 (*jiá jǐ*) (T6~L5)

[Nursing and Prevention]

(1) Don't overwork. Do appropriate functional exercise. Keep a good mindset and have confidence.

(2) Myasthenia gravis is a chronic progressive disease. With proper prompt early treatment, work ability and viability to some extent may be preserved for a longer time.

11. Primary Hypertension

[Overview]

It is characterized by dizziness, dim eyesight, or accompanied by headache and high blood pressure. In traditional Chinese medicine, it is in the category of "vertigo" or "headache".

[Cause and Mechanism of Disease]

(1) Ascendant hyperactivity of liver yang: It is caused by deficiency of liver yin or kidney yin, or by anger and unsmooth flow of liver qi. Stagnated qi transforms into fire. After a long period, liver yin consumes and liver yang becomes hyperactive as it fails to be checked. Liver yang disturbs the upper orifices, causing dizziness and headache from malnutrition of channels.

(2) Both qi and blood deficiency: It is caused by a chronic disease,or the loss of blood without recovery, or insufficient qi and blood in the spleen and stomach. Finally the brain and channels fail to be nourished, the condition occurs.

(3) Kidney essence deficiency: It is caused by poor constitution or consumption of yin essence from over-strain and excessive sexual activities. Bone marrow fails to produce. The brain is the sea of marrow, which is not sufficient, and deficiency in the upper and lower portion results in dizziness.

(4) Turbid phlegm obstructing middle-*jiao*: It is caused by phlegm or improper diet, or imbalance of rest and work. The spleen fails to transport and then phlegm produces, which suppresses yang to rise and yin to descend. When upper orifices are obstructed, phlegm and stasis combine. The brain, the channels are not nourished well, and essence does not get replenishment, so dizziness occurs.

[Types of Syndromes]

Main manifestations: Dizziness, headache.

(1) Ascendant hyperactivity of liver yang: Dizziness, tinnitus, distending pain in the head, aggravated by anger, flushed cheeks, red eyes, irritability, insomnia, dream-disturbed sleep, bitter taste in the mouth, dry pharynx, red tongue with yellow fur, and wiry pulse.

(2) Both qi and blood deficiency: Dizziness, aggravated when active, pale complexion, lusterless lips and nails, palpitation, lassitude, disinclination to talk, anorexia, loose stools, pale tongue with tooth marks on the edge, and thready weak pulse.

(3) Kidney essence deficiency: Dizziness, tinnitus, lassitude, dream-disturbed sleep, poor memory, aching pain in the lower back and knees, seminal emission, night sweating, red tongue with scanty coating, thready rapid pulse, or cold limbs, pale tender-soft tongue with thin and white fur, and deep thready pulse.

(4) Turbid phlegm obstructing middle-*jiao*: Dizziness, or headache as if the head was bound up, constriction and fullness in the chest, nausea, vomiting, poor appetite, white greasy tongue fur and slippery pulse.

[Syndrome Differentiation and Treatment]

Treatment: To pacify the liver, subdue yang, invigorate the spleen and kidney.

Point combination 1:

GB 20 (*fēng chí*)	DU 16 (*fēng fǔ*)	EX-HN1 (*sì shén cōng*)
LI 4 (*hé gǔ*)	LV 3 (*tài chōng*)	

Secondary points:

Ascendant hyperactivity of liver yang:

EX-HN5 (*tài yáng*)	SJ 5 (*wài guān*)	LV 2 (*xíng jiān*)
BL 18 (*gān shù*)	KI 3 (*tài xī*)	

Both qi and blood deficiency:

ST 36 (*zú sān lǐ*)	SP 6 (*sān yīn jiāo*)	BL 20 (*pí shù*)
BL 17 (*gé shù*)	RN 6 (*qì hǎi*)	

Kidney essence deficiency:

RN 4 (*guān yuán*)	BL 23 (*shèn shù*)	BL 18 (*gān shù*)
KI 3 (*tài xī*)	GB 39 (*xuán zhōng*)	

Turbid phlegm obstructing middle-*jiao*:

RN 12 (*zhōng wǎn*)	ST 40 (*fēng lóng*)	SP 9 (*yīn líng quán*)
BL 20 (*pí shù*)		

Point combination 2:

GB 20 (*fēng chí*)	LI 11 (*qū chí*)	LI 4 (*hé gǔ*)
ST 36 (*zú sān lǐ*)	LV 3 (*tài chōng*)	

Point combination 3:

Ear point: EX-HN6 (*ěr jiān*) or veins on the back of the ear

Operation: After routine sterilization, gentle or moderate tapping is applied, once every two to three days and ten treatments make a course. Give strict sterilization to the skin in ear acupuncture.

[Nursing and Prevention]

(1) Take light diet, avoid rich and spicy foods. Quit smoking and alcohol dependence.

(2) Keep a good mindset. Don't be agitated.

(3) Maintain a proper balance between rest and work. Check blood pressure regularly.

12. Diabetes

[Overview]

It is a disease characterized by hyperdiuresis, polydipsia, polyphagia, emaciation and sweet urine. In traditional Chinese medicine it is in the category of "wasting and thirst disorder".

[Cause and Mechanism of Disease]

(1) Poor constitution: It is caused by poor constitution, especially suffering from yin deficiency.

(2) Improper diet: It is caused by long overeating rich sweet pungent fragrant and dry foods, and alcohol dependence, leading to impairment to the spleen and stomach and dysfuction of them. Internal heat is then accumulated and transformed into dryness which injures body fluids, resulting in diabetes.

(3) Mental disorder: It is caused by long irritation, such as stagnation of liver qi due to anger that impairs the liver, or constant worry which generates fire. Flaming of fire scorches yin fluids of the lung and stomach, causing diabetes.

(4) Indulging in sexual activities: It is caused by excessive sexual activities, resulting in consumption of kidney essence and the production of deficiency-fire. Finally, kidney deficiency, dryness in the lung and heat in the stomach bring about this condition.

Prolonged diabetes injures qi and fluids, leading to deficiency of both qi and yin. If yin impairment has yang involved, there is deficiency of both yin and yang. The lesion is in the lung, stomach and kidney, especially the kidney. In pathological condition one particular organ may be severely diseased, but they are mutually agitated too.

[Types of Syndromes]

Main manifestations: Polydipsia, polyphagia, hyperdiuresis, emaciation, general debilitation, turbid urine, or sweet urine.

(1) Lung heat consuming fluids: Thirst with a desire for drinks, no relief of thirst, dry mouth or nose, frequent micturition, profuse urine, red tip and edge of the tongue with thin yellow fur, and surging rapid or thready rapid pulse.

(2) Intense stomach fire: Hyperorexia, emaciation, fatigue, dry stools, yellow fur, and slippery replete powerful pulse.

(3) Kidney yin deficiency: Frequent micturition, profuse urine as turbid as cream or sweet urine, tidal fever, night sweating, weakness of the lower back, red tongue, and deep thready rapid pulse.

(4) Both yin and yang deficiency: Frequent micturition, urine as turbid as cream, or passing urine immediately after drinking water, dark complexion, dry helix, aching pain and weakness of the lower back and knees, aversion to cold, cold limbs, impotence, pale tongue with white fur, and deep thready or deep and slow pulse.

(5) Both qi and yin deficiency: Dry mouth with a desire for drinks, spontaneous sweating or night sweating, listlessness, shortness of breath, lassitude, tender-soft tongue or fissured tongue with less coating, and thready rapid pulse.

[Syndrome Differentiation and Treatment]

Treatment: To reinforce healthy qi, eliminate pathogenic factors, replenish yin and remove dryness.

Point combination 1:

Main points:

ST 36 (*zú sān lǐ*)	LI 11 (*qǔ chí*)	SI 4 (*wàn gǔ*)
SP 6 (*sān yīn jiāo*)	RN 6 (*qì hǎi*)	

Secondary points:

Lung heat consuming fluids:

LU 5 (*chǐ zé*)	LU 10 (*yú jì*)	BL 13 (*fèi shù*)
LU 1 (*zhōng fǔ*)		

Intense stomach fire:

BL 21 (*wèi shù*)	RN 12 (*zhōng wǎn*)	ST 25 (*tiān shū*)
ST 44 (*nèi tíng*)	LI 4 (*hé gǔ*)	

Kidney yin deficiency:

BL 23 (*shèn shù*)	KI 3 (*tài xī*)	KI 7 (*fù liū*)

Both yin and yang deficiency:

BL 23 (*shèn shù*)	RN 4 (*guān yuán*)	ST 36 (*zú sān lǐ*)
KI 3 (*tài xī*)		

Both qi and yin deficiency:

RN 6 (*qì hǎi*)	DU 20 (*bǎi huì*)	KI 10 (*yīn gǔ*)
KI 7 (*fù liū*)		

Point combination 2:

Main points:

LI 11 (*qū chí*)	GB 34 (*yáng líng quán*)	RN 4 (*guān yuán*)
SP 6 (*sān yīn jiāo*)		

(Li Donglin's prescription, from *Acupuncture Therapy for Diabetes*)

Secondary points:

Lung heat consuming fluids: LU 10 (*yú jì*), KI 7 (*fù liū*)

Intense stomach fire: RN 12 (*zhōng wǎn*), ST 44 (*nèi tíng*)

Kidney yin deficiency: GB 26 (*dài mài*)

Both yin and yang deficiency: GB 26 (*dài mài*), KI 7 (*fù liū*)

Both qi and yin deficiency: RN 12 (*zhōng wǎn*), RN 6 (*qì hǎi*)

Profuse sweating:

DU 14 (*dà zhuī*)	BL 67 (*zhì yīn*)	LI 4 (*hé gǔ*)
KI 7 (*fù liū*)		

Point combination 3:

BL 13 (*fèi shù*)	BL 20 (*pí shù*)	BL 21 (*wèi shù*)
KI 3 (*tài xī*)	LU 9 (*tài yuān*)	SP 3 (*tài bái*)

Operation: After routine sterilization, gentle or moderate tapping is used once every two to three days and ten treatments make a course.

[Nursing and Prevention]

(1) Diabetes patients are prone to infection so it is important to have strict sterilization.

(2) Reduce body weight of the diabetes patients if they are obese.

(3) Control diet.

(4) Early discover and treat to avoid complications.

(5) Check blood glucose regularly. Take hypoglycemic drugs under the instruction of doctors.

13. Coronary Heart Disease

It is caused by insufficient healthy qi, phlegm, stagnation of qi and blood and cold retention, resulting in obstruction of the Heart Channel, characterized by a fit of suffocative pain in the middle or left chest due to over-strain, eating too much food or emotional problems, or without any reason. In a mild case, there is only a fit of transient slight oppression or dull pain in the chest, or vague discomfort at RN 17 (*tán zhōng*) or left chest.In a severe case, there is severe pain or colicky pain, or rather, angina pectoris, usually accompanied by palpitations, shortness of breath, difficult breathing, even panting breathing, panic, pale complexion, cold spontaneous sweating, etc.

Coronary heart disease is a cardiac condition which endangers the life of the middle-aged and geriatrics. With the change of life-style and food structure in modern society, its incidence tends to increase. Therefore, it attracts more and more attention. In traditional Chinese medicine it is in the category of "chest impediment," "real hearty pain," or "heart-impediment".

[Cause and Mechanism of Disease]

(1) Senility and weakness: It is often seen in the middle-aged and geriatric patients, as their health condition is declining due to deficiency of kidney qi. Insufficient kidney yin fails to agitate the yang of the five *zang* organs, leading to deficiency of heart qi or heart yang. Therefore, blood vessels are not warmed. Since they are short of blood flow, the condition occurs. These patients suffer from kidney yin deficiency, which fails to nourish the five *zang* organs, leading to exhaustion of heart yin and unmoistened vessels, or they have excessive heart fire which scorches the fluids into phlegm and obstructs the Heart Channel, then the condition occurs.

(2) Improper diet: It is caused by impairment of the spleen and stomach due to improper diet, such as overeating of sweet, greasy, raw foods for a long period, which causes failure of transportation and transformation, and accumulated phlegm-dampness goes upward to attack the heart area and chest, leading to insufficiency of yang, disturbance of qi movement and obstruction of the Heart Channel, or by long retention of phlegm accompanied by stasis. Impairment of qi due to overeating makes the qi fail to transport, leading to unsmooth flow of qi and blood.

(3) Disorder emotion: It is also caused by emotional problems and pensiveness, which impairs the spleen and its function. Body fluids fail to distribute properly and phlegm produces. Phlegm in conjunction with stagnation of qi and blood leads to blockage of the heart vessels, causing this condition. Another reason is rage because it impairs the liver, making liver qi fail to flow smoothly. The stagnated qi turns into fire and scorches body fluids into phlegm. When the heart vessels are obstructed by phlegm, the condition occurs. Emotional excitation is a trigger too. As liver qi communicates with heart qi, stagnation of liver qi makes deficiency of heart qi, followed by the condition.

(4) Inword invasion of cold: It is also due to invasion of the body by cold when yang is deficient. Cold congeals and qi stagnates, then chest yang declines. There is impeded blood circulation, finally this condition occurs.

[Types of Syndromes]

Main manifestations: Pain in the front of the chest. In a mild case, there is a feeling of constriction in the chest, but in a severe case, the pain involves the shoulder, back and medial arm.

(1) Cold coagulation in blood vessels: Heart pain radiating to the back, aggravated by cold, feeling of constriction in the chest, shortness of breath, palpitation, pale complexion, cold limbs, white or white thick fur, and deep tight pulse.

(2) Qi stagnation and blood stasis: Fixed stabbing heart pain, palpitation, shortness of breath, purplish tongue or with petechia or ecchymoses and thready rough or intermittent or knotted pulse.

(3) Turbid phlegm obstruction: Feeling of pain and constriction in the chest, or with the shoulder and back involved, shortness of breath, obesity, sluggishness, nausea or vomiting of thin phlegm, white greasy fur and slippery pulse.

(4) Heart blood insufficiency: Feeling of constriction and dull pain in the chest, palpitation, shortness of breath, dizziness, insomnia, pale complexion, pale tongue with white fur, and deep thready pulse.

(5) Heart yang insufficiency: Pain in the heart area, radiating to the back, feeling of constriction, shortness of breath, palpitation, sweating, dark or pale complexion, cold limbs, cyanotic or pale lips and nails, purplish or pale tongue, and deep thready pulse or faint pulse.

[Syndrome Differentiation and Treatment]

Treatment: To warm yang, disperse cold, replenish qi, activate blood, remove impediment and relieve pain.

Point combination 1:

Main points:

BL 15 (*xīn shù*)	BL 14 (*jué yīn shù*)	RN 14 (*jù quē*)
PC 4 (*xì mén*)		

Secondary points:

Cold coagulation in blood vessels:

RN 4 (*guān yuán*)	DU 4 (*mìng mén*)	ST 36 (*zú sān lǐ*)

Qi stagnation and blood stasis:

BL 17 (*gé shù*)	RN 17 (*shàn zhōng*)	PC 6 (*nèi guān*)

Turbid phlegm obstruction:

RN 12 (*zhōng wǎn*)	ST 40 (*fēng lóng*)	PC 6 (*nèi guān*)
SP 4 (*gōng sūn*)		

Both qi and blood deficiency:

BL 18 (*gān shù*)	BL 20 (*pí shù*)	ST 36 (*zú sān lǐ*)
RN 17 (*dàn zhōng*)		

Heart yang insufficiency:

DU 26 (*shuǐ gōu*)	ST 36 (*zú sān lǐ*)	DU 20 (*bǎi huì*)
RN 4 (*guān yuán*)	RN 6 (*qì hǎi*)	

Point combination 2:

RN 17 (*shàn zhōng*)	PC 6 (*nèi guān*)	HT 7 (*shén mén*)

Point combination 3:

RN 14 (*jù quē*)	DU 26 (*shuǐ gōu*)	PC 4 (*xì mén*)

Point combination 4:

BL 15 (*xīn shù*)	BL 14 (*jué yīn shù*)	BL 16 (*dū shù*)

Operation: After routine sterilization, gentle or moderate tapping is applied, once every other day and ten treatments make a course.

[Nursing and Prevention]

(1) In a severe case Western medical therapy is employed, while in a mild case the integrated Western and traditional Chinese medicine is used. Acupuncture is only an adjunctive therapy.

(2) Don't overeat. Have light meals. Keep free bowels movement.

(3) Patients of severe cases should take complete bed rest. Get fresh air and a quiet environment.

14. Arrhythmia

[Overview]

It refers to variation from the normal rhythm of the heartbeat, tachycardia, bradycardia, premature systole, atrial fibrillation, atrial flutter, atrioventricular block, sick sinus syndrome, pre-excitation syndrome, cardiac insufficiency, cardiac neurosis, etc. In traditional Chinese medicine, it is in the category of "palpitation," "fright palpitation" or "fearful throbbing."

[Cause and Mechanism of Disease]

It is caused by deficiency of qi, blood, yin and yang, or by phlegm-fluid retention and stasis of blood, which leads to malnutrition of the heart and obstruction of the heart vessels, followed by irregular heartbeat. Palpitations are often accompanied by shortness of breath, constriction in the chest, dizziness, panting and syncope. The pulse may be rapid, or slow, or irregular. It is usually triggered by fright, panic or over-strain. Patients are in a normal state without attack. In a mile case fright palpation is the chief complaint. In a severe case continuous palpitations are found, aggravated by over-strain.

Palpitations are a common symptom in cardiac diseases. It may be caused by pathological changes of the heart itself associated with disorders of other organs. The majority is a deficiency syndrome. A deficiency syndrome may also turn to an excess syndrome or rather, a deficiency-excess complexity.

(1) Heart blood deficiency: It is caused by deficiency of heart blood, and the heart fails to be nourished, which affects the mind, causing palpitation, or by pensiveness, that impairs the heart and spleen, and impedes production of qi and blood. Then the upper portion of the body is undernourished.

(2) Heart deficiency with timidity: It is caused by feeling diffident, timidity and insufficient endowment, or debility or a protracted illness, or over-strain, indulgent sexual activities, leading to consumption of qi, blood, yin and yang. When one is exposed to danger or terror, he could not control himself causing the condition to occur.

(3) Yin deficiency with effulgent fire: It is caused by kidney yin deficiency. A disharmony between the heart and kidney leads to blazing of fire that disturbs the mind and causes the condition.

(4) Insufficiency of heart yang: It is caused by insufficiency of spleen and kidney yang, which fails to produce fluid. The retained fluid goes upward, attacking the heart, followed by contained heart yang and blockage of blood vessels, and the condition occurs.

(5) Drug poisoning: It is also caused by overdose of drugs, or poisonous drugs and herbs, such as Radix Aconiti Lateralis Preparata, Radix Linderae, antimonial, digitalis, conquinine, epinephrine, atropine, etc. Drug overdose or improper administering of drugs results in palpitations and intermittent or knotted pulse.

[Types of Syndromes]

Main manifestations: Paroxysms of palpitation, restlessness.

(1) Heart blood deficiency: Palpitation, aggravated on exertion, dizziness, lusterless complexion, feeling of constriction in the chest, shortness of breath, light red tongue, and thready weak pulse.

(2) Heart deficiency with timidity: Palpitation, shortness of breath, being in a state of apprehension, restlessness, insomnia, dream-disturbed sleep, thin white fur, and deficient intermittent or knotted pulse.

(3) Yin deficiency with effulgent fire: Palpitation, feeling of constriction in the chest, restlessness, irritability, insomnia, dizziness, feverish sensation in palms and soles, tinnitus, red tongue with less coating, and thready rapid pulse.

(4) Inactivity of heart yang: Palpitation, feeling of constriction in the chest, shortness of breath, pale complexion, chills, cold limbs, pale and tender-soft tongue with slippery fur, and deep slow pulse.

[Syndrome Differentiation and Treatment]

Treatment: To anchor the mind

Point Combination:

Main points:

PC 6 (*nèi guān*)	SP 4 (*gōng sūn*)	HT 7 (*shén mén*)

Secondary points:

Heart blood deficiency:

BL 15 (*xīn shù*)	BL 20 (*pí shù*)	RN 17 (*dàn zhōng*)

Heart deficiency with timidity:

BL 15 (*xīn shù*)	BL 19 (*dǎn shù*)	GB 40 (*qiū xū*)

Yin deficiency with effulgent fire:

LU 1 (*zhōng fǔ*)	GB 40 (*qiū xū*)	KI 1 (*yǒng quán*)

Inactivity of heart yang:

RN 17 (*dàn zhōng*)	RN 4 (*guān yuán*)	ST 36 (*zú sān lǐ*)

Operation: After routine sterilization, gentle tapping is used once every two to three days and ten treatments make a course.

[Nursing and Prevention]

(1) Have a quiet clean and comfortable environment. Avoid over-strain, stress and emotional excitation.

(2) Have low salt, low fat, nutritous diet.

(3) Patients in a severe condition should confine in bed. Be prepared with an oxygen tank. Watch closely the heart rate, pulse and blood pressure.

15. Insomnia

[Overview]

It refers to abnormal wakefulness during sleep, in which tiredness is not removed and physical strength is not restored. In a mild case, it is difficult to fall asleep or fall asleep again after waking up, or go into a deep sleep or it is easy to wake frequently, and in a severe case, there is no sleep through all night. For this reason, one feels lassitude, dizzy, headache, palpitation, poor memory and restless.

As a frequently seen disorder, it is caused by malnourishment of the heart or restlessness. Though it is not a critical condition, it often disturbs people's normal life, work and study;and it is harmful to health, which aggravates or triggers palpitation, chest impediment, dizziness, headache, stroke, etc. Refractory insomnia brings long suffering to patients, even brings about dependence on hypnotics, but long-term taking hypnotics may result in iatrogenic disease.

Insomnia due to other diseases is beyond this discussion. Treatment of insomnia present in menopausal syndrome can consult this section.

[Cause and Mechanism of Disease]

(1) Deficiency of both heart and spleen: It is caused by pensiveness, which impairs the heart and spleen, exhausts heart blood, and causes perception of uncontrollability. While blood production is impeded from insufficiency of spleen qi, the heart is undernourished.

(2) Heart-gallbladder qi deficiency: It is caused by poor constitution, leading to feeling diffident, timid, panicky reaction, being out of wits, and disturbed sleep.

(3) Non-interaction between the heart and kidney: The kidney fails to suppress heart fire, causing its hyperactivity, or by excessive liver fire from yin deficiency of the liver-kidney. Hyperactivity of liver yang disturbs the mind and non-interaction between the heart and kidney occurs.

(4) Upward disturbance of liver fire: It is caused by emotional problems, leading to stagnation of liver qi, which transforms into fire. Blazing of fire disturbs the mind, and insomnia follows, or by five emotions in excess, which causes excessive heart fire. The mind is disturbed and insomnia follows.

(5) Retention of food: It is caused by improper diet, which impairs the spleen and stomach, and causes production of phlegm-heat in the mddle-*jiao*, and in turn, dysfunction of stomach qi is seen. Then yang floats and the condition occurs.

[Types of Syndromes]

Main manifestations: Inability to have normal sleep, in a mild case, difficulty in falling asleep, or no deep sleep, or inability to fall asleep after waking up, or no sleep at all at night.

(1) Deficiency of both heart and spleen: Insomnia, palpitation, dream-disturbed sleep, being easy to wake up, dizziness, lassitude, lusterless complexion, anorexia, pale tongue with thin white fur, and thready weak pulse.

(2) Heart-gallbladder qi deficiency: Dream-disturbed sleep, nightmare, timidity and palpitation, panicky reaction, lassitude, pale complexion, pale tongue with thin white fur,and weak pulse.

(3) Non-interaction between the heart and kidney: Restlessness, inability to fall asleep, palpitations, feverish sensation in the chest, palms and soles, dizziness, tinnitus, aching pain and weakness of the lower back and knees, dry mouth, tidal fever, night sweating, red tongue with scanty coating, and wiry thready and rapid pulse.

(4) Upward disturbance of liver fire: Restlessness, insomnia, irritability, distending pain in the costal region, anorexia, red eyes, bitter taste in the mouth, constipation, yellow urine, red tongue with yellow fur, and wiry rapid pulse.

(5) Retention of food: Superficial sleep, fullness in the epigastric region, belching or vomiting, acid regurgitation, anorexia, bowels movement problems, thick greasy fur, and slippery replete pulse.

[Syndrome Differentiation and Treatment]

Treatment: To anchor the mind.

Point combination 1:

Main points:

DU 24 (*shén tíng*)	HT 7 (*shén mén*)	SP 6 (*sān yīn jiāo*)

Secondary points:

Deficiency of both heart and spleen:

BL 15 (*xīn shù*)	BL 20 (*pí shù*)	SP 3 (*tài bái*)
ST 36 (*zú sān lǐ*)		

Heart-gallbladder qi deficiency:

BL 15 (*xīn shù*)	BL 19 (*dǎn shù*)	GB 40 (*qiū xū*)
RN 6 (*qì hǎi*)	DU 20 (*bǎi huì*)	

Non-interaction between the heart and kidney:

BL 15 (*xīn shù*)	GB 40 (*qiū xū*)	HT 8 (*shào fǔ*)
KI 6 (*zhào hǎi*)	KI 7 (*fù liū*)	

Upward disturbance of liver fire:

BL 18 (*gān shù*)	LV 2 (*xíng jiān*)	GB 20 (*fēng chí*)
GB 40 (*qiū xū*)		

Retention of food:

BL 21 (*wèi shù*)	RN 12 (*zhōng wǎn*)	ST 25 (*tiān shū*)
ST 36 (*zú sān lǐ*)	ST 44 (*nèi tíng*)	

Point combination 2:

Main points:

HT 7 (*shén mén*)	PC 6 (*nèi guān*)	ST 36 (*zú sān lǐ*)
EX (*ān mián*)		

Secondary points:

Deficiency of both heart and spleen:

GB 40 (*qiū xū*)	SP 6 (*sān yīn jiāo*)	BL 15 (*xīn shù*)
BL 20 (*pí shù*)		

Heart-gallbladder qi deficiency:

BL 44 (*shén táng*)	BL 47 (*hún mén*)	BL 42 (*pò hù*)
BL 15 (*xīn shù*)		

Non-interaction between the heart and kidney:

DU 4 (*mìng mén*)	BL 23 (*shèn shù*)	RN 6 (*qì hǎi*)
RN 4 (*guān yuán*)	KI 7 (*fù liū*)	

Upward disturbance of liver fire:

GB 20 (*fēng chí*)	EX-HN5 (*tài yáng*)	GB 34 (*yáng líng quán*)
LV 3 (*tài chōng*)		

Operation: After routine sterilization, for the deficiency syndrome gentle tapping is used, while for the excess syndrome moderate tapping is used once every two to three days and ten treatments make a course.

Point combination 3:

Along the 1st and 2nd lines of the Bladder Channel on the back.

Operation: After routine sterilization, for the deficiency syndrome tapping is performed along the traveling course of the channel, while for the excess syndrome tapping is performed against the traveling course of the channel, until skin becomes flushed. Treatment is given once a day or every other day and ten treatments make a course.

[Nursing and Prevention]

(1) Have good life style and regular daily life.

(2) Keep a pleasant mood and away from agitation.

(3) Do not drink strong tea or coffee and watch exciting TV programs before sleep. Do not eat too much in supper. Have a cup of milk before sleeping at night.

16. Forgetfulness

[Overview]

It refers to lack of memory or inability to remember past experience. In traditional Chinese medicine, it is in the category of "tendency of forgetfulness," usually as a symptom of dementia praecox.

[Cause and Mechanism of Disease]

(1) Deficiency of both heart and spleen: It is caused by pensiveness, which impairs the heart and spleen, consumes yin blood, and makes poor production of blood. The brain is undernourished, causing the condition to occur.

(2) Insufficiency of kidney essence: It is caused by yin of the body from consumption of kidney yin due to excessive sexual activities. As the kidney dominates essence and marrow, kidney essence insufficiency leads to brain problem. When the brain is undernourished, the condition occurs.

[Types of Syndromes]

Main manifestations: Diminished function of the brain, poor memory, inability to remember past experience.

(1) Deficiency of both heart and spleen: Amnesia, insomnia, dizziness, palpitation, dream-disturbed sleep, listlessness, anorexia, lusterless complexion, pale tongue with thin white fur, and thready weak pulse.

(2) Insufficiency of kidney essence: Amnesia, humming in the brain, dizziness, tinnitus, deafness, aching pain and weakness of the lower back and knees, tidal fever, night sweating, seminal emission, red tongue with scanty coating, and thready rapid pulse.

[Syndrome Differentiation and Treatment]

Treatment: To reinforce the heart, invigorate the spleen and kidney and supplement the marrow.

Point Combination:

Main points:

EX-HN1 (*sì shén cōng*)	DU 24 (*shén tíng*)	HT 7 (*shén mén*)
DU 20 (*bǎi huì*)	GB 39 (*xuán zhōng*)	

Secondary points:

Deficiency of both heart and spleen:

BL 15 (*xīn shù*)	BL 20 (*pí shù*)	ST 36 (*zú sān lǐ*)
SP 6 (*sān yīn jiāo*)		

Insufficiency of kidney essence:

BL 23 (*shèn shù*)	RN 4 (*guān yuán*)	KI 3 (*tài xī*)
KI 10 (*yīn gǔ*)	LV 3 (*tài chōng*)	

Operation: After routine sterilization, gentle tapping is used once every two to three days and ten treatments make a course.

[Nursing and Prevention]

(1) Read books and periodicals frequently. Chat with others or do some games of puzzle.

(2) Put a memorandum with family members' telephone number and family address in pocket in case losing one's way.

17. Epilepsy

[Overview]

It is characterized by a sudden seizure, temporary loss of consciousness with foaming at the mouth, screaming, eyes staring upward and convulsions of the limbs. The patient returns to normal after the episode.

[Cause and Mechanism of Disease]

(1) Excess Syndrome

(i) Wind-phlegm obstruction: It is due to six excesses, or improper diet, or other diseases that impair the *zang-fu* organs and phlegm produces. Too much work and irregular daily life disturb qi movement and cause phlegm to go upward. When the mind is clouded and channels are blocked, this condition occurs.

(ii) Upward disturbance of liver fire: It is due to terror which disturbs qi flow and impairs the *zang-fu* organs, liver and kidney, leading to failure of yin to be checked. As a result, heat and wind produce.

(iii) Obstruction of the orifices by blood stasis: It is due to blood stasis, caused by falling or striking or difficult labor, which impairs the brain, leading to confused mind and loss of consciousness, when channels are obstructed by stagnated blood, convulsion of limbs and epilepsy occur.

(2) Deficiency Syndrome

(i) Liver-kidney yin deficiency: It is caused by liver-kidney yin deficiency starting from childhood, or with innate factors, so there is a saying that "the disease originates from the fetus' qi." In olden times, people attributed this condition to the terrified mother, resulting in disturbed qi movement and impairment to essence and kidney qi. It is in consistent with the saying that "terror leads to consumption of essence." Fetal abnormality is caused by impairment of mother's qi and essence, or constant kidney yin deficiency that impedes blood production. When blood fails to nourish the liver, liver wind is stirred up.

(ii) Spleen-stomach deficiency: It is caused by spleen-stomach deficiency, which impedes distribution of refined nutritious substances and phlegm accumulates. With any trigger factor, phlegm goes upward with the reversed flow of qi or fire, or wind, and clouds the mind, causing the condition to occur. The *zang-fu* organs of children are delicate, and the original qi is still insufficient. Vigor is not full too. With wind-phlegm it is easier to bring about the disease when they are terrified.

[Types of Syndromes]

(1) Excess Syndrome

Main manifestations: Falling down in a fit, loss of consciousness, eyes staring upward, locked jaw with foam at the mouth, convulsions of limbs, screaming like the cries of pig or sheep, urinary and fecal incontinence.

(i) Wind-phlegm obstruction: Accompanied by dizziness, anorexia, chest oppression, white and greasy fur, and slippery or wiry pulse.

(ii) Upward disturbance of liver fire: Accompanied by irritability, restlessness, bitter taste in the mouth, dry pharynx, constipation, yellow urine, red tongue with yellow greasy fur, and wiry slippery rapid pulse.

(iii) Obstruction of the orifices by blood stasis: Due to traumatic injury to the head, accompanied by stabbing pain in the head, purplish tongue or with ecchymosis, and rough or tight pulse.

(2) Deficiency Syndrome

(i) Liver-kidney yin deficiency: Accompanied by feverish sensation in the chest, palms and soles, tidal fever, night sweating, tinnitus, dizziness, red tongue with scanty coating and thready rapid pulse.

(ii) Spleen-stomach deficiency: Accompanied by sallow complexion, anorexia, abdominal distension, loose stools, pale tongue with tooth-marks on the edge and thin white fur,and soggy moderate pulse.

[Syndrome Differentiation and Treatment]

Treatment: To dispel phlegm, extinguish wind, support healthy qi, induce resuscitation to stop convulsions.

Point combination 1:

Main points:

RN 15 (*jiū wěi*)	DU 14 (*dà zhuī*)	EX-B9 (*yāo qí*)
DU 26 (*shuǐ gōu*)		

Secondary points:

Wind-phlegm obstruction:

RN 12 (*zhōng wǎn*)	ST 40 (*fēng lóng*)	DU 16 (*fēng fǔ*)
BL 10 (*tiān zhù*)		

Upward disturbance of liver fire:

ST 44 (*nèi tíng*)	LV 2 (*xíng jiān*)	PC 8 (*láo gōng*)

Obstruction of the orifices by blood stasis:

BL 17 (*gé shù*)	SP 6 (*sān yīn jiāo*)	LI 4 (*hé gŭ*)
LV 3 (*tài chōng*)		

Liver-kidney yin deficiency:

BL 23 (*shèn shù*)	KI 3 (*tài xī*)	KI 10 (*yīn gŭ*)

Spleen-stomach deficiency:

SP 3 (*tài bái*)	SP 6 (*sān yīn jiāo*)	BL 20 (*pí shù*)

Epilepsy onset at night: KI 6 (*zhào hăi*)

Epilepsy onset at daytime: BL 62 (*shēn mài*)

Operation: After routine sterilization, gentle tapping is applied for the deficiency syndrome, while moderate tapping for the excess syndrome. Treatment is given once every two to three days and ten treatments make a course.

Point combination 2:

In the period of attack:

DU 26 (*shuĭ gōu*)	LI 4 (*hé gŭ*)	LV 3 (*tài chōng*)
PC 6 (*nèi guān*)	DU 14 (*dà zhuī*)	KI 1 (*yŏng quán*)

Remission stage:

GB 20 (*fēng chí*)	EX-B9 (*yāo qí*)	DU 24 (*shén tíng*)
DU 20 (*băi huì*)	EX-HN1 (*sì shén cōng*)	ST 36 (*zú sān lĭ*)

Operation: After routine sterilization, gentle tapping is used in the period of attack, while moderate tapping is used in the remission stage. Treatment is given once every two to three days and ten treatments make a course.

[Differential Diagnosis]

(1) Primary epilepsy mostly attacks in teenagers. Electroencephalogram helps to make an accurate diagnosis.

(2) Secondary epilepsy mostly attacks in people over 30. It may be triggered by cerebrovascular disease, cerebral tumor, or brain cysticercosis. The skull CT can help diagnosis.

[Nursing and Prevention]

(1) Avoid over-strain and emotional stress. Keep a pleasant mood. Have light

meals and avoid fat, sweet and greasy foods.

(2) Assist the patient to lie down on attack. Unbutton his collar. Take out the false teeth. Put a tongue depressor wrapped with absorbent gauze into the mouth to avoid biting the tongue. Don't press the limbs forcefully when the patient has convulsion to avoid bone fracture.

(3) After the episode, turn the patient's head laterally to eliminate phlegm.

18. Neurosis

[Overview]

Neurosis is in the category of hysteria, depression and globus hystericus in traditional Chinese medicine. Depressive disease results from emotional problems and stagnation of qi, characterized by depression, restlessness, fullness and distress in the chest, hypochondriac distension and pain, irritability, prone to worry, or feeling of a lump lodged in the throat. In addition, for depressive symptoms that occur during menopausal syndrome and reactive psychosis, this section can be consulted for treatment.

[Cause and Mechanism of Disease]

(1) Stagnation of liver qi: It is caused by anger, disgust or hatred, which impedes free flow of liver qi. Stagnation of liver qi is the main mechanism of a depressive disease. Since qi is the commander of blood, qi flows followed by blood circulation. Qi stagnation leads to impeded circulation of blood. Long-standing qi stagnation must affect blood and cause stagnation of blood.

(2) Excessive liver fire: Long-standing qi stagnation leads to production of fire. Consquently, blazing of liver fire brings about accumulation of fire.

(3) Qi stagnation and phlegm obstruction: It is caused by worry, pensiveness and stress, resulting in stagnation of spleen qi or liver qi that encroachs the spleen, leading to failure of the spleen in transportation, and impairment to the spleen's digestive function. When they can't flow freely, body fluids retain in the *zang-fu* organs and channels and turn into phlegm, forming retention of phlegm.

(4) Deficiency of both heart and spleen: It is caused by stagnation fire injuring the spleen. Less intake of food forms poor source of qi and blood, leading to deficiency in the heart and spleen. When the spleen fails to transport well, food retention is the result.

(5) Yin deficiency with effulgent fire: It is caused by yin deficiency with effulgent fire, resulting in consumption of blood, which leads to deficiency of liver yin.

Emotional problem is another trigger factor. The condition is not only related to the intensity or duration of mental stress, but also to the physical condition.

[Types of Syndromes]

(1) Stagnation of liver qi: Depression, suspiciousness, hypochondriac distending pain, belching, hiccups, irregular bowels movement, and thin white fur and wiry pulse.

(2) Excessive liver fire: Irritability, gastric upset, acid regurgitation, bitter taste in the mouth and dryness of the throat, headache or dizziness, red eyes, tinnitus, constipation, brown urine, red tongue with yellow fur, and wiry rapid pulse.

(3) Qi stagnation and phlegm obstruction: Feeling of a lump lodged in the throat, hard to spit it out or to swallow it, fullness and distress in the chest, hypochondriac pain, frequent deep sighing, white greasy fur, and wiry slippery pulse.

(4) Deficiency of both heart and spleen: Wearing a faraway, grief to tears, pensiveness, worry beyond measure, insomnia, dream-disturbed sleep, shallow complexion, general lassitude, poor appetite, abdominal distension, pale tongue with thin white fur, and deep slow pulse.

(5) Yin deficiency with effulgent fire: Dizziness, tinnitus, irritability, moodiness, aching pain and weakness of the lower back and knees, red tongue with scanty or no fur, and thready rapid pulse.

[Syndrome Differentiation and Treatment]

Treatment: To soothe the liver, remove depression, invigorate the spleen, kidney, heart, and calm the mind.

Point combination:

Main points:

HT 7 (*shén mén*)	PC 6 (*nèi guān*)	LV 3 (*tài chōng*)
RN 17 (*dàn zhōng*)		

Secondary points:

Stagnation of liver qi:

BL 18 (*gān shù*)	LV 14 (*qī mén*)	GB 34 (*yáng líng quán*)

Excessive liver fire:

LV 2 (*xíng jiān*)	GB 43 (*xiá xī*)	PC 8 (*láo gōng*)

Qi stagnation and phlegm obstruction:

RN 12 (*zhōng wǎn*)	ST 40 (*fēng lóng*)	LI 4 (*hé gǔ*)

Deficiency of both heart and spleen:

BL 15 (*xīn shù*)	BL 20 (*pí shù*)	ST 36 (*zú sān lǐ*)

Yin deficiency with effulgent fire:

KI 10 (*yīn gǔ*)	KI 2 (*rán gǔ*)	BL 23 (*shèn shù*)
BL 18 (*gān shù*)		

Feeling of a lump lodged in the throat:

LU 7 (*liè quē*)	KI 6 (*zhào hǎi*)	RN 22 (*tiān tū*)

Operation: After routine sterilization, moderate tapping is used. Gentle tapping is applied to the Back-*Shu* points. Treatment is given once two to three days, and ten treatments make a course.

[Nursing and Prevention]

Patients should consult a doctor of psychology and keep a good mood.

19. Spasm of Diaphragm

[Overview]

Diaphragmatic spasm is a condition characterized by involuntary hiccups. There are simple diaphragmatic spasm and secondary diaphragmatic spasm due to gastrointestinal neurosis, gastritis, gastrectasia, gastric cancer, cirrhosis at the late stage, cerebrovascular disease, uremia, and postoperative reaction of the gastric and esophageal surgery. This section may be consulted for the treatment of hiccups caused by above disorders.

[Cause and Mechanism of Disease]

(1) Cold stagnation in stomach: It is caused by improper diet, eating too much or too fast, or eating too many raw and cold foods or administering overdose of medicinal herbs cold in nature, leading to retained cold in the stomach, which goes along the Lung Channel upward to affect the diaphragm, where qi movement is disturbed. The reversed qi rushes upward to the throat, triggering repeated hiccups.

(2) Up-flaming of stomach fire: It is caused by overeating of hot or spicy food, resulting in excessive internal dryness-heat and the excess syndrome of the *yangming-fu* organ. Finally, stomach qi rushes upward instead of downward.

(3) Stagnation of liver qi: It is caused by depression or fury that injures the liver. Liver qi attacks the stomach, and disturbs the descending function

of stomach qi and the diaphragm, or it is caused by stagnant liver qi which attacks the spleen, or by impairment of the spleen due to pensiveness, leading to dysfunction of the spleen in transportation and transformation and production of phlegm, or it is caused by retention of phlegm and fluid and fury that brings qi upward together with phlegm to the diaphragm, then hiccups occur.

(4) Spleen-stomach yang deficiency: It is caused by poor health, being worn out with age, or a chronic or severe illness when healthy qi has not restored, or by excessive vomiting or purging, or wrong use of purgation in a deficiency syndrome, which results in impairment of the middle-*jiao* qi, yang deficiency of the spleen and stomach, failure of stomach qi to descend, or it is due to a serious disease with the kidney involved, leading to failure of the kidney to receive qi. When kidney qi goes upward together with stomach qi, affecting the diaphragm, hiccups occur.

(5) Stomach yin deficiency: It is caused by deficiency of stomach yin, which impedes descending of stomach qi, instead, it goes upward and affects the diaphragm, giving rise to hiccups.

[Types of Syndromes]

Main manifestations: Repeated involuntary hiccups

(1) Retention of cold in the stomach: Slow and forceful hiccups, discomfort in the stomach, relieved by heat and aggravated by cold, tastelessness in the mouth, absence of thirst, white moist fur, and slow pulse.

(2) Blazing of stomach fire: Loud and forceful hiccups, aggravated by heat, gastric upset, acid regurgitation, flushed face, foul breath, thirst with a desire for cold drinks, dry stools, concentrated urine, red tongue with yellow fur, and rapid slippery pulse.

(3) Stagnation of liver qi: Repeated hiccups, epigastric and hypochondriac fullness, caused or aggravated by emotional problems, poor appetite, borborygmus, farting, thin white fur, and wiry pulse.

(4) Deficiency of spleen and stomach yang: Low and weak hiccups, shortness of breath, lassitude, sallow complexion, cold limbs, anorexia, loose stools, pale tongue with white fur, and deep thready pulse.

(5) Deficiency of stomach yin: Quick, low and weak hiccups, dry mouth and tongue, restlessness, insomnia, red tongue with scanty fluid, or cracked tongue with less fur or no fur, and deep or rapid thready pulse.

[Syndrome Differentiation and Treatment]

Treatment: To disperse cold, purge heat, warm yang, nourish yin, harmonize the stomach and bring stomach qi downward.

Point combination 1:

Main points:

RN 12 (*zhōng wǎn*)	ST 36 (*zú sān lǐ*)	PC 6 (*nèi guān*)
BL 46 (*gě guān*)	BL 2 (*cuán zhú*)	

Secondary points:

Retention of cold in the stomach:

ST 21 (*liáng mén*)	RN13 (*shàng wǎn*)	BL21 (*wèi shù*)

Blazing of stomach fire:

ST 44 (*nèi tíng*)	SP 5 (*shāng qiū*)	LI 11 (*qū chí*)

Stagnation of liver qi:

RN17 (*dàn zhōng*)	LV14 (*qī mén*)	LV 3 (*tài chōng*)

Deficiency of spleen and stomach yang:

RN 11 (*jiàn lǐ*)	RN 6 (*qì hǎi*)	BL 20 (*pí shù*)
BL 21 (*wèi shù*)		

Deficiency of stomach yin:

ST 41 (*jiě xī*)	BL 21 (*wèi shù*)	SP 6 (*sān yīn jiāo*)
KI 7 (*fù liū*)		

Point combination 2: PC 6 (*nèi guān*), SP 4 (*gōng sūn*), (Senior Dr. Jiang Ji-jun's prescription, Dongzhimen Hospital Affiliated to the Beijing University of Chinese Medicine)

Operation: After routine sterilization, moderate tapping is used for the excess syndrome, while gentle tapping for the deficiency syndrome. Treatment is given once one to two days and ten treatments make a course.

[Nursing and Prevention]

Keep warm and avoid raw and cold foods. Do not take spicy food in case of deficiency of stomach yin.

20. Acute and Chronic Gastritis

[Overview]

It is characterized by epigastric pain, often accompanied by nausea, vomiting, epigastric distress, belching, irregular bowels movement, etc. Consult this section in the treatment of peptic ulcer, gastric spasm, gastroptosis, prolapse of gastric mucosa and gastric neurosis with the above symptoms. Syndrome differentiation and treatment offered in this part can be taken as reference. But when gastric pain occurs in these diseases such as hepatitis, cholecystitis, pancreatitis, pneumonia, appendicitis, myocardiac infarction and nephritis, the primary disease should be treated first. In traditional Chinese medicine, it is in the category of "epigastric pain" or "vomiting".

[Cause and Mechanism of Disease]

(1) Excess Syndrome

(i) Pathogenic cold invading stomach: It is caused by overeating of cold stuff which injures the middle-*jiao*, impeding qi movement. Disturbance of stomach qi brings about this condition.

(ii) Improper diet damaging stomach: It is caused by improper diet or crapulence that injures the spleen and stomach, leading to retention of food, impeded qi movement in the stomach and failure of stomach qi to descend, causing pain.

(iii) Liver qi invading stomach: It is caused by moodiness, anger and emotional stress, resulting in failure of liver qi to flow freely. When liver qi transversely attacks the stomach, leading to failure of stomach qi to descend, gastric pain occurs.

(iv) Heat stagnation in liver and stomach: It is caused by heat accumulated in the liver, which turns to fire, attacking the stomach. When stomach qi is disturbed, gastric pain occurs.

(v) Stagnation of static blood: It is caused by stagnation of blood and impeded flow of qi, resulting in gastric pain.

(2) Deficiency Syndrome

(i) Stomach yin deficiency: It is caused by yin impaired in a febrile disease, or excessive stomach heat, which injures stomach yin, or by administering overdose of medicinal herbs aromatic in flavor and dry in nature, serving to promote qi flow, which impairs stomach yin and makes the stomach undernourished, resulting in gastric pain.

(ii) Deficiency-cold of spleen and stomach: It is caused by poor health, or over-strain, or improper diet, or impairment of the spleen and stomach in a chronic illness, or kidney yang deficiency that fails to warm the stomach. It is also caused by administering overdose of medicinal herbs cold in nature, that injures stomach and spleen yang, resulting in gastric pain.

[Types of Syndromes]

Main manifestations: Epigastric pain, nausea and vomiting.

(1) Excess syndrome

(i) Pathogenic cold invading stomach: Sudden onset of gastric cold pain, aggravated by cold and relieved by warmth, nausea, vomiting, absence of thirst, preference for hot drinks, white fur, and wiry tight pulse.

(ii) Improper diet damaging stomach: Distending pain in the epigastrium, aggravated by pressure, acid regurgitation, belching with fetid odour, nausea, vomiting, pain relieved after vomiting, fetid stools, thick greasy fur, and slippery pulse.

(iii) Liver qi invading stomach: Distending pain in the epigastrium, radiating to the hypochondriac region, aggravated when angry, frequent belching, anorexia, acid regurgitation, thin white fur, and deep wiry pulse.

(iv) Heat stagnation in liver and stomach: Burning pain in the gastric region, aggravated by heat and pressure, irritability, thirsty, red tongue with yellow fur, and wiry rapid pulse.

(v) Stagnation of static blood: Fixed epigastric pain, aggravated by pressure, or stabbing pain, aggravated after meals, purplish tongue and rough pulse.

(2) Deficiency Syndrome

(i) Stomach yin deficiency: Continous burning pain in the gastric region, dry mouth and tongue, thirst without a desire for drinks, dry stools, red tongue with scanty fur, and thready rapid and weak pulse.

(ii) Deficiency-cold of spleen and stomach: Dull pain in the epigastrium, relieved by pressure and warmth, aggravated by cold and hunger, lassitude, loose stools, pale and swollen tongue with tooth marks on its edge, and slow or soggy and weak pulse.

[Syndrome Differentiation and Treatment]

Treatment: To harmonize the stomach, relieve pain, ease adverse rise of qi and stop vomiting.

Point combination 1:

Main points:

RN 12 (*zhōng wǎn*)	ST 36 (*zú sān lǐ*)	PC 6 (*nèi guān*)
SP 4 (*gōng sūn*)		

Secondary points:

Pathogenic cold invading stomach:

RN 11 (*jiàn lǐ*)	ST 21 (*liáng mén*)	RN 4 (*guān yuán*)

Improper diet damaging stomach: ST 20 (*chéng mǎn*), ST 25 (*tiān shū*)

Liver qi invading stomach:

RN 17 (*dàn zhōng*)	GB 34 (*yáng líng quán*)	SP 5 (*shāng qiū*)

Heat stagnation in liver and stomach:

LV 2 (*xíng jiān*)	ST 44 (*nèi tíng*)	SJ 6 (*zhī gōu*)

Stagnation of static blood:

BL 17 (*gé shù*)	LV 3 (*tài chōng*)	LI 4 (*hé gǔ*)

Stomach yin deficiency:

BL 20 (*pí shù*)	BL 21 (*wèi shù*)	KI 7 (*fù liū*)

Deficiency-cold of spleen and stomach:

RN 6 (*qì hǎi*)	RN 13 (*shàng wǎn*)	SP 3 (*tài bái*)

Point combination 2:

RN 12 (*zhōng wǎn*)	ST 36 (*zú sān lǐ*)	BL 21 (*wèi shù*)
BL 20 (*pí shù*)		

Operation: After routine sterilization, for the excess syndrome moderate tapping is used, while for the deficiency syndrome gentle tapping is used. Treatment for acute gastritis is given once a day and five treatments make a course. Treatment for chronic gastritis is given once every two to three days and ten treatments make a course.

[Differential Diagnosis]

(1) Acute gastritis is mostly caused by improper diet or unsanitary food and chronic gastritis is characterized by its recurrence.

(2) It is essential to distinguish chronic gastritis from gastric and duodenal ulcer and gastric tumor. Gastroscopy should be performed in time to confirm diagnosis and avoid delaying treatment.

[Nursing and Prevention]

(1) Have light meals, less greasy food and quit smoking and alcohol dependence.

(2) Keep good mood. Avoid anger and fatigue.

21. Bacillary Dysentery

[Overview]

It is a frequently seen intestinal epidemic disease clinically marked by abdominal pain, diarrhea, tenesmus and passing stools containing blood and mucus. It may occur in any season, but more common in summer and autumn. It is highly infectious among males, females, old and young. It causes coma and death in children and aged people as it has a sudden onset with high fever, convulsion and collapse, so effective measures must be taken to prevent and treat the disease actively. Consult this section in the treatment of amebic dysentery and ulcerative colitis with the above symptoms.

[Cause and Mechanism of Disease]

It is due to invasion of the body by summer-heat, pestilent toxins or improper diet that injure the intestines, leading to stagnation of qi and blood, disturbance of transmission. The main mechanism of dysentery is resident of pathogenic factors in the intestines and stagnation of qi and blood, leading to dysfunction in transmission of intestinal contents and injury to blood vessels. The decayed tissues turn to pus and blood mixed in the stools and dysentery occurs. Another cause is epidemic toxins or improper diet, that retain in the intestines. As a result, there is stagnation of qi and blood integrated with pathogens, leading to qi stagnation in the intestines and disturbance of transmission, so abdominal pain, irregular bowels movement and tenesmus occur.

It is also caused by accumulation of heat and stagnated qi and blood in the intestines, which injures the blood vessels, manifested itselt as frequent stool discharge containing blood and mucus. Excessive heat impairs blood and much blood with less mucus is found in stools. But if dampness dominates qi, more mucus with less blood is in stools. Cold-damp dysentery is caused by spleen deficiency and stomach and exposure to cold, then cold-dampness takes the advantages to invade. When dampness-heat retains in the stomach and intestines, stomach qi fails to descend, leading to nausea, vomiting and complete loss of appetite. It is known as food-denying dysentery. Prolonged dysentery results in middle-*jiao* qi deficiency and lowered body resistance. Then exposure to cold and improper diet may cause recurrence of dysentery, known as intermittent dysentery.

[Types of Syndromes]

Main manifestations: Fever, abdominal pain, frequent stools containing blood and mucus and tenesmus.

(1) Damp-heat dysentery: Stools containing more blood and less pus, tenesmus, burning sensation in the anus, fever, restlessness, thirst, concentrated urine, yellow greasy fur, and slippery rapid pulse.

(2) Cold-damp dysentery: Stools containing more mucus and less blood, tenesmus, distension and fullness in the epigastrium and abdomen, anorexia, tastelessness in the mouth, white greasy fur, and soggy slow pulse.

(3) Epidemic toxic dysentery: Sudden onset, stools containing purplish bloody pus, tenesmus, severe abdominal pain, fever, thirst, headache, restlessness, or even coma or convulsion, crisom tongue with yellow dry fur, and slippery rapid pulse.

(4) Food-denial dysentery: Frequent stools containing blood and mucus, tenesmus, complete loss of appetite, nausea and vomiting after eating, abdominal pain, constriction in the chest, lassitude, yellow greasy fur, and soggy rapid pulse.

(5) Yin-deficiency dysentery: Stools containing blood and pus, or bright thick blood, burning pain in the navel and abdomen, anorexia, dry mouth, restlessness, insomnia, red tongue with scanty coating or saliva, and thready rapid pulse.

(6) Recurrent dysentery: Repeated attack, anorexia, lassitude, aversion to cold, abdominal pain and tenesmus on attack, stools containing blood and mucus, pale tongue or with tooth marks on its edge and greasy fur, soggy soft or empty rapid pulse.

(7) Deficiency-cold dysentery: Watery stools containing white jelly-like mucus, even prolapse of rectum, dull pain in the abdomen, aversion to cold, cold limbs, lassitude, anorexia, pale tongue with thin white fur, and thready weak pulse.

[Syndrome Differentiation and Treatment]

Treatment: To clear heat, resolve dampness, invigorate the spleen, disperse cold, regulate the intestines and stop dysentery.

Point combination 1:

Main points:

ST 25 (*tiān shū*)	ST 37 (*shàng jù xū*)	SP 8 (*dì jī*)

Secondary points:

Damp-heat dysentery:

LI 11 (*qū chí*)	SP 9 (*yīn líng quán*)	LI 4 (*hé gū*)

Cold-damp dysentery:

ST 36 (*zú sān lǐ*)	RN 4 (*guān yuán*)	DU 4 (*mìng mén*)

Food-denial dysentery:

RN 12 (*zhōng wǎn*)	ST 44 (*nèi tíng*)	PC 6 (*nèi guān*)

Epidemic toxin dysentery:

LI 11 (*qū chí*)	DU 14 (*dà zhuī*)	EX-UE11 (*shí xuān*)

Yin-deficiency dysentery:

KI 3 (*tài xī*)	KI 6 (*zhào hǎi*)	BL 23 (*shèn shù*)

Recurrent dysentery:

Yang deficiency:

BL 20 (*pí shù*)	BL 21 (*wèi shù*)	BL 23 (*shèn shù*)

Yin deficiency:

KI 6 (*zhào hǎi*)	SP 6 (*sān yīn jiāo*)	SP 9 (*yīn líng quán*)

Deficiency-cold dysentery:

RN 4 (*guān yuán*)	ST 36 (*zú sān lǐ*)	BL 20 (*pí shù*)

Prolapse of rectum in long-standing dysentery:

DU 20 (*bǎi huì*)	RN 6 (*qì hǎi*)	ST 36 (*zú sān lǐ*)

Tenesmus: BL 29 (*zhōng lǚ shù*)

Point combination 2:

Main points:

ST 37 (*shàng jù xū*)	ST 39 (*xià jù xū*)	ST 36 (*zú sān lǐ*)
BL 39 (*wěi yáng*)		

Secondary points:

High fever:

DU 14 (*dà zhuī*)	LI 11 (*qū chí*)	LI 4 (*hé gǔ*)

Abdominal pain: ST 25 (*tiān shū*), BL 25 (*dà cháng shù*)

Tenesmus: BL 29 (*zhōng lǚ shù*)

More blood in stools:

SP 10 (*xuè hǎi*)	BL 20 (*pí shù*)	BL 17 (*gé shù*)

More mucus in stools: BL 20 (*pí shù*), RN 4 (*guān yuán*)

Operation: After routine sterilization, moderate tapping is used for the excess syndrome, while gentle tapping is used for the deficiency syndrome. Treatment is given once a day or every other day and five 5 treatments make a course. For patients with epidemic toxin dysentery, tapping is applied to LI 11 (*qŭ chí*) and DU 14 (*dà zhuī*), followed by cupping.

[Nursing and Prevention]

(1) Pay attention to food hygiene. Do not eat unsanitary or contaminated food, and have a good personal sanitary habit.

(2) Take light meals and avoid greasy food when one has dysentery. Besides, patients must be strictly isolated.

(3) Prevention: Take half to one bulb of garlic twice a day. Chinese herbal decoction: *Herba Portulacae* and *Radix Pulsatillae*, twice a day.

22. Acute and Chronic Enteritis

[Overview]

It is a disease characterized by frequent diarrhea, or with undigested food, even watery diarrhea. It occurs in any season, but more common in summer and autumn. Consult this section in the treatment of diarrhea due to functional or organic changes of the digestive system, such as intestinal tuberculosis, irritable bowel syndrome, or malabsorption syndrome. It is in the category of diarrhea, in traditional Chinese medicine.

[Cause and Mechanism of Disease]

Acute and chronic enteritis, a commonly seen fundctional disorder of the spleen, stomach and intestines, is usually caused by excessive dampness and dysfunction of the spleen and stomach.

(1) Acute Diarrhea

(i) Invasion of exogeneous pathogenic factors: It is due to invasion of the body by exogeneous pathogenic factors, mostly summer-heat, cold, dampness-heat, especially dampness. The spleen likes dryness and dislikes dampness, which is prone to disturb the spleen, leading to impeded digestion and absorption of food essence. When undigested food and water are pouring, diarrhea occurs. It is also divided into cold-dampness diarrhea and dampness-heat diarrhea according to different conditions.

(ii) Indigestion: It is caused by indigestion due to overeating and food retention. Excessive intake of rich and sweet food, or raw, cold stuff injures the spleen and stomach, or contaminated food impairs the spleen and stomach. Then indigestion together with cold-dampness or dampness-heat disturbs their ascending and descending function, diarrhea occurs.

(2) Chronic Diarrhea

(i) Spleen-stomach deficiency: It is caused by spleen deficiency and stomach due to long-term improper diet, or over-strain, or general debility in a prolonged illness, or hypofunction of the spleen and stomach, which fails to normally receive food and water, transport and transform them into refined substances. When interior dampness and undigested stuff go downward, the condition occurs.

(ii) Depressive liver invading spleen: It is caused by depressive liver invading spleen. Agitation and irascibility impede free flow of liver qi, which attacks the spleen and impairs the spleen's function in transportation, as well as its ascending and descending function, or it is caused by worry beyond measure, that disturbs spleen's normal function, or by spleen deficiency and eating when angry, which injures the spleen, and diarrhea occurs.

(iii) Kidney yang deficiency: It is caused by wearing out with age, deficiency of kidney qi, or by impairment of kidney yang in a prolonged illness, or by indulgence in sexual activities and diminished fire of the life gate, failure of the spleen to be warmed and perform normal digestion, finally diarrhea occurs. The kidney is the pass of the stomach and dominates passing of urine. If kidney qi is insufficient, the pass is insecure and diarrhea occurs.

[Types of Syndromes]

(1) Acute Diarrhea

Main manifestations: Sudden onset with increased bowels movement.

(i) Cold-dampness diarrhea: Loose stools or watery diarrhea, abdominal pain and borborygmus, abdominal distension and anorexia, chills and fever, general aching pain, thin greasy or white greasy fur, and soggy slow pulse.

(ii) Dampness-heat diarrhea: Yellow fetid stools, urgent difficult bowels movement, burning sensation in the anus, thirst, restlessness, concentrated urine, yellow greasy fur, and soggy rapid pulse.

(iii) Indigestion diarrhea: Fetid stools, abdominal pain, relieved after bowels movement, borborygmus, epigastric and abdominal fullness, belching with fetid odor, acid regurgitation, white, thick greasy fur, and slippery full pulse.

(2) Chronic Diarrhea

Main manifestations: Slow onset, recurrence with a prolonged duration.

(i) Spleen-stomach deficiency: Occasional loose stools with undigested food, repeated attack, increase of bowels movement soon after improper diet, lassitude, sallow complexion, aversion to cold, preference for warmth, pale tongue with tooth marks on its edge, thin white fur, and deep weak pulse.

(ii) Depressive liver invading spleen: Difficult diarrhea due to anger or emotional stress, abdominal pain radiating to the hypochondriac region, belching, anorexia, pale-red tongue and wiry pulse.

(iii) Kidney yang deficiency: Diarrhea occurring at dawn, abdominal dull pain, relieved after bowels movement, borborygmus, cold limbs, aching pain and weakness in the lower back and knees, pale tongue with white fur, and deep thready pulse.

[Syndrome Differentiation and Treatment]

(1) Acute Diarrhea

Treatment: To eliminate pathogenic factors, remove food retention, regulate the intestinal function and stop diarrhea.

Point combination 1:

Main points:

ST 25 (*tiān shū*)	ST 37 (*shàng jù xū*)	ST 39 (*xià jù xū*)

Secondary points:

Cold-dampness: RN 4 (*guān yuán*), KI 16 (*huāng shù*)

Dampness-heat:

LI 2 (*èr jiān*)	ST 44 (*nèi tíng*)	SP 6 (*sān yīn jiāo*)

Indigestion diarrhea:

ST 21 (*liáng mén*)	RN 11 (*jiàn lǐ*)	ST 44 (*nèi tíng*)

(2) Chronic Diarrhea

Treatment: To soothe the liver, invigorate the spleen, warm yang and stop diarrhea.

Point combination 2:

Main points:

ST 25 (*tiān shū*)	RN 12 (*zhōng wǎn*)	ST 36 (*zú sān lǐ*)
SP 9 (*yīn líng quán*)		

Secondary points:

Spleen-stomach deficiency:

BL 20 (*pí shù*)	BL 21 (*wèi shù*)	LV 13 (*zhāng mén*)
RN 6 (*qì hǎi*)		

Depressive liver invading spleen:

BL 18 (*gān shù*)	LV 14 (*qī mén*)	BL 20 (*pí shù*)

Kidney yang deficiency:

BL 23 (*shèn shù*)	DU 4 (*mìng mén*)	KI 3 (*tài xī*)

Point combination 3: RN 8 (*shén què*), EX (*sì biān*) (around the umbilicus)

Point combination 4:

Main points:

BL 25 (*dà cháng shù*)	ST 25 (*tiān shū*)	ST 36 (*zú sān lǐ*)
SP 3 (*tài bái*)		

Secondary points:

Dampness-heat: BL 22 (*sān jiāo shù*), SP 9 (*yīn líng quán*)

Indigestion: BL 21 (*wèi shù*), RN 12 (*zhōng wǎn*)

Liver qi depression: BL 18 (*gān shù*), GB 34 (*yáng líng quán*)

Kidney deficiency: BL 23 (*shèn shù*), LV 8 (*qū quán*)

Point combination 5: BL 40 (*wěi zhōng*), LI 1 (*shāng yáng*) (for acute diarrhea due to dampness-heat)

Operation: After routine sterilization, moderate or strong tapping is used for the excess syndrome, and gentle tapping for the deficiency syndrome. Treatment for acute diarrhea is given once a day and three treatments make a course. Treatment for chronic diarrhea is given once two to three days and ten treatments make a course. Bloodletting with cupping is applied to BL 40 (*wěi zhōng*).

[Nursing and Prevention]

(1) Pay attention to dietetic hygiene, avoid raw, cold, contaminated or rotten food, cultivate the habit of hygiene.

(2) Have light meals when one suffers from diarrhea.

(3) Chronic diarrhea patients should have confidence and insist on treatment.

23. Constipation

[Overview]

It is caused by the disturbed transmitting function of the large intestine, manifested itself as infrequent or difficult evacuation of feces, or a desire for bowels movement but with difficult evacuation. This section deals with diseases marked by constipation, including constipation, irritable bowel syndrome, enteritis in its convalescent period, constipation due to rectal or anal disorders, drug-induced constipation, endocrine and metabolic disorders, and declined muscular strength.

[Cause and Mechanism of Disease]

(1) Accumulated heat in stomach and intestines: It is caused by excessive yang of the body, or the remnant heat after some febrile diseases, or the heat and dryness in the lung, which descends to the large intestine, or alchol dependence and eating more spicy greasy food or administering overdose of herbal medicines hot in nature, leading to accumulated heat and dryness in the stomach and intestines, impairing body fluids, and dry feces difficult to evacuate. It is known as "heat constipation".

(2) Drepression and stagnation of qi movement: It is caused by to anxiety and pensiveness, resulting in injury to the spleen, or by depression and anger, leading to stagnation of liver qi, or by lack of moving about and unsmooth flow of qi, resulting in stagnation of qi of the *fu*-organs, which disturbes the descending and ascending function of the large intestine, and triggers accumulation of water. This condition is called qi constipation.

(3) Cold accumulation: It is caused by accumulation of cold in the stomach and intestines due to overeating of raw and cold food, or contraction of cold or administering overdose of herbal medicines cold in nature, leading to retention of cold in the stomach and intestines, that impairs the transmitting function. When wastes are unable to evacuate, cold constipation occurs.

(4) Yang qi deficiency: It is caused by qi deficiency, declined yang, improper diet or fatigue, which impair the spleen and stomach, or by poor health and deficiency of yang qi, or by wearing out with age, deficiency of qi and yang, or it occurs after a long illness or childbirth when healthy qi has not restored. It is also caused by overeating of raw and cold food or administering overdose of herbal medicines cold in nature and bitter in flavor, that impair yang and qi, leading to qi deficiency and yang decline. Qi deficiency impairs transmission while yang decline results in failure of the intestines to be warmed. Accumulation of cold in the interior triggers difficult evacuation of feces.

(5) Yin-blood deficiency: It is caused by deficiency of yin and blood, insufficient body fluids, or by deficiency of blood after an illness, or by loss of blood and sweating, or wearing out with age and deficiency of blood, or by administering overdose of purgent herbal medicines dry-hot in nature and aromatic in flavor, leading to deficiency of yin and blood. When the large intestine fails to be moistened, constipation occurs.

[Types of Syndromes]

Main manifestations: Infrequent bowels movement, once every three to five days, or a desire for bowels movement but with difficulty of evacuation of feces.

(1) Excess Syndrome

(i) Heat constipation: Dry stools, difficult to pass, flushed face, feverish sensation, thirst, foul breath, concentrated urine, or abdominal distending pain, red tongue with yellow or dry yellow fur, and rapid pulse.

(ii) Qi constipation: Difficult evacuation of feces, fullness and distension in the chest and hypochondriac region, frequent belching, abdominal distension after meals, thin or greasy fur, and wiry pulse.

(iii) Cold accumulation: Difficult bowels movement, chills, preference for warmth, cold limbs, profuse urine, pale tender-soft tongue with white moist fur, and deep slow pulse.

(2) Deficiency Syndrome

(i) Yang qi deficiency: Normal stools, a desire for defecation but lack of strength, sweating, shortness of breath durings bowels movement, listlessness, pale complexion after bowels movement, pale tender-soft tongue with thin fur, and empty pulse.

(ii) Yin-blood deficiency: Dry stools, lusterless complexion, dizziness, palpitation, pale tongue, and thready pulse.

[Syndrome Differentiation and Treatment]

Treatment: To soothe the liver, clear the intestines, warm the kidney, invigorate the spleen, regulate the intestines and promote bowels movement.

Point combination 1:

Main points: ST 25 (*tiān shū*), ST 37 (*shàng jù xū*)

Secondary points:

Heat constipation:

LI 11 (*qǔ chí*)	LI 4 (*hé gǔ*)	SP 14 (*fù jié*)
ST 44 (*nèi tíng*)	SP 15 (*dà héng*)	

Qi constipation:

LV 3 (*tài chōng*)	GB 34 (*yáng líng quán*)	KI 4 (*dà zhōng*)

Deficiency constipation:

Qi deficiency:

BL 20 (*pí shù*)	BL 21 (*wèi shù*)	ST 36 (*zú sān lǐ*)
BL 23 (*shèn shù*)		

Blood deficiency:

SP 6 (*sān yīn jiāo*)	BL 18 (*gān shù*)	BL 17 (*gé shù*)

Cold constipation:

RN 6 (*qì hǎi*)	BL 23 (*shèn shù*)	BL 26 (*guān yuán shù*)
ST 36 (*zú sān lǐ*)		

Point combination 2: BL 57 (*chéng shān*).

Operation: After routine sterilization, moderate tapping is used for the excess syndrome and gentle tapping for the deficiency syndrome. Treatment is given once two to three days and ten treatments make a course.

[Nursing and Prevention]

(1) Cultivate a habit to have bowels movement regularly. As soon as there is a desire for defecation, go to the toilet. Don't read newspapers and books during bowels movement.

(2) Take more fruits, vegetables and coarse cereals.

(3) Do physical exercises and massage the abdomen frequently.

24. Urinary Infection

[Overview]

It is characterized by frequent, urgent, dribbling and painful urination, spasm of the lower abdomen, pain in the lumbar region and abdomen. In the treatment of urolithiasis, urinary tumor and chylous urine marked by stranguria, consult this section. In traditional Chinese medicine, it is in the category of "stranguria".

[Cause and Mechanism of Disease]

It is caused by dysfunction of the kidney and urinary bladder, inability of qi activity and obstruction of the water passage.

(1) Bladder dampness-heat: It is caused by dampness-heat in the urinary bladder due to overeating spicy, hot, greasy or sweet food, or liquor addiction, that leads to accumulation of dampness-heat in the urinary bladder, or by pathogenic factors from unsanitary genitals that attack the urinary bladder, leading to retention of dampness-heat, finally stranguria occurs. Heat stranguria is marked by urination with burning and stabbing pain. Urolithic stranguria is marked by urinary calculi due to accumulation of dampness-heat and impurifies in the urine. Chylous stranguria is marked by painful discharge of turbid substances, milky urine like rice-water due to heat accumulation in the lower-

jiao, disturbed qi activity and inseparability of usables from unusables.

(2) Heat damaging blood vessels: It is caused by injury to blood vessels by heat, which forces the blood to extravasate, characterized by difficult painful urination with blood. It is bloody stranguria. Another reason of bloody stranguria is kidney yin deficiency, invasion of the channels by deficiency-heat, marked by bloody urine.

(3) Liver depression and qi stagnation: It is caused by liver depression and qi stagnation due to impairment of the liver from rage, stagnated qi turning to fire, or by accumulation of qi and fire in the lower-*jiao* and impeded qi activity of the bladder, leading to distension of the lower abdomen, difficult, painful and dribbling urination, known as qi stranguria. This is an excess syndrome.

(4) Deficiency of both spleen and kidney: In a chronic disease, healthy qi is consumed by dampness-heat. Aged people in poor health, over-strain and indulgent sexual activities all trigger insufficiency in the spleen and kidney, leading to sinking of middle-*jiao* qi and insecurity of the lower origin, therefore, dribbling urination occurs. If stranguria recurs on over-strain, it is known as strain stranguria. Deficiency and sinking of middle-*jiao* qi bring about qi stranguria. Deficiency of kidney qi leads to insecurity of the lower origin and failure to check the flow of chylous fluid, then chylous stranguria occurs.

[Types of Syndromes]

Main manifestations: Frequency of urination, painful dribbling urination, spasm of the lower abdomen, mostly seen in women.

(1) Bladder dampness-heat: Frequent painful urination with concentrated urine, spasm and bloated pain in the lower abdomen, nausea, vomiting, anorexia, constipation, red tongue with yellow or yellow greasy fur, and slippery rapid pulse.

(2) Heat damaging blood vessel: Burning painful urination, bloody urine, or urine with blood clots. In the excess-heat syndrome, it is accompanied by restlessness, red tongue with yellow fur and slippery rapid pulse, while in the yin deficiency syndrome, it is accompanied by lassitude, aching pain and weakness in the lower back and knees, dizziness, tinnitus, pale red tongue with scanty fur, and thready rapid pulse.

(3) Liver depression and qi stagnation: Frequent, urgent and difficult urination with buring pain, hypochondriac distension and pain, irritability, bitter taste in the mouth, dark tongue, and wiry or thready wiry pulse.

(4) Deficiency of both spleen and kidney: Dribbling urination, occurring off and on, worse after over-strain, aching pain and weakness in the lower back and

knees, lassitude, pale tongue with thin white fur, and deep thready weak pulse.

[Syndrome Differentiation and Treatment]

Treatment: To clear heat, cool blood, promote urination and relieve stranguria.

Point combination 1:

Main points:

BL 28 (*páng guāng shù*)	RN 3 (*zhōng jí*)	SP 9 (*yīn líng quán*)
BL 40 (*wěi zhōng*)	BL 66 (*zú tōng gǔ*)	

Secondary points:

Bladder dampness-heat: BL 32 (*cì liáo*), BL 39 (*wěi yáng*)

Heat damaging blood vessel:

Excess syndrome: BL 17 (*gé shù*), DU 14 (*dà zhuī*)

Deficiency syndrome: KI 7 (*fù liū*), SP 6 (*sān yīn jiāo*)

Liver depression and qi stagnation: LV 2 (*xíng jiān*), LV 14 (*qī mén*)

Deficiency of both spleen and kidney:

BL 20 (*pí shù*)	BL 23 (*shèn shù*)	ST 36 (*zú sān lǐ*)

Point combination 2:

Main points:

RN 3 (*zhōng jí*)	ST 28 (*shuǐ dào*)	SP 6 (*sān yīn jiāo*)
SJ 5 (*wài guān*)		

Secondary points:

Urethralgia: LV 5 (*lǐ gōu*)

General debility: RN 6 (*qì hǎi*), ST 36 (*zú sān lǐ*);

[Nursing and Prevention]

(1) Take more rest after onset, drink more water and pass water regularly. Have light meals and avoid spicy food.

(2) Pay attention to personal hygiene.

Section 2 External and Bone Diseases

1. Deep Root Boil

[Overview]

It is a dangerous disease which gets worse quickly, and occurs anywhere, mostly on the face, hands and feet. If it isn't treated properly, the lesion on the face may easily develop to pyosepticemia, and endangers the life. The lesion on hands and feet may damage tendons and bones, and affect their function.

[Cause and Mechanism of Disease]

It is mostly caused by overeating greasy or pungent food or by liquor addiction, leading to accumulation of heat in the *zang-fu* organs and fire-toxin; or by stinging of insects, bringing about invasion of the muscles and skin by toxins, which results in stagnation of qi and blood, then the condition occurs.

[Types of Syndromes]

At the early stage it is red or purple in color, like a millet-grain with a hard base. There is a numbly itching with a little pain. Then a burning pain follows and a white pus spot appears, mostly accompanied by fever or chills, extreme thirst with a desire for drinks, brown urine and dry stools. If irritability or loss of consciousness occurs, it's a critical condition of pyosepticemia. Red lines in the affected parts of limbs found is called "red-streaked boil", or acute lymphangitis.

[Syndrome Differentiation and Treatment]

Treatment: To clear heat and toxicity

Point Combination:

Main points:

DU 12 (*shēn zhù*)	DU 10 (*líng tái*)	DU 14 (*dà zhuī*)
BL 17 (*gé shù*)	BL 40 (*wěi zhōng*)	PC 8 (*láo gōng*)

Secondary points:

On the face:

LI 4 (*hé gǔ*)	ST 44 (*nèi tíng*)	ST 43 (*xiàn gǔ*)

On the arms:

LI 11 (*qǔ chí*)	SJ 5 (*wài guān*)	SJ 4 (*yáng chí*)
LU 11 (*shào shāng*)		

On the legs:

GB 34 (*yáng líng quán*)	SP 10 (*xuè hǎi*)	LV 2 (*xíng jiān*)

Pyosepticemia: DU 26 (*shuǐ gōu*), EX-UE11 (*shí xuān*)

Operation: After routine sterilization, strong tapping is applied to the main points in strong patients and moderate tapping in weak and aged patients.

Collateral-puncturing and cupping are applied to DU 14 (*dà zhuī*), DU 12 (*shēn zhù*) and BL 17 (*gé shù*); but the amout of bloodletting is controlled. Treatment is given once a day or every other day and ten treatments make a course.

[Nursing and Prevention]

(1) At the early stage, never squeeze or prick the boil or use moxibusion, cupping or needling. Surgical treatment is necessary when pus forms.

(2) Pyosepticemia should be treated in time. Take bed rest when there are general symptoms.

(3) Do not eat fish, seafood, meat, or drink liquor, quit smoking. Keep a pleasant mood.

2. Hyperplasia of Mammary Glands

[Overview]

It is a frequently seen benign disease, manifested itself as breast pain and nodules. Nodules may occur on one or both sides, pain and the size of the nodules vary with menstrual cycle and emotional changes. Nodules are moveable and soft, different in size and shapes with unclear margin. In traditional Chinese medicine, it is in the category of "nodular mass in the breast".

[Cause and Mechanism of Disease]

(1) Liver depression and qi stagnation: It is caused by qi stagnation and emotional stress, which triggers unsmooth flow of liver qi and disturbance of qi movement. When stagnated qi retains in the collaterals of the breasts, this condition occurs.

(2) Union of phlegm and qi: It is caused by liver depression and qi stagnation which then attacks the spleen and impairs the function of the spleen and stomach in transportation and transformation, there produce dampness and phlegm. When they get united and block the collaterals of the breasts, the condition occurs.

[Types of Syndromes]

Main manifestations: One or several different-sized, movable nodules with unclear margin in one or both breast.

(1) Liver depression and qi stagnation: Accompanied by distending pain in the breast, fullness and constriction in the chest and hypochondrium, worse with emotional changes, before menstrual cycle, and alleviated after it, bitter taste in the mouth, anorexia, white fur, and wiry pulse.

(2) Union of phlegm and qi: Accompanied by dizziness, fullness in the chest and epigastric region, frequent deep sighing, or feeling of a lump lodged in the throat, white greasy fur, and slippery or wiry pulse.

[Syndrome Differentiation and Treatment]

Treatment: To soothe the liver, regulate qi, resolve phlegm and dissipate nodules

Point combination 1:

Main points:

ST 18 (*rŭ gēn*)	RN 17 (*dàn zhōng*)	ST 40 (*fēng lóng*)

Secondary points:

Liver depression and qi stagnation:

LV 14 (*qī mén*)	GB 34 (*yáng líng quán*)	GB 41 (*zú lín qì*)

Union of phlegm and qi:

LV 2 (*xíng jiān*)	RN 12 (*zhōng wăn*)	SP 6 (*sān yīn jiāo*)

Point combination 2:

RN 17 (*dàn zhōng*)	ST 36 (*zú sān lĭ*)	LV 3 (*tài chōng*)
GB 41 (*zú lín qì*)		

Point combination 3:

GB 21 (*jiān jĭng*)	BL 18 (*gān shù*)	BL 20 (*pí shù*)
LV 14 (*qī mén*)		

Point combination 4: RN 17 (*dàn zhōng*), ST 18 (*rŭ gēn*), local nodules

Operation: After routine sterilization, moderate tapping is used. Treatment is given once two to three days and ten treatments make a course.

[Differential Diagnosis]

It is essential to distinguish hyperplasia of mammary glands from mammary cancer, as the latter has no symptoms at the early stage, characterized by single small hard unsmooth and unmovable mass seen occasionally with no pain and unclear margin, while the former usually presents multiple soft movable nodules.

[Nursing and Prevention]

(1) Keep a pleasant mood, avoid emotional stress and greasy food.

(2) Treat menstrual irregularity and chronic disorders of the uterus and uterine appendages in time.

3. Cholecystitis and Cholelithiasis

[Overview]

Cholecystitis and cholelithiasis have the same symptoms, i.e., pain in the right upper abdomen or radiating to the right shoulder and back, nausea and vomiting. The former is mostly caused by cholelithiasis. In traditional Chinese medicine, it is in the category of "hypochondriac pain", "jaundice", or "epigastric pain".

[Cause and Mechanism of Disease]

(1) Liver depression and qi stagnation: Depression triggers poor circulation of qi in the Liver Channel and obstruction of gallbladder qi, which accumulates in the hypochondriac region, resulting in hypochondriac pain.

(2) Liver-gallbladder dampness-heat: It is caused by dampness-heat contraction, or overeating greasy food, leading to internal accumulation of dampness-heat, that impairs qi movement and impedes smooth flow of liver and gallbladder qi. When dampness and heat get united, cholecystitis or cholelithiasis occurs.

(3) Qi stagnation and blood stasis: When liver qi fails to flow freely, there occurs stagnation of qi and blood, which obstructs the Liver and Gallbladder Channels, leading to failure of gallbladder qi to descend and the stomach attacked by liver qi, followed by these conditions.

[Types of Syndromes]

Main manifestations: Pain in the right hypochondriac region, or radiating to the right shoulder and back.

(1) Liver depression and qi stagnation: Accompanied by distending pain or dull pain in the right hypochondriac region, radiating to the right shoulder and back, intensified by pressure, usually induced or aggravated by anger, fullness in the chest and hypochondriac region, nausea, belching, poor appetite, white fur, and wiry pulse.

(2) Liver-gallbladder dampness-heat: Accompanied by continuous pain in the right hypochondriac region, radiating to the right shoulder and back, nausea, vomiting, bitter taste in the mouth, dry throat, yellow coloration of eyes and body, poor appetite, constipation, brown urine, red tongue with yellow greasy fur, and rapid slippery pulse.

(3) Qi stagnation and blood stasis: Fixed distending or stabbing pain in the right hypochondriac region, hiccups, belching, dark purple tongue, and wiry or rough pulse.

(4) Accumulation of heat-toxin: Acute onset, severe pain in the upper abdomen, chills, high fever, vomiting, restlessness, thirst, yellow coloration of the whole body, scanty and brown urine, dry stools, deep-red tongue with yellow dry fur, and surging large pulse.

[Syndrome Differentiation and Treatment]

Treatment: To soothe the liver, promote smooth flow of gallbladder qi and relieve pain.

Point combination 1:

GB 34 (*yáng líng quán*)	GB 24 (*rì yuè*)	PC 6 (*nèi guān*)

Secondary points:

Liver depression and qi stagnation:

LV 14 (*qī mén*)	LV 3 (*tài chōng*)	RN 17 (*dàn zhōng*)

Liver-gallbladder dampness-heat:

EX-LE6 (*dăn náng*)	SP 9 (*yīn líng quán*)	GB 43 (*xiá xī*)

Qi stagnation and blood stasis:

BL 17 (*gé shù*)	LI 4 (*hé gŭ*)	LV 3 (*tài chōng*)

Accumulation of heat-toxin:

DU 14 (*dà zhuī*)	LV 2 (*xíng jiān*)	GB 43 (*xiá xī*)

Point combination 2:

EX-LE6 (*dăn náng*)	SJ 5 (*wài guān*)	GB 41 (*zú lín qì*)
BL 18 (*gān shù*)	BL 19 (*dăn shù*)	GB 24 (*rì yuè*)

Operation: After routine sterilization, moderate tapping is applied. Collateral-puncturing with cupping is applied to DU 14 (*dà zhuī*), BL 17 (*gé shù*), GB 34 (*yáng líng quán*) and EX-LE6 (*dăn náng*). Treatment is given once a day or every other day and ten treatments make a course.

[Nursing and Prevention]

(1) It is advised not to eat greasy and high-fat food. Have regular diet and pay attention to diet hygiene. Don't eat contaminated food to prevent biliary infection.

(2) Tapping is applied to BL 19 (*dăn shù*) and BL 18 (*gān shù*) on the back during acute onset of colicky pain in the gallbladder. If colicky pain is caused

by gallstones, appropriate therapeutic measures should be taken to give prompt treatment.

4. Acute Appendicitis

[Overview]

It is a frequently seen acute abodomen, manifested itself as a shifting pain at the right lower abdomen. In traditional Chinese medicine, it is in the category of "intestinal abscess".

[Cause and Mechanism of Disease]

It is caused by crapulence or overeating raw, cold and greasy foods, that injures the intestines and stomach, leading to internal accumulation of dampness-heat and decayed flesh, which develops to periappendicular abscess, or by running about after a big meal, giving rise to unsmooth circulation of qi in the intestines and stomach and stagnation of qi and blood, then the condition occurs.

[Types of Syndromes]

At the early stage, there is a pain in the epigastrium or around the umbilicus. Soon paroxysmal pain becomes severe and moves to the right lower abdomen, aggravated by pressure, or accompanied by chills, fever, nausea, vomiting, brown urine, constipation, yellow greasy fur, and rapid forceful pulse.

[Syndrome Differentiation and Treatment]

Treatment: To clear heat, dissipate mass, move qi and relieve pain

Point combination 1:

ST 36 (*zú sān lǐ*)	EX-LE7 (*lán wěi*)	ST 25 (*tiān shū*)
ST 39 (*xià jù xū*)		

Secondary points:

Fever: DU 14 (*dà zhuī*), LI 11 (*qū chí*)

Nausea and vomiting: PC 6 (*nèi guān*), SP 4 (*gōng sūn*)

Point combination 2:

ST 36 (*zú sān lǐ*)	ST 37 (*shàng jù xū*)	EX-LE7 (*lán wěi*)

Secondary points:

Fever: LI 11 (*qū chí*), LI 4 (*hé gǔ*)

Point combination 3: EX-LE (*xī sì*) (4 *cun* above the laterosuperior border of the right patella when the patient lies on his back with his knee flexed), SP 15 (*dà héng*)

Operation: After routine sterilization, moderate tapping is used. Treatment is given once a day and ten treatments make a course.

[Nursing and Prevention]

(1) Don't do fierce sports after meals. Avoid crapulence to prevent this disease.

(2) Acupuncture is only effective to simple appendicitis. Surgical operation must be performed for those with severe symptoms.

5. Urinary Stone

[Overview]

It is characterized by paroxysmal colic or distending pain in the lower back and abdomen and hematuria. In traditional Chinese medicine, it is in the category of "urolithic stranguria" and "bloody stranguria".

[Cause and Mechanism of Disease]

(1) Dampness-heat in the lower-*jiao*: It is caused by improper diet, which impairs the spleen's function of transportation, leading to production of dampness, which turns to heat when it exists in a long period. Dampness-heat goes downward to scorch impurities in urine into calculi.

(2) Qi stagnation and blood stasis: It is caused by depression. Long retained qi turns to fire, which goes downward to scorch impurities in urine into calculi.

(3) Spleen-kidney deficiency: It is caused by hematuzia, or passing too much urine, that consums kidney yin and yang. Deficiency of original yang brings about inadequate warming of the *zang-fu* organs, leading to deficiency of spleen yang, then the condition occurs.

[Types of Syndromes]

Main manifestation: Hematuria, renal colic pain, distending pain in the lower abdomen.

(1) Dampness-heat in the lower-*jiao*: Accompanied by calculi in urine, hesitant urination or interruption of urination, urethral pain, or intolerable colic pain of the lower back and abdomen, blood in urine, dry mouth without a desire for drinks, irregular bowels movement, red tongue with yellow greasy fur, and slippery rapid pulse.

(2) Qi stagnation and blood stasis: Retention of calculi, vague pain or dull pain in the lower back and abdomen, aggravated when the calculi move, fullness in the lower abdomen, scanty brown urine, dark red tongue with ecchymosis, thin white fur, and deep tight pulse.

(3) Spleen-kidney deficiency: Occasional dull pain, drooping and fullness in the lower back and abdomen, aggravated after overwork, aching pain and weakness in the lower back and knees, lassitude, aversion to cold, cold limbs, frequency of urination at night, pale tongue with thin white fur, and deep or rapid thready pulse.

[Syndrome Differentiation and Treatment]

Treatment: To clear heat and dampness, invigorate the spleen and kidney, remove stones and relieve stranguria.

Point combination 1:

BL 23 (*shèn shù*)	BL 28 (*páng guāng shù*)	GB 25 (*jīng mén*)
RN 3 (*zhōng jí*)		

Secondary points:

Dampness-heat in the lower-*jiao*:

LV 5 (*lǐ gōu*)	SP 9 (*yīn líng quán*)	BL 39 (*wěi yáng*)

Qi stagnation and blood stasis:

LV 2 (*xíng jiān*)	SP 10 (*xuè hǎi*)	LV 3 (*tài chōng*)

Spleen-kidney deficiency:

BL 20 (*pí shù*)	BL 23 (*shèn shù*)	RN 4 (*guān yuán*)

Point combination 2:

RN 6 (*qì hǎi*)	ST 28 (*shuǐ dào*)	SP 6 (*sān yīn jiāo*)
LV 5 (*lǐ gōu*)		

Secondary points:

Calculus of the kidney: BL 23 (*shèn shù*), GB 25 (*jīng mén*)

Calculus of the upper ureter: ST 25 (*tiān shū*)

Calculus of the middle and lower ureter:

BL 32 (*cì liáo*)	BL 25 (*dà cháng shù*)	BL 27 (*xiǎo cháng shù*)
RN 3 (*zhōng jí*)		

Vesical and urethral calculus:

BL 28 (*páng guāng shù*)	BL 33 (*zhōng liáo*)	LV 3 (*tài chōng*)
RN 2 (*qǔ gǔ*)	LV 8 (*qǔ quán*)	

Colicky pain:

BL 23 (*shèn shù*)	LI 4 (*hé gǔ*)	GB 25 (*jīng mén*)

Deficiency syndrome: RN 4 (*guān yuán*), KI 3 (*tài xī*)

Blood in urine: SP 10 (*xuè hǎi*)

Operation: After routine sterilization, moderate tapping is used for the excess syndrome while gentle tapping for the deficiency syndrome. Strong tapping is for colicky pain. Treatment is given once one to two days and ten treatments make a course.

[Differential Diagnosis]

Urinary stone is usually confused with cholecystitis, cholelithiasis and acute appendicitis. Accurate diagnosis is made based on the quality of pain, hematuria combined with B-ultrasonic examination and laboratory tests.

(1) The pain caused by cholecystitis and cholelithiasis has a sudden onset, confined to the upper abdomen and epigastrium with local tenderness. It is a paroxysmal severe colicky or distending pain, radiating to the right shoulder and back, accompanied by chills, fever, nausea and vomiting. Jaundice may occur. But nephrocolic is paroxysmal colicky pain from the lower back radiating down along the ureter and hematuria presents.

(2) It is essential to tell acute appendicitis from calculus of the right lower ureter with nephrocolic. The former is mostly marked by persisted dull pain in gradual aggravation. Severe colicky pain is found in obstructive appendicitis. Tenderness, rebound tenderness or muscular tension can be seen at the McMurray point. Most patients have no change in urine quality. The pain of the latter may radiate to the medial side of the thigh, groin, penis and scrotum or lip of pudendum, accompanied by hematuria.

[Nursing and Prevention]

(1) Drink more water to maintain urine in a dilute state and eat more fruits and vegetables.

(2) When the stone can't be removed, surgery must be performed to avoid delaying treatment.

6. Acute and Chronic Prostatitis

[Overview]

It is a disease of the reproductive system in men, usually triggered by infection of staphylococcus, streptococcus or colibacillus. The main symptoms are frequent, urgent and painful urination and sperm in the meatus urinarius. In traditional Chinese medicine, it is in the range of "chylous stranguria" and "strain stranguria".

[Cause and Mechanism of Disease]

(1) Dampness-heat in the lower-*jiao*: It is caused by improper diet, such as overeating greasy sweat food and liquor addiction, which causes production of dampness-heat. When it goes downward to the lower-*jiao*, or when external dampness-heat invades and gathers in the lower-*jiao*, the condition occurs.

(2) Qi stagnation and blood stasis: It is caused by indulgence in sexual activities, leading to the sperm pathway attacked by dampness-heat. When dampness-heat accumulates in the lower-*jiao*, qi stagnation and blood stasis occur, followed by this condition.

(3) Kidney deficiency: It is caused by poor health or a chronic illness or indulgence in sexual activities, leading to consumption of kidney yin and hyperactivity of ministerial fire. When yang is impaired by yin and kidney yang becomes insufficient, the condition occurs.

[Types of Syndromes]

Main manifestations: Pain in the lower abdomen, perineum, testis and lumbosacral region, frequent and painful urination, or burning sensation in the urethra, urethral dribbling of white substances.

(1) Dampness-heat in the lower-*jiao*: Frequent, urgent, painful and hesitant urination, whitish or turbid substances dripping from the urethra at the end of urination, heat and pain in the penis, distending pain in the lumbosacral area, perineum and testis, constipation, brown urine, red tongue with yellow or greasy fur,and rapid slippery pulse.

(2) Qi stagnation and blood stasis: Distending pain in the lower abdomen, perineum or testis, or difficult, hesitant and painful urination, dark tongue or with ecchymosis, and deep rough or wiry tight pulse.

(3) Kidney yin deficiency: Hesitant urination, whitish and turbid substances dripping from the urethra at the end of urination, accompanied by dizziness, tinnitus, insomnia, dream-disturbed sleep, nocturnal emission, night sweating, red tongue with little fur, and thready rapid pulse.

(4) Kidney yang deficiency: Dribbling urination, whitish and turbid substances from the urethra during urination, listlessness, aching pain and weakness of the lower back and knees, aversion to cold, cold limbs, or impotence, premature ejaculation, pale enlarged tongue with thin white fur, and deep thready pulse.

[Syndrome Differentiation and Treatment]

Treatment: To clear heat, relieve stranguria, reinforce the kidney and activate blood circulation

Point combination 1:

BL 23 (*shèn shù*)	BL 28 (*páng guāng shù*)	RN 3 (*zhōng jí*)
SP 6 (*sān yīn jiāo*)		

Secondary points:

Dampness-heat in the lower-*jiao*:

BL 22 (*sān jiāo shù*)	BL 39 (*wěi yáng*)	BL 32 (*cì liáo*)

Qi stagnation and blood stasis:

SP 9 (*yīn líng quán*)	SP 10 (*xuè hǎi*)	RN 17 (*dàn zhōng*)

Kidney yin deficiency: KI 3 (*tài xī*), LV 8 (*qū quán*)

Kidney yang deficiency:

BL 23 (*shèn shù*)	RN 4 (*guān yuán*)	ST 36 (*zú sān lǐ*)

Point combination 2:

Main points:

BL 23 (*shèn shù*)	BL 28 (*páng guāng shù*)	RN 3 (*zhōng jí*)
SP 6 (*sān yīn jiāo*)		

Secondary points:

Acute prostatitis:

LV 5 (*lǐ gōu*)	LV 2 (*xíng jiān*)	KI 12 (*dà hè*)
SP 9 (*yīn líng quán*)		

Chronic prostatitis:

KI 3 (*tài xī*)	RN 4 (*guān yuán*)	BL 18 (*gān shù*)
ST 36 (*zú sān lǐ*)		

Operation: After routine sterilization, moderate tapping is used for the excess syndrome,while gentle tapping for the deficiency syndrome. Treatment is given once two to three days and ten treatments make a course.

[Differential Diagnosis]

(1) Chronic epididymitis has dull pain in the groin and scrotum, which is

similar to that in chronic prostatitis. But thickened and painful nodules can be touched in chronic epididymitis.

(2) When seminal vesiculitis and prostatitis occur simultaneously, there are symptoms similar to those of prostatitis but accompanied by hematuria and pain in ejaculation.

(3) Prostatic hyperplasia is mostly found in old people. Its main manifestations are frequent urination accompanied by dysuria and increased residual urine in the bladder.

[Nursing and Prevention]

(1) Never give massage to the prostate in acute prostatitis to prevent spreading of inflammation.

(2) Have a good life habit. Quit liquor addiction and spicy food.

(3) Drink more water and urinate more to douche the urethra.

(4) Don't ride bicycle too long.

7. Prostatic Hyperplasia

[Overview]

It is one of the commonly encountered diseases in old male patients, marked by difficult urination. In traditional Chinese medicine, it is in the category of "retention of urine" and "hypertrophy of prostate". In the treatment of uroschesis after surgery this section can be referred to.

[Cause and Mechanism of Disease]

(1) Excess syndrome: If the lung is attacked, and lung fluid is impaired. The lung's dispersing function is impeded and the water passage is blocked. Dampness-heat in the middle-*jiao* goes downward to the bladder, then the condition occurs. Traumatic injury causes qi stagnation and blood stasis, which impedes the activity of bladder qi and leads to retention of urine, then the condition occurs.

(2) Deficiency syndrome: If declined kidney yang fails to produce more water, which impedes the activity of bladder qi. Deficient qi in the middle-*jiao* impedes the transportation of dampness, which impairs qi movement in the lower-*jiao*. Retention of urine occurs, followed by this condition.

[Types of Syndromes]

Main manifestations: Difficult urination, or even retention of urine, distending pain in the lower abdomen.

(1) Deficiency syndrome: Difficult urination, or hesitant dribbling urination, even no urine passing, distending pain of the lower abdomen.

(i) Kidney yang deficiency: Accompanied by aching pain and weakness in the lower back and knees, cold limbs, pale enlarged tongue,and deep slow pulse.

(ii) Spleen qi deficiency: Accompanied by listlessness, lack of strength, poor appetite, disinclination to talk, loose stools, pale tongue or with tooth marks on its edge, and soggy moderate pulse.

(2) Excess syndrome: No urine passing or hesitant dribbling urination, distending fullness and pain in the lower abdomen, thirst, restlessness, red face and rough voice.

(i) Lung heat and qi stagnation: Accompanied by cough, panting, restlessness, thirst with a desire for drinks, red tongue with thin yellow fur and rapid pulse.

(ii) Dampness-heat in the bladder: Accompanied by thirst but without a desire for drinks, fullness in the lower abdomen, urethral pain, difficult bowels movement.

(iii) Traumatic injury: Having a history of trauma and surgery, dark purple tongue or with ecchymosis and rough pulse.

[Syndrome Differentiation and Treatment]

Treatment: To replenish qi, get rid of retained urine, clear heat, resolve dampness and promote urination

Point combination 1:

RN 3 (*zhōng jí*)	SP 6 (*sān yīn jiāo*)	BL 28 (*páng guāng shù*)
KI 3 (*tài xī*)		

Secondary points:

Kidney yang deficiency:

BL 23 (*shèn shù*)	KI 16 (*huāng shù*)	ST 28 (*shuǐ dào*)
RN 4 (*guān yuán*)		

Spleen qi deficiency:

BL 20 (*pí shù*)	SP 6 (*sān yīn jiāo*)	ST 36 (*zú sān lǐ*)
RN 6 (*qì hǎi*)		

Lung heat and qi stagnation:

BL 13 (*fèi shù*)	LU 5 (*chǐ zé*)	BL 22 (*sān jiāo shù*)

Dampness-heat in the bladder:

BL 66 (*zú tōng gǔ*)	BL 40 (*wěi zhōng*)	SP 9 (*yīn líng quán*)

Traumatic injury:

BL 32 (*cì liáo*)	BL 17 (*gé shù*)	LV 3 (*tài chōng*)
LI 4 (*hé gǔ*)		

Point combination 2:

SP 9 (*yīn líng quán*)	SP 6 (*sān yīn jiāo*)	LV 6 (*zhōng dū*)
LV 5 (*lǐ gōu*)	RN 3 (*zhōng jí*)	KI 3 (*tài xī*)

Operation: After routine sterilization, moderated tapping is used for the excess syndrome while gentle tapping for the deficiency syndrome. Treatment is given once two to three days and ten treatments make a course.

[Nursing and Prevention]

(1) Pass water in time and avoid over-filling of the bladder.

(2) Avoid wind-cold and quit liquor addiction, strong tea and spicy food.

8. Impotence

[Overview]

It is a male sexual disorder, characterized by failure of the penis to erect, or weak erection.

[Cause and Mechanism of Disease]

(1) Deficiency syndrome: It is caused by indulgence in sexual activities, which injures kidney qi, or by poor born gifts and declined fire of the life gate, resulting in malnourished genitals. Worry beyond measure impairs the heart and spleen and triggers deficiency of qi and blood and undernourishment of the genitals, then the condition occurs.

(2) Excess syndrome: It is caused by overeating greasy food, which promotes production of internal dampness-heat, or by spleen deficiency and prolonged retained dampness, which turns ino heat. When it goes downward, dampness-heat schorches the penis and makes it unable to erect.

[Types of Syndromes]

Main manifestations: Failure of the penis to erect, or weak erecttion.

(1) Deficiency Syndrome

(i) Declined fire of the life gate: Accompanied by thin sperm, listlessness, cold limbs, pallor, pale tongue with white and moist fur, and deep slow pulse.

(ii) Deficiency of both heart and spleen: Accompanied by palpitation, forgetfulness, lassitude, sallow complexion, shortness of breath, spontaneous sweating, poor appetite, loose stools, pale tongue with tooth marks on its edge, thin white fur, and soggy thready pulse.

(iii) Impairment of the kidney due to terror: Accompanied by timidity, oversentiveness, palpitation, insomnia, pale tongue with white fur, and thready wiry pulse.

(2) Excess Syndrome

Downward pouring of dampness-heat: Accompanied by wet itching scrotum with a drooping and distending sensation, or bloated aching pain, swollen and painful scrotum, bitter taste and slimy sensation in the mouth, yellow greasy fur, and rapid soggy pulse.

[Syndrome Differentiation and Treatment]

Treatment: To warm the kidney, strengthen yang, invigorate the heart and kidney, clear heat and resolve dampness.

Point combination 1:

BL 23 (*shèn shù*)	SP 6 (*sān yīn jiāo*)	BL 32 (*cì liáo*)
LV 3 (*tài chōng*)		

Secondary points:

Declined fire of the life gate:

RN 4 (*guān yuán*)	DU 4 (*mìng mén*)	KI 3 (*tài xī*)

Deficiency of both heart and spleen:

BL 15 (*xīn shù*)	BL 20 (*pí shù*)	ST 36 (*zú sān lǐ*)

Impairment of the kidney due to terror:

HT 7 (*shén mén*)	BL 15 (*xīn shù*)	RN 6 (*qì hǎi*)
KI 3 (*tài xī*)		

Downward pouring of dampness-heat:

BL 28 (*páng guāng shù*)	SP 9 (*yīn líng quán*)	RN 2 (*qū gǔ*)

Itching vulva:

SP 9 (*yīn líng quán*)	LV 5 (*lǐ gōu*)	LV 12 (*jí mài*)

Point combination 2: BL 23 (*shèn shù*), EX-B (*yáng wěi*) (2.5 *cun* above BL 23 (*shèn shù*) and 1 *cun* lateral to the *Du* Vessel), RN 3 (*zhōng jí*)

Secondary points: SP 6 (*sān yīn jiāo*), ST 36 (*zú sān lǐ*)

Point combination 3:

RN 4 (*guān yuán*)	SP 6 (*sān yīn jiāo*)	BL 31, 32, 33, 34 (*bā liáo*)

Operation: After routine sterilization, moderate tapping is used for the excess syndrome while gentle tapping for the deficiency syndrome. Treatment is given once two to three days and ten treatments make a course.

[Nursing and Prevention]

(1) If impotence is related to indulgence in sexual activities, it is necessary to have less sexual activities and quit masturbation.

(2) If impotence is related to over-strain, stress or depression, it is necessary to have enough rest, get rid of anxiety and keep a pleasant mood.

9. Seminal Emission

[Overview]

It refers to discharge of seminal fluid without sexual intercourse. In traditional Chinese medicine, it is in the category of "nocturnal emission" and "spermatorrhea". The former occurs during dreamful sleep and the latter occurs when one is awake.

[Cause and Mechanism of Disease]

(1) Non-interaction between heart and kidney: It is caused by constant liver-kidney yin deficiency, or indulgence in sexual activities, which consume kidney yin. When kidney water fails to ascend to supplement the heart, heart fire is stirred up and it disturbs the sperm chamber, causing the condition to occur.

(2) Inability of the kidney to store sperm: It is caused by poor born gifts, or by a chronic illness that injures the kidney. Deficiency of kidney qi and insecurity of the sperm chamber leads to this condition.

(3) Downward pouring of dampness-heat: It is caused by spleen deficiency and dampness when one lives in a damp place for years. Dampness turns into heat, which goes downward to the lower-*jiao* and disturbs the sperm chamber, then the condition occurs.

[Types of Syndromes]

(1) Non-interaction between heart and kidney: Seminal emission in dreams, insomnia, dizziness, tinnitus, feverish sensation in the chest, palms and soles, tidal fever, night sweating, red tongue with scanty fur, and thready rapid pulse.

(2) Inability of the kidney to store sperm: Frequent seminal emission, even spermatorrhea, lusterless complexion, listlessness, aching pain and cold in the lower back and knees, pale tongue with white fur, and deep thready pulse.

(3) Downward pouring of dampness-heat: Frequent seminal emission, white sticky substances in urine, or turbid fluid from the balanus, brown urine, dribbling urination or with burning sensation, thirst without a desire for drinks, red tongue with yellow and greasy fur, and soggy rapid pulse.

[Syndrome Differentiation and Treatment]

Treatment: To restore normal coordination between the heart and kidney, reinforce the kidney, astringe semen, clear heat and resolve dampness.

Point combination 1:

Main points:

BL 15 (*xīn shù*)	BL 52 (*zhì shì*)	RN 3 (*zhōng jí*)
HT 7 (*shén mén*)	SP 6 (*sān yīn jiāo*)	

Secondary points:

Non-interaction between heart and kidney: PC 8 (*láo gōng*), KI 7 (*fù liū*)
Inability of the kidney to store sperm: RN 4 (*guān yuán*), DU 4 (*mìng mén*)
Downward pouring of dampness-heat: SP 9 (*yīn líng quán*), SP 2 (*dà dū*)
Point combination 2:

BL 23 (*shèn shù*)	BL 52 (*zhì shì*)	RN 3 (*zhōng jí*)
KI 12 (*dà hè*)	KI 3 (*tài xī*)	ST 36 (*zú sān lǐ*)

(for inability of the kidney to store sperm)

Secondary points:

Frequent urination: SP 6 (*sān yīn jiāo*), SP 9 (*yīn líng quán*)

Operation: After routine sterilization, moderate tapping is used for the excess syndrome while gentle tapping for the deficiency syndrome. Treatment is given once two to three days and ten treatments make a course.

[Nursing and Prevention]

(1) Adjust emotional state, be pure of the heart and have few desires.

(2) Have temperate sexuality, quit masturbation and have a habit of lying on one's side. Bedclothes should not be too thick and the underpants should not be too tight.

(3) Avoid spicy and irritating foods.

10. Hemorrhoids

[Overview]

It refers to a soft venous ball formed by dilation and varicosis of the venous plexus below the mucous membrane of the rectal end and the skin of the anal canal. It occurs in males or females, young or old as a commonly encountered chronic anal disease. Its clinical manifestations are hematochezia, prolapse of hemorrhoids, and discomfort of the anus. In accordance with different locations, it's divided into internal hemorrhoids, external hemorrhoids and complicated hemorrhoids.

[Cause and Mechanism of Disease]

(1) Internal accumulation of dryness-heat: It is caused by preference for spicy food. When dryness-heat descends through the large intestine and to the anus, the condition occurs.

(2) Qi stagnation and blood stasis: Prolonged sitting or standing, or overloading in a long journey impedes free flow of qi and blood. Blood stasis gathers in the anus, resulting in hemorrhoids.

[Types of Syndromes]

(1) Internal accumulation of dryness-heat: Bright red blood in stools, burning sensation around the anus, thirst, foul breath, dry stools, scanty brown urine, red tongue with yellow fur, and rapid slippery or wiry pulse.

(2) Qi stagnation and blood stasis: Dark purple blood in stools, feeling of a foreign body in the anus, difficult bowels movement or with severe pain, dark tongue with thin white fur, and deep or wiry pulse.

[Syndrome Differentiation and Treatment]

Treatment: To clear heat, move qi, resolve stasis and stop bleeding.

Point combination 1:

BL 57 (*chéng shān*)	BL 32 (*cì liáo*)	DU 1 (*cháng qiáng*)
BL 17 (*gé shù*)		

Secondary points:

Internal accumulation of dryness-heat:

ST 25 (*tiān shū*)	ST 37 (*shàng jù xū*)	ST 44 (*nèi tíng*)

Qi stagnation and blood stasis:

BL 18 (*gān shù*)	LV 14 (*qī mén*)	SP 6 (*sān yīn jiāo*)
BL 40 (*wěi zhōng*)		

Point combination 2:

EX-UE2 (*èr bái*)	DU 2 (*yāo shù*)	BL 57 (*chéng shān*)
ST 25 (*tiān shū*)		

Operation: After routine sterilization, moderate tapping is used. Treatment is given once a day and ten treatments make a course.

Point combination 3:

BL 31 (*shàng liáo*)	BL 32 (*cì liáo*)	BL 33 (*zhōng liáo*)
BL 34 (*xià liáo*)		

Operation: Gentle tapping is applied to BL 31, 32, 33, 34 (*bā liáo*) until congestion. Apply *Flos Caryophylli and Ramulus Cinnamomi* Powder (*Dīng Guì Săn*) and *Guan Jie Zhi Tong Oilment* to the points. Then suspending or pecking moxibustion is used, ten to fifteen minutes each time, once every other day.

[Differential Diagnosis]

It is essential to distinguish hemorrhoids from anal fistula and rectal cancer. Hemorrhoids are characterized by hematochezia, but anal fistula by pain, hematochezia and dry stools, and rectal cancer by hematochezia mixed with mucus and usually accompanied by change of defecation habit at the early stage. It is not difficult to make an accurate diagnosis with appropriate examinations.

[Nursing and Prevention]

(1) Have a good habit of bowels movement. Don't read books, newspapers or magazines during bowels movement. Don't sit too long. Stand up and walk around regularly.

(2) Take less spicy food and more fruits and vegetables to maitain free bowels movement.

(3) Surgery is necessary for hemorrhoid incarceration.

11. Erysipelas

[Overview]

It is an acute infectious disease characterized by sudden emergence of red skin, mostly caused by streptococcus. Erysipelas which occurs on the head and face is called "head erysipelas", on the lower limbs "leg erysipelas" and on the feet "foot erysipelas".

[Cause and Mechanism of Disease]

(1) Dampness-heat immersion: It is caused by overeating fat, sweat and spicy foods, or by spleen deficiency. Long retention of dampness produces heat. When skin is scorches, the condition occurs.

(2) Invasion of exogenous pathogenic toxins: It is due to exogenous pathogenic toxins and blood heat, which get united and reside in the skin, then the condition occurs.

[Types of Syndromes]

Main manifestations: Rapid onset, red swollen skin in the shape of cloud, hot pain.

(1) Dampness-heat immersion: Red, swollen skin with a hot feeling, or with yellow blisters, that erupt and ooze fluid, itching and pain, aversion to cold, low grade fever, red tongue with yellow greasy fur, and soggy rapid pulse.

(2) Invasion of exogenous pathogenic toxins: Red swollen skin with pain, restlessness, thirst, fever, dry stools, brown urine, red tongue with yellow fur, and surging large pulse.

[Syndrome Differentiation and Treatment]

Treatment: To clear heat, relieve toxicity, resolve dampness and alleviate swelling.

Point Combination:

SP 10 (*xuè hǎi*)	BL 40 (*wěi zhōng*)	EX-LE3 (*bǎi chóng wō*)
LU 5 (*chǐ zé*)	SP 6 (*sān yīn jiāo*)	

Secondary points:

Dampness-heat immersion:

ST 44 (*nèi tíng*)	SP 9 (*yīn líng quán*)	ST 40 (*fēng lóng*)

Invasion of exogenous pathogenic toxins:

DU 10 (*líng tái*)	DU 14 (*dà zhuī*)	LI 11 (*qū chí*)

Operation: After routine sterilization, moderate tapping is used. Collateral-puncturing and cupping are applied to DU 14 (*dà zhuī*), DU 10 (*líng tái*), BL 40 (*wěi zhōng*) and EX-LE3 (*bǎi chóng wō*) (1 *cun* above SP 10 (*xuè hǎi*)). Treatment is given once a day and ten treatments make a course.

[Nursing and Prevention]

(1) When the skin and mucous membrane are ruptured, treat the wound properly to avoid infection.

(2) Pay attention to the primary disease. If erysipelas is due to Athlete's foot, that should be treated too.

(3) Drink more water and sleep alone. Raise the infected leg in an angle of 30~40° if erysipelas is on the lower limbs.

12. Costal Chondritis

[Overview]

It is caused by periosteal fibrous thickening of the costal cartilage or hyperplasia of the soft tissues, characterized by idiopathic painful nonsuppurative swelling of one or more costal cartilages with obvious tenderness, aggravated by deep breathing or raise of the arm. In traditional Chinese medicine, this category is called, "impediment disease".

[Cause and Mechanism of Disease]

(1) **Contraction of external wind-cold:** It is caused by poor health and insufficient healthy qi. When wind-cold obstructs the channels and induces pain, the condition occurs.

(2) **Qi stagnation and blood stasis:** It is caused by traumatic injuries or sprain of the ribs, which impedes free flow of qi and blood, leading to blockage of channels and the condition.

[Types of Syndromes]

(1) **Contraction of external wind-cold:** Pain in the costal and hypochondriac regions, relieved by heat, aversion to wind and cold, pale-red tongue with thin white fur, and floating tense or wiry pulse.

(2) **Qi stagnation and blood stasis:** Fixed stabbing pain in the hypochondriac region, intensified by pressure and depression, and dark tongue with thin white fur and wiry pulse.

[Syndrome Differentiation and Treatment]

Treatment: To dissipate wind, expel cold, move qi, activate blood circulation, and unblock channels to stop pain.

Point Combination:

PC 6 (*nèi guān*)	SP 4 (*gōng sūn*)	*Ashi* points

Secondary points:

Contraction of external Wind-cold: BL 12 (*fēng mén*), GB 20 (*fēng chí*)

Qi stagnation and blood stasis:

LV 3 (*tài chōng*)	LV 14 (*qī mén*)	BL 17 (*gé shù*)

Operation: After routine sterilization, strong tapping is applied to *Ashi* points, followed by collateral-puncturing and cupping. Mild moxibustion can also be used. Tapping is applied to other points. Treatment is given once two to three days and five treatments make a course.

13. Ganglionic Cyst

[Overview]

It is a cystic mass at joints or tendon sheaths, usually caused by mucunous degeneration of the tendon sheaths. The cyst is mostly connected to the joint cavity or tendon sheath, almost found near the joint cavity or tendon sheath, especially at the dorsum of the wrist and foot. It occurs often in young and middle-aged people, more females than males. In traditional Chinese medicine, it is categorized as "musculotendinous nodulation" and "varix".

[Cause and Mechanism of Disease]

It is caused by over-strain that impairs tendons, or cold-dampness attacking tendons, leading to qi stagnated in channels and causing this condition to occur.

[Types of Syndromes]

Cysts at the dorsum of the wrist and foot are soft, smooth and round in shape with clear-cut margins. Symptoms are not obvious. There are only occasional aching pain, weakness, or discomfort, aggravated by cold or over-strain.

[Syndrome Differentiation and Treatment]

Treatment: To dissipate swelling and nodulation, unblock channels and stop pain

Point Combination: *Ashi* points

Operation: After routine sterilization, strong tapping starts from the centre of the cyst to outside in the shape of a circle ringlikely until congestion or presence of blood dots. Mild moxibustion is used too. Treatment is given once two to three days and five treatments make a course.

[Nursing and Prevention]

Reduce cold water irritation to the hands and feet. Avoid tiredness of the hands and feet.

14. Acute Lumbar Sprain

[Overview]

It is caused by improper movement, falling, or injury to the lower back, that impairs the local muscles and fascia. In traditional Chinese medicine it is categorized as "lower back pain" or "impediment disease".

[Cause and Mechanism of Disease]

It is usually caused by improper movement, falling, or traumatic injury, that impedes local free flow of qi and blood, leading to stagnation of qi and blood and the condition.

[Types of Syndromes]

There is local swelling and pain. Bruise or red skin is seen. Normal joint motion is impeded owing to severe pain.

[Syndrome Differentiation and Treatment]

Treatment: To soothe the tendons, activate channels and stop pain.

Point combination 1: SI 3 (*hòu xī*), *Ashi* points, EX-UE7 (*yāo tòng diǎn*) (on the dorsum of the hand, midway between the transverse wrist crease and metacarpophalangeal joint, between the second and third metacarpal bones and between the fourth and fifth metacarpal bones, four points in all on both sides)

Point combination 2: *Ashi* points, SI 6 (*yǎng lǎo*)

Point combination 3: BL 40 (*wěi zhōng*)

Operation: After routine sterilization, strong tapping is used. Moderate tapping is used for the weak, aged patients and children. Collateral-puncturing and cupping are applied to BL 40 (*wěi zhōng*) and *Ashi* points. Treatment is given once a day and three treatments make a course.

[Nursing and Prevention]

Don't do fierce exercise and exert oneself in physical labor. If sprain has been cured, take great care not to do the same movement that would trigger recurrence.

15. External Humeral Epicondylitis

[Overview]

It is a chronic strain, characterized by repeated attack of pain in the elbow joint. It is also called "tennis elbow". In traditional Chinese medicine it is categorized as "injury to muscles and tendons".

[Cause and Mechanism of Disease]

It is usually caused by repeated strains, or contraction of wind-cold that leads to unsmooth circulation of qi and blood in the local channels and collaterals, resulting in stagnation of qi and blood and undernourishment of channels.

[Types of Syndromes]

Fixed distending aching pain in the elbow, occurring off and on, aggravated by cold or tiredness.

[Syndrome Differentiation and Treatment]

Treatment: To unblock collaterals and stop pain.

Point combination 1:

LI 11 (*qū chí*)	LI 10 (*shǒu sān lǐ*)	SJ 10 (*tiān jǐng*)
SI 8 (*xiǎo hǎi*)	LI 4 (*hé gǔ*)	

Point combination 2: *Ashi* points, LI 4 (*hé gǔ*)

Operation: After routine sterilization, moderate tapping is used. Apply cupping or moxibustion to the tender spots after tapping. Treatment is given once every two days and five treatments make a course.

[Nursing and Prevention]

(1) Do not do rotatory movement of the elbow and forearm during treatment. Avoid overloading.

(2) Hot compress and massage can be combined. Avoid contraction of wind-cold.

16. Stiff Neck

[Overview]

It is a simple stiff neck pain with difficult motion. In traditional Chinese medicine, it is in the category of "injury to muscles and tendons". It often occurs in middle-aged and old people. It is spontaneously cured in four to five days if it is a mild condition. However, a severe condition may last for several weeks. Repeated attack of stiff neck usually indicates cervical spondylopathy.

[Cause and Mechanism of Disease]

It is triggered by contraction of wind-cold, which blocks the channels and collaterals, leading to disturbed circulation of qi and blood and the condition.

[Types of Syndromes]

Stiff painful neck, deviation of the head to the affected side with motor impairment, even with the back involved, aggravated by pressure or wind-cold.

[Syndrome Differentiation and Treatment]

Treatment: To disperse cold, unblock channels and stop pain

Point combination 1:

SI 14 (*jiān wài shù*)	BL 10 (*tiān zhù*)	DU 14 (*dà zhuī*)
BL 60 (*kūn lún*)	SI 3 (*hòu xī*)	

Point combination 2: EX-UE8 (*lào zhěn*), GB 39 (*xuán zhōng*)

Secondary points:

Painful neck which fails to move up and down: BL 60 (*kūn lún*), BL 10 (*tiān zhù*)

Painful neck which fails to turn round: SI 3 (*hòu xī*), SI 12 (*bǐng fēng*)

Painful neck with the shoulder involved: GB 21 (*jiān jǐng*), SI 3 (*hòu xī*)

Contraction of Wind-cold: BL 12 (*fēng mén*), GB 20 (*fēng chí*)

Point combination 3: SI 3 (*hòu xī*), GB 20 (*fēng chí*)

Point combination 4: RN 24 (*chéng jiāng*), *Ashi* points

Operation: After routine sterilization, moderate tapping is used. Apply cupping to tender spots after tapping. Treatment is given once a day and five treatments make a course.

[Differential Diagnosis]

Painful neck is also seen in cervical spondylopathy, but usually there is no difficult motion of the neck. It is often accompanied by arm pain, numbness or dizziness. Painful stiff neck impedes its motion. If it often occurs with other symptoms, cervical spondylopathy is suspected. Appropriate examinations may confirm diagnosis.

[Nursing and Prevention]

Avoid contraction of wind-cold during sleep. Choose a pillow of proper height. If stiff neck is triggered by cervical spondylopathy, the primary disease should be treated first.

17. Arthritis

[Overview]

In general, arthritis refers to rheumatic arthritis, rheumatoid arthritis and osteoarthrosis, characterized by pain of joints. In the treatment of gout this section can be referred to. It is called "impediment disease" or "multiple arthritis" in traditional Chinese medicine.

[Cause and Mechanism of Disease]

It is caused by exposure to wind in sweating, rain or walk through water, living in a damp place, or contraction of exogenous wind-cold and dampness, leading to obstruction of the channels and impeded flow of qi and blood. When wind is the chief pathogenic factor, it is called"migratory arthralgia". When cold is the chief pathogenic factor, it is called "agonizing arthralgia". When dampness is the chief pathogenic factor, it is called "detained arthralgia". "Heat arthralgia" occurs in people with excessive yang and contraction of pathogenic cold-dampness, which transforms into heat.

[Types of Syndromes]

Main manifestations: Pain or numbness of the limbs and joints, swollen joints and motion difficulties

(1) Migratory arthralgia: Migratory pain in joints, aversion to wind, preference for warmth, thin white fur, and floating tense pulse.

(2) Agonizing arthralgia: Severe fixed pain in joints, alleviated by warmth and aggravated by cold, with fixed localization, thin white fur, and wiry tense pulse.

(3) Detained arthralgia: Aching pain and heaviness sensation of limbs and joints, or swollen joints, motion difficulties, numbness, pain aggravated on cloudy and wet days, white greasy fur, and soggy slippery pulse.

(4) Heat arthralgia: Burning pain, red swollen joints, hot skin, pain alleviated by cold and aggravated by heat or touch, fever, dry mouth, thirst with a desire for cold drinks, yellow dry fur and rapid slippery pulse.

[Syndrome Differentiation and Treatment]

Treatment: To dissipate wind and cold, clear heat, resolve dampness, unblock channels and stop pain.

Point combination 1:

Lower jaw:

ST 7 (*xià guān*)	ST 6 (*jiá chē*)	SJ 17 (*yì fēng*)
LI 4 (*hé gŭ*)		

Neck:

EX-B2 (*jiá jĭ*)(on the neck)	GB 20 (*fēng chí*)	DU 14 (*dà zhuī*)
BL 10 (*tiān zhù*)	SI 14 (*jiān wài shù*)	LU 7 (*liè quē*)

Shoulder and back:

SI 11 (*tiān zōng*)	SI 12 (*bĭng fēng*)	LI 15 (*jiān yú*)
SJ 14 (*jiān liáo*)	SI 9 (*jiān zhēn*)	LI 16 (*jù gŭ*)

Elbow and arm:

LI 11 (*qŭ chí*)	LI 10 (*shŏu sān lĭ*)	SJ 10 (*tiān jĭng*)
LI 12 (*zhŏu liáo*)	SI 8 (*xiăo hăi*)	SJ 5 (*wài guān*)
LI 4 (*hé gŭ*)		

Wrist:

SJ 4 (*yáng chí*)	LI 5 (*yáng xī*)	SI 4 (*wàn gŭ*)
LI 4 (*hé gŭ*)		

Palms and fingers: EX-UE9 (*bā xié*) (on the dorsum of the hand, between the 2nd and 3rd metacarpal bone, and 0.5 *cun* proximal to the metacarpophalangeal joint)

Fingers: EX-UE6 (*xiǎo gǔ kōng*), EX-UE4 (*zhōng kuí*)

Lumbosacral portion:

EX-B2 (*jiá jǐ*) (on the lower back)	DU 3 (*yāo yáng guān*)	BL 23 (*shèn shù*)
BL 25 (*dà cháng shù*)	BL 32 (*cì liáo*)	

Buttocks:

GB 30 (*huán tiào*)	BL 54 (*zhì biān*)	BL 36 (*chéng fú*)
GB 29 (*jù liáo*)	ST 31 (*bì guān*)	GB 31 (*fēng shì*)

Knees:

EX-LE5 (*nèi xī yǎn*)	ST 35 (*wài xī yǎn*)	ST 34 (*liáng qiū*)
SP 10 (*xuè hǎi*)	GB 34 (*yáng líng quán*)	GB 33 (*xī yáng guān*)
ST 36 (*zú sān lǐ*)	LV 7 (*xī guān*)	BL 40 (*wěi zhōng*)

Ankles:

BL 62 (*shēn mài*)	KI 6 (*zhào hǎi*)	BL 60 (*kūn lún*)
GB 40 (*qiū xū*)	ST 41 (*jiě xī*)	KI 3 (*tài xī*)

Feet and toes:

EX-LE10 (*bā fēng*)	LV 3 (*tài chōng*)	GB 41 (*zú lín qì*)

Secondary points:

Migratory arthralgia:

BL 13 (*fèi shù*)	BL 12 (*fēng mén*)	GB 31 (*fēng shì*)

Agonizing arthralgia:

BL 23 (*shèn shù*)	RN 6 (*qì hǎi*)	DU 4 (*mìng mén*)

Detained arthralgia:

BL 20 (*pí shù*)	SP 9 (*yīn líng quán*)	ST 36 (*zú sān lǐ*)

Heat arthralgia: DU 14 (*dà zhuī*), LI 11 (*qǔ chí*)

Operation: After routine sterilization, moderate tapping is used. Cupping is applied to the tender spots and DU 14 (*dà zhuī*) after tapping, which is especially for heat arthralgia. Treatment is given once a day or every other day and ten treatments make a course.

[Nursing and Prevention]

(1) Do exercise to improve health.

(2) Avoid living in a damp place. Don't sit or lie on damp or cold places.

(3) Keep warm, avoid wind-cold and exposure to wind in sweating and prevent invasion of the body by exogenous pathogenic factors.

18. Cervical Spondylopathy

[Overview]

It is a syndrome of the intervetebral disc disorder and cervical hyperplasia. It's divided into the nerve root type, Barre-Lieou syndrome, vertebral artery type and myeloid form according to the site of the lesion. It is one of the commonly seen diseases in the middle-aged and old people. In traditional Chinese medicine it is in the category of "impediment diseases"," headache" and "dizziness".

[Cause and Mechanism of Disease]

(1) Invasion of the channels by exogenous pathogenic factors: It is due to insuffiicient healthy qi and dysfunction of the muscular striae, leading to diminished defensive qi, invasion of the channels by wind, cold and dampness and stagnation of channel qi and pain.

(2) Qi stagnation and blood stasis: It is due to bending over a desk writing, improper posture of the neck, or trauma and contusion, leading to impeded flow of qi and blood, and pain and numbness.

(3) Liver-kidney yin deficiency: It is due to being worn out with age, or by a prolonged illness that consumes yin essence and marrow, followed by undernourishment of channels. Dizziness, painful neck or numbness of the upper limbs occurs.

(4) Spleen deficiency with dampness retention: It is due to improper diet, that impairs the stomach and spleen and the spleen's function in transportation and transformation, leading to internal accumulation of dampness-phlegm, which suppresses yang ascending, resulting in poor nourishment of the seven orifices, then dizziness and pain occur due to obstruction of channels.

[Types of Syndromes]

Main manifestations: Painful neck, painful or numb shoulder, back, arm and hand, headache, dizziness, or tinnitus, walking haltingly, even paralysis of limbs in severe cases.

(1) Invasion of the channels by exogenous pathogenic factors: Aching pain in the neck, shoulder and arm, motion difficulties of the neck, aggravation by cold or even numbness of the arm, pale-red tongue with thin white fur, and floating pulse.

(2) Impairment of tendons and bones by over-strain, qi stagnation and blood stasis: Constant improper posture of the neck, or trauma of the neck, pain and numbness in the neck, shoulder, even with the forearm and hand involved, aggravation when tired, dark purple tongue or with ecchymosis and rough pulse.

(3) Liver-kidney yin deficiency and undernourishment of tendons and vessels: Painful neck, motion difficulties, numbness and weakness of limbs, accompanied by dizziness, blurred vision, tinnitus, deafness, tidal fever, sweating, aching pain and weakness of the lower back and knees, urinary and fecal incontinence in severe cases, red tongue with little fur and thready pulse.

(4) Spleen deficiency with dampness retention and obstruction of the channels by phlegm-dampness: dizziness, head-binding feeling, oppression in the chest, palpitation, sluggishness, lassitude, somnolence, nausea, vomiting, anorexia, loose stools, white greasy tongue and moderate pulse.

[Syndrome Differentiation and Treatment]

Treatment: To unblock channels and stop pain

Point combination 1:

EX-B2 (*jiá jǐ*) (on the neck)	GB 20 (*fēng chí*)	DU 14 (*dà zhuī*)
LU 7 (*liè quē*)	LI 4 (*hé gǔ*)	

Secondary points:

Wind-cold invasion:

BL 12 (*fēng mén*)	SJ 5 (*wài guān*)	GB 21 (*jiān jǐng*)

Qi stagnation and blood stasis:

GB 21 (*jiān jǐng*)	BL 10 (*tiān zhù*)	BL 17 (*gé shù*)

Liver-kidney yin deficiency:

BL 18 (*gān shù*)	BL 23 (*shèn shù*)	KI 3 (*tài xī*)
SP 6 (*sān yīn jiāo*)		

CHAPTER 2 Treatment

Obstruction of the channels by phlegm-dampness:

ST 40 (*fēng lóng*)	ST 36 (*zú sān lǐ*)	BL 20 (*pí shù*)

Dizziness and vomiting: PC 6 (*nèi guān*), RN 12 (*zhōng wǎn*)
Numb fingers: EX-UE9 (*bā xié*)
Treatment: To soothe the tendons and activate channels
Point combination 2: EX-B2 (*jiá jǐ*) (on the neck)
Secondary points:
Nerve root type:

LI 15 (*jiān yú*)	SJ 14 (*jiān liáo*)	LI 11 (*qū chí*)
SJ 5 (*wài guān*)	SI 6 (*yáng lǎo*)	LI 4 (*hé gǔ*)

Vertebral artery type:

DU 20 (*bǎi huì*)	GB 20 (*fēng chí*)	ST 8 (*tóu wéi*)
EX-HN1 (*sì shén cōng*)		

Myeloid form:

LI 15 (*jiān yú*)	LI 11 (*qū chí*)	SJ 5 (*wài guān*)
GB 30 (*huán tiào*)	GB 39 (*xuán zhōng*)	GB 34 (*yáng líng quán*)

Barre-Lieou syndrome:

RN 17 (*dàn zhōng*)	RN 12 (*zhōng wǎn*)	BL 15 (*xīn shù*)
HT 7 (*shén mén*)	PC 6 (*nèi guān*)	

Point combination 3: DU 14 (*dà zhuī*)
Secondary points:
Painful back: SI 6 (*yǎng lǎo*), SI 3 (*hòu xī*)
Swollen painful neck: LU 7 (*liè quē*), SI 3 (*hòu xī*)
Pain in the tendons of the neck: GB 20 (*fēng chí*), LV 3 (*tài chōng*)
Point combination 4:

DU 14 (*dà zhuī*)	BL 12 (*fēng mén*)	SI 11 (*tiān zōng*)
SI 12 (*bǐng fēng*)	SI 14 (*jiān wài shù*)	SI 15 (*jiān zhōng shù*)

Operation: After routine sterilization, moderate tapping is used. Tapping is applied to the tender spots, followed by cupping. Treatment is given once two to three days and five treatments make a course.

[Nursing and Prevention]

(1) Do not move the head too quickly or too fiercely in patients with cervical spondylopathy.

(2) Give massage to the neck and do therapeutic excercises every day. Do not work over a desk too long, have a rest for a while and move the neck backward or left and right to relieve tiredness of the muscles of the neck.

(3) Adjust the height of pillows. Pillows are not too hard or too soft.

19. Scapulohumeral Periarthritis

[Overview]

It is characterized by shoulder joint pain and motion difficulties. In traditional Chinese medicine it is in the category of "frozen shoulder" or "fifty years old shoulder".

[Cause and Mechanism of Disease]

It is due to being worn out with age, deficiency of healthy qi, dysfunction of the nutrient and defensive aspects and void channels, or to invasion of the body by wind-cold and dampness, leading to obstruction of the channels, or to overstrain and contusion, resulting in qi stagnation and blood stasis and obstruction of the channels, then the condition occurs.

[Types of Syndromes]

Main manifestations: Aching pain and heaviness sensation in one or both shoulder joints, alleviated in daytime and aggravated at night, motion difficulties of joints.

(1) Medial shoulder pain due to disorders of the Spleen Channel: Pain involving the supraclavicular fossa, supine difficulties of the shoulder.

(2) Anterior shoulder pain due to disorders of the Large Intestine Channel: Pain with the elbow and arm involved, abducting and raising difficulties of the shoulder.

(3) Lateral shoulder pain due to disorders of the Sanjiao Channel: Pain with the neck involved, abducting and raising difficulties of the shoulder.

(4) Posterior shoulder pain due to disorders of the Small Intestine Channel: Pain with the back involved, abducting and intorsing difficulties of the shoulder.

[Syndrome Differentiation and Treatment]

Treatment: To dispel wind, dissipate cold, activate channels and stop pain.

Point combination 1:

LI 15 (*jiān yú*)	SJ 14 (*jiān liáo*)	SI 9 (*jiān zhēn*)

Secondary points:

Disorders of the Spleen Channel:

EX-UE (*jiān nèi líng*)	LU 5 (*chǐ zé*)	LU 9 (*tài yuān*)

Disorders of the Large Intestine Channel:

LI 11 (*qū chí*)	LI 10 (*shǒu sān lǐ*)	LI 4 (*hé gǔ*)

Disorders of the *Sanjiao* Channel:

GB 21 (*jiān jǐng*)	SJ 13 (*nào huì*)	SJ 5 (*wài guān*)
GB 34 (*yáng líng quán*)		

Disorders of the Small Intestine Channel:

SI 12 (*bǐng fēng*)	SI 11 (*tiān zōng*)	SI 8 (*xiǎo hái*)
SI 3 (*hòu xī*)		

Excessive wind: GB 20 (*fēng chí*), LV 3 (*tài chōng*)
Excessive cold: ST 36 (*zú sān lǐ*), RN 4 (*guān yuán*)
Excessive dampness: ST 40 (*fēng lóng*), SP 6 (*sān yīn jiāo*)
Point combination 2: ST 38 (*tiáo kǒu*), BL 57 (*chéng shān*)
Point combination 3: *Ashi* points

Operation: After routine sterilization, moderate tapping is used. Tapping is applied to the tender spots followed by cupping. Treatment is given once every two days and ten treatments make a course.

[Nursing and Prevention]

(1) Strengthen activities of the shoulder joints when treatment is given.

(2) If there are sprains or trauma of the shoulder joint, prompt treatment is given.

20. Sciatica

[Overview]

It is characterized by a radiating pain along the pathway of the sciatica nerves. In traditional Chinese medicine, it is in the category of "impediment diseases". Please consult this section in the treatment of prolapse of lumbar intervertebral disc, piriformis syndrome and hyperosteogeny of lumbar vertebrae.

[Cause and Mechanism of Disease]

(1) Contraction of wind-cold: It is caused by contraction of wind-cold, which obstructs the channels, leading to stagnation of channel qi, then there occurs pain of the lower back and leg.

(2) Qi stagnation and blood stasis: It is caused by traumatic injuries, which impair the tendons and vessels, leading to qi stagnation and blood stasis, and obstruction of channels, then pain occurs.

(3) Deficiency of both qi and blood: It is caused by poor health or by over-strain that consumes qi and blood, leading to undernourishment of channels, then the conditon occurs.

[Types of Syndromes]

Main manifestations: Radiating pain in a part of or the whole pathway of the sciatic nerves.

(1) Contraction of wind-cold: Severe pain in the affected lower back and leg, flexion difficulties, scurrying pain along the channel, alleviated by warmth, aggravated by cold and at night, thin white fur, and wiry pulse.

(2) Qi stagnation and blood stasis: Traumatic injury to the lower back, severe stabbing pain in the lower back and leg, aggravated at night, alleviated when active, dark tongue or with ecchymosis, and wiry rough pulse.

(3) Deficiency of both qi and blood: Recurrence of pain in the leg,, aggravated after coughing, sneezing or exertion, alleviated after rest, thin white fur and deep thready pulse.

Syndromes according to the traveling course of channels:

Disorders of the Bladder Channel: Pain radiating from the buttocks to the posterior thigh and leg and the dorsum of the foot.

Disorders of the Gallbladder Channel: Pain radiating from the buttocks to the lateral thigh and leg, the dorsum of the foot and little toe.

[Syndrome Differentiation and Treatment]

Treatment: To soothe the tendons, activate channels, move qi and stop pain.

Point combination 1:

Disorders of the Bladder Channel:

BL 23 (*shèn shù*)	BL 25 (*dà cháng shù*)	BL 54 (*zhì biān*)
BL 40 (*wěi zhōng*)	BL 60 (*kūn lún*)	

Disorders of the Gallbladder Channel:

GB 30 (*huán tiào*)	GB 31 (*fēng shì*)	SP 9 (*yīn líng quán*)
GB 36 (*wài qiū*)	GB 41 (*zú lín qì*)	

Secondary points:

Contraction of Wind-cold:

DU 14 (*dà zhuī*)	BL 12 (*fēng mén*)	DU 3 (*yāo yáng guān*)

Qi stagnation and blood stasis:

LV 3 (*tài chōng*)	SP 10 (*xuè hǎi*)	BL 40 (*wěi zhōng*)

Deficiency of both qi and blood: ST 36 (*zú sān lǐ*), RN 6 (*qì hǎi*)

Point combination 2:

GB 30 (*huán tiào*)	BL 54 (*zhì biān*)	*Ashi* points (on the buttocks)

Operation: After routine sterilization, modreate tapping is used. Tappings are applied to BL 40 (*wěi zhōng*) followed by tapping for qi stagnation and blood stasis. Treatment is given once every two days and ten treatments make a course.

[Nursing and Prevention]

(1) Keep warm and avoid wind-cold.

(2) Define the cause of sciatica and treat the primary disease.

21. Lateral Femoral Neuritis

[Overview]

It is characterized by localized numbness of the lateral thigh, or accompanied by stabbing burning pain and formication. Sometimes there are no subjective symptoms except hot pain and tactile hypoesthesia.

[Cause and Mechanism of Disease]

(1) Contraction of external cold-dampness: It is caused by exposure to wind when sweating, or by residing in a wet place, leading to the condition by obstruction of the channels and impeded circulation of qi and blood, and undernourishment of the skin.

(2) Qi deficiency and blood stasis: Constant qi deficiency may fail to promote blood circulation or traumatic injury impedes qi movement and makes blood stagnate. Consequently, when the skin is not sufficiently nourished, this condition occurs.

[Types of Syndromes]

Main manifestations: Lateral and anterior femoral burning pain, numbness and formication.

(1) Obstruction of the channels by wind-cold: Muscular pain and formication, aggravated by cold, relieved when active, aversion to wind, thin white fur, and floating pulse.

(2) **Obstruction of the channels by dampness:** Muscular numbness and sluggishness, difficult to cure, aggravated on wet days, greasy white fur, and slippery soggy pulse.

(3) **Qi deficiency and blood stasis:** Stabbing fixed pain in muscles, aggravated by over-strain, light tongue with thin and white fur, and thready rough pulse.

[Syndrome Differentiation and Treatment]

Treatment: Replenish qi, activate blood circulation, disperse cold and unblock channels.

Point combination 1:

GB 31 (*fēng shì*)	ST 32 (*fú tù*)	ST 34 (*liáng qiū*)

Secondary points:

Obstruction of the channels by Wind-cold:

GB 20 (*fēng chí*)	BL 12 (*fēng mén*)	LU 7 (*liè quē*)

Obstruction of the channels by dampness:

SP 9 (*yīn líng quán*)	ST 36 (*zú sān lǐ*)	SP 6 (*sān yīn jiāo*)

Qi defiency and blood stasis:

SP 10 (*xuè hǎi*)	BL 17 (*gé shù*)	BL 20 (*pí shù*)
RN 6 (*qì hǎi*)		

Point combination 2: Areas of abnormal sensation

Operation: After routine sterilization, gentle tapping is used for obstruction of the channels by wind-cold, while moderate tapping for obstruction of the channels by dampness. Moderate tapping is applied to the local points, SP 10 (*xuè hǎi*), BL 17 (*gé shù*) in qi deficiecy and blood stasis. For areas of abnormal sensation, collateral-puncturing and cupping are followed after tapping. Treatment is given once every two to three days and ten treatments make a course.

Section 3 Dermatosis

1. Herpes Zoster

[Overview]

It is characterized by severe neuralgic pain along the distribution area of the affected nerve and crops of clustered vesicles over the area of the corresponding dermatome, usually seen in the hypochrondrium, waist and face in spring and autumn due to viral infection.

[Cause and Mechanism of Disease]

(1) Liver-gallbladder retained heat: It is caused by moodiness. Long retained stagnated liver qi turns into fire, which disturbs the liver and gallbladder and accumulates in the muscles, resulting in this condition.

(2) Spleen deficiency with excessive dampness: This condition is caused by deficiency and dampness in the spleen, or improper diet, that impairs the spleen and stomach, or by constant spleen deficiency, leading to dysfunction of spleen's transportation and transformation, and interior production of dampness, which retains and turns into heat to scorch the muscles.

(3) Qi stagnation and blood stasis: This condition is caused by being worn out with age, or insufficiency of healthy qi and excessive dampness-heat, which obstructs the channels and impedes smooth flow of qi and blood.

[Types of Syndromes]

Main manifestations: At the early stage, scattered bright red or dark red patches, itching or painful, subsequently, clusters of vesicles on erythema with burning pain.

(1) Liver-gallbladder retained heat: Herpes mostly seen in the hypochondrium with dark red skin around and burning pain, accompanied by a bitter taste in the mouth, dry throat, headache, dizziness, restlessness, irritability, brown urine, dry stools, red tongue with yellow fur, and wiry rapid pulse.

(2) Spleen deficiency with excessive dampness: Herpes mostly seen on the head, face, chest and abdomen, light red skin, fullness plump vesicles, bloated pain, oozing after eruption, lassitude, fullness in the stomach and abdomen, poor appetite, loose stools, greasy white fur or scanty coating and soggy pulse.

(3) Qi stagnation and blood stasis: Occasionally stabbing and fixed pain after diminition of herpes, dark red tongue with thin white fur, and thready wiry or rough pulse.

[Syndrome Differentiation and Treatment]

(1) Liver-gallbladder retained heat:

Treatment: To clear and purge the liver and gallbladder

Point combination 1:

Ashi points	LV 14 (*qī mén*)	GB 24 (*rì yuè*)
LV 2 (*xíng jiān*)		

Secondary points:

Headache and dizziness: SJ 5 (*wài guān*), GB 20 (*fēng chí*)

(2) Spleen Channel dampness-heat:

Treatment: To clear heat and resolve dampness

Point combination 2:

Ashi points	ST 36 (*zú sān lǐ*)	ST 44 (*nèi tíng*)
SP 6 (*sān yīn jiāo*)	GB 20 (*fēng chí*)	

Secondary points:

Fullness of stomach and abdomen:

ST 21 (*liáng mén*)	RN 12 (*zhōng wǎn*)	ST 20 (*chéng mǎn*)

(3) Qi stagnation and blood stasis

Treatment: To activate blood and resolve stasis

Point Combination 3:

Ashi points	LI 4 (*hé gǔ*)	LV 3 (*tài chōng*)
BL 17 (*gé shù*)	EX-B2 (*jiá jǐ*) (the corresponding part of the lesion)	

Point combination 4:

LI 4 (*hé gǔ*)	SJ 6 (*zhī gōu*)	GB 34 (*yáng líng quán*)
The regions around the lesion		

Point combination 5: EX-B2 (*jiá jǐ*) (the region around the lesion); bilateral LI 4 (*hé gǔ*), LI 11 (*qǔ chí*), SJ 5 (*wài guān*) when the lesion is above the waist, or homolateral LV 3 (*tài chōng*), GB 43 (*xiá xī*), ST 36 (*zú sān lǐ*) when the lesion is below the waist; GB 2 (*tīng huì*), EX-HN5 (*tài yáng*), BL 2 (*cuán zhú*) when the lesion is on the distribution area of the trigeminal nerve.

Operation: After routine sterilization, moderate tapping is used once a day or every two days and ten treatments make a course.

[Nursing and Prevention]

(1) Avoid seafood, beef and mutton, spicy food, eat more vegetables and fruits during the course of the disease.

(2) Keep the skin clean after eruptions of herpes to avoid inflammation.

2. Urticaria

[Overview]

It is a common allergic dermatosis characterized by sudden localized edema with intense itching. An acute case has short duration but a chronic case has repeatedly attacks.

[Cause and Mechanism of Disease]

(1) Invasion of the body by external wind: It is due to insufficient healthy qi, or to insecurity of the defensive aspect, affliction from wind-heat or wind-cold, which resides in the skin and obstructs the channels, then the condition occurs.

(2) Dampness-heat of Intestines and stomach: It is due to poor born gifts, preference for greasy and sweet food or to intestinal roundworms or hookworms, which leads to disharmony between the spleen and stomach and engenders dampness-heat. Retained dampness-heat scorches the skin, resulting in the condition.

(3) Deficiency of both qi and blood: It is due to obstinate disease, which consumes qi and blood, or to constant spleen deficiency and stomach, which fails to produce enough qi. Wind is stirred up from deficiency of blood, followed by this condition.

(4) Disorder of the Thoroughfare Vessel and *Ren* Vessel: It is due to excitation of the seven emotions that impairs blood and causes liver-kidney yin deficiency, generation of dryness and wind. When the skin is disturbed by them, the condition occurs.

[Types of Syndromes]

(1) Wind-heat: Red wheals, itching and hot, aggravated by heat, relieved by cold, or aggravated in summer and relieved in winter, hot sensation, thin yellow fur, and floating rapid pulse.

(2) Wind-cold: Pale wheals, itching, aggravated by cold and wind, relieved by heat, aggravated in winter and relieved in summer, thin white fur, and floating tight pulse.

(3) Dampness-heat of intestine and stomach: Red higher wheals, bloated itching, aggravated by eating seafood, accompanied by fullness and distension in the abdomen, nausea and vomiting, constipation, diarrhea, yellow greasy fur,and slippery rapid pulse.

(4) Deficiency of both qi and blood: Repeated attack by wheals, itching, onset when tired and aggravated by overworking, pale complexion, lassitude, dizziness, insomnia, bloated abdomen, anorexia, pale red tongue with thin fur, and thready weak pulse.

(5) Disharmony between the Thoroughfare Vessel and *Ren* Vessel: Wheals appearing several days before the menstrual cycle, itching, disappearing in the end of menstruation, accompanied by menstrual irregularity or dysmenorrhea, pale tongue with scanty fur, and thready weak pulse.

[Syndrome Differentiation and Treatment]

Treatment: To disperse cold, release the exterior, clear heat, resolve dampness, replenish qi and nourish blood.

Point combination 1:

SP 10 (*xuè hǎi*)	SP 6 (*sān yīn jiāo*)	LI 11 (*qū chí*)
LI 4 (*hé gǔ*)		

Secondary points:

Wind-heat:

DU 14 (*dà zhuī*)	LU 5 (*chǐ zé*)	LI 5 (*yáng xī*)

Wind-cold: BL 13 (*fèi shù*), BL 12 (*fēng mén*)

Dampness-heat of intestine and stomach:

ST 44 (*nèi tíng*)	LI 2 (*èr jiān*)	ST 25 (*tiān shū*)
RN 12 (*zhōng wǎn*)		

Deficiency of both qi and blood: RN 6 (*qì hǎi*), ST 36 (*zú sān lǐ*)

Disharmony between the Thoroughfare Vessel and *Ren* Vessel:

RN 4 (*guān yuán*)	BL 32 (*cì liáo*)	BL 23 (*shèn shù*)

Point combination 2:

Upper body: LI 11 (*qū chí*), PC 6 (*nèi guān*)

Lower body:

SP 10 (*xuè hǎi*)	ST 36 (*zú sān lǐ*)	SP 6 (*sān yīn jiāo*)

Whole body:

GB 31 (*fēng shì*)	GB 20 (*fēng chí*)	ST 25 (*tiān shū*)
BL 25 (*dà cháng shù*)		

Point combination 3:

SI 3 (*hòu xī*)	LI 11 (*qŭ chí*)	ST 36 (*zú sān lĭ*)

Point combination 4:

DU 14 (*dà zhuī*)	SJ 10 (*tiān jĭng*)	SP 10 (*xuè hăi*)
GB 39 (*xuán zhōng*)	LI 11 (*qŭ chí*)	PC 3 (*qŭ zé*)
BL 40 (*wĕi zhōng*)		

(for obstinate urticaria)

Operation: After routine sterilization, moderate tapping is used for dampness-heat in the intestine and stomach, while gentle tapping for wind-heat, wind-cold and deficiency of qi and blood. Treatment is given once a day or every two days and ten treatments make a course.

[Nursing and Prevention]

(1) Do not eat seafood and greasy food when it attacks to avoid deterioration.

(2) Patients having repeated attacks should avoid wind while sweating. Do not have food or drugs that induce the illness.

(3) Emergency measures are taken when dyspnea presents.

(4) Do exercise to build up health. Pay attention to weather change.

3. Neurodermatitis

[Overview]

It is a chronic dermatosis, characterized by itching and thick hard skin. The lesion is in patches formed by flat pimples in round or poly shape. After scratching the skin becomes thicker with deepening sulci, and the skin is prone to lichenification. As the affected skin feels like oxhide, in traditional Chinese medicine it is called "oxhide tinea", or "cervical sore". Since it is difficult to cure, it is also known as "obstinate tinea".

[Cause and Mechanism of Disease]

(1) Wind-dampness-heat: It is caused by exogenous wind, dampness and heat, which reside in the skin, or by profuse sweating around the neck, which impedes smooth circulation of qi and blood, and triggers malnutrition of the skin.

(2) Hyperactivity of liver fire: It is caused by moodiness or stress, or tiredness, leading to stagnation of liver qi and generation of fire. When qi and blood flow is impeded, the condition occurs.

(3) Blood deficiency with wind-dryness: It is caused by chronic disease, which consumes yin and blood, or by hyperactivity of heart and liver fire that impairs yin and blood too. Insufficient blood triggers wind-dryness and malnutrition of the skin, finally, this condition.

[Types of Syndromes]

Main manifestations: Itching of the skin, flat round and polymorphic lesions into patches in a longer period, growing thickening of the skin as hard as oxhide.

(1) Wind-dampness-heat: Red eruptions, wet or scab formation after scratching, thirst without a desire for drinks, red tongue with thin yellow or yellow greasy fur, and slippery or slippery rapid pulse.

(2) Hyperactivity of liver fire: Red skin lesions, irritability, fullness in the chest and hypochondrium, bitter taste in the mouth, dry throat, dizziness, insomnia, red tongue edge, thin yellow fur, and wiry rapid or rapid pulse.

(3) Blood deficiency with wind-dryness: Long disease course, pale red eruptions as hard as oxhide, or restlessness, insomnia, thin pale light red or red tongue with thin white fur, and thready pulse.

[Syndrome Differentiation and Treatment]

Treatment: To disperse wind, clear heat, nourish blood, remove dryness, and purge fire.

Point combination 1:

DU 14 (*dà zhuī*)	LI 11 (*qū chí*)	SP 10 (*xuè hǎi*)
LU 5 (*chǐ zé*)		

Secondary points:

Wind-dampness-heat:

GB 20 (*fēng chí*)	BL 12 (*fēng mén*)	SP 9 (*yīn líng quán*)

Hyperactivity of liver fire:

LV 2 (*xíng jiān*)	GB 43 (*xiá xī*)	DU 14 (*dà zhuī*)

Blood deficiency with wind-dryness:

ST 36 (*zú sān lǐ*)	SP 6 (*sān yīn jiāo*)	BL 20 (*pí shù*)
BL 21 (*wèi shù*)		

Operation: After routine sterilization, moderate tapping is used for the excess syndrome. Collatral-puncturing is applied to DU 14 (*dà zhuī*), LV 2 (*xíng jiān*) after tapping. Gentle tapping is used for the deficiency syndrome. Treatment is given once every two to three days and 10 treatments make a course.

Point combination 2:

Head, face and neck:

Tender spots on both sides of the neck and cords of the lesion, affected areas	PC 6 (*nèi guān*)	LI 11 (*qŭ chí*)
LU 9 (*tài yuān*)	LI 4 (*hé gŭ*)	

Point combination 3:

Dermatitis of the upper limbs:

Tender spots between the 4th vertical vertebra to the 5th thoracic vertebra and cords of the lesion, affected areas	PC 6 (*nèi guān*)	LI 11 (*qŭ chí*)
BL 13 (*fèi shù*)	BL 15 (*xīn shù*)	

Point combination 4:

Dermatitis of the lower limbs:

Cords in the lumbosacral region and vesicular masses of the lesion, affected areas	SP 10 (*xuè hăi*)	ST 36 (*zú sān lĭ*)
BL 23 (*shèn shù*)		

Point Combination 5:

Dermatitis of the abdominal and perineal region:

Both sides of the 10th to 12th thoracic vertebrae	Tender spots of the lumbo-sacral region and cords of the lesion, affected areas	BL 20 (*pí shù*)
BL 23 (*shèn shù*)	RN 4 (*guān yuán*)	SP 6 (*sān yīn jiāo*)
ST 36 (*zú sān lĭ*)		

Operation: After routine sterilization, tapping is applied with different manipulations to the regions and points according to the physique condition once every two days and fifteen treatments make a course.

[Nursing and Prevention]

(1) Adjust the mental state and avoid stress and lassitude. Have enough sleep.

(2) Avoid wearing any clothes which are allergic to skin.

(3) Do not scratch and wash the lesion in hot water.

4. Psoriasis

[Overview]

It is a chronic recurrent dermatosis, characterized by repeated presence of multilayer silver dry scales or desquamation by scratching.

[Cause and Mechanism of Disease]

(1) Blood heat: It is caused by moodiness and stagnation of liver qi and generation of fire when it lasts for days, or by eating too much spicy food, leading to interior excessive fire, which disturbs blood and scorches the skin, then the condition occurs.

(2) Blood stasis: It is caused by deficiency of qi and blood from poor health. Qi fails to move actively, followed by unsmooth flow of blood, resulting in blood stasis. When it resides in the skin, the condition occurs.

(3) Blood dryness: It is caused by a chronic disease, which consumes qi and blood, or by poor born gifts, leading to deficiency of essence and blood. Dryness and wind are triggered, resulting in malnutrition of the skin and the condition.

(4) Disharmony of the Thoroughfare Vessel and *Ren* Vessel: This condition is caused by disorder of the Thoroughfare Vessel and *Ren* Vessel, and deficiency in the liver and kidney, leading to disharmony of the nutrient and blood aspects.

[Types of Syndromes]

Main manifestations: Multilayer silver dry scales, repeated attack, desquamation with scratching, pine-bark lesion, itching.

(1) Blood heat: Sudden attack, general eruptions, flush red in color, excessive scales, itching, bleeding after scratching, bright red in color, restlessness, irritability, dry stools, brown urine, red or dark red tongue with thin yellow fur, and wiry rapid or slippery rapid pulse.

(2) Blood stasis: Unhealed eruptions, dark red in color, or pain in joints, or pustules (aseptic), dark red tongue with ecchymosis, and rough or wiry pulse.

(3) Blood dryness: Diminished red lesion, less scales adhered tightly to the skin, pale red tongue with wiry greasy or greasy rapid pulse.

(4) Disharmony of the Thoroughfare Vessel and *Ren* Vessel: Change of the lesion related to the menstrual cycle or pregnancy, accompanied by menatrual irregularity or dysmenorrhea, pale red tongue with thin or scanty fur and

thready pulse.

[Syndrome Differentiation and Treatment]

Treatment: To cool blood and activate blood,circulation, remove dryness and stop itching.

Point combination 1:

SP 10 (*xuè hǎi*)	LI 11 (*qǔ chí*)	BL 13 (*fèi shù*)

Secondary points:

Blood heat:

DU 14 (*dà zhuī*)	LV 2 (*xíng jiān*)	ST 44 (*nèi tíng*)
LU 10 (*yú jì*)		

Blood dryness:

SP 6 (*sān yīn jiāo*)	ST 36 (*zú sān lǐ*)	GB 31 (*fēng shì*)
GB 20 (*fēng chí*)		

Blood stasis:

BL 17 (*gé shù*)	LV 3 (*tài chōng*)	LI 4 (*hé gǔ*)

Disharmony of the Thoroughfare Vessel and *Ren* Vessel:

SP 6 (*sān yīn jiāo*)	RN 3 (*zhōng jí*)	BL 26 (*guān yuán shù*)
BL 32 (*cì liáo*)		

Pustules:

SP 9 (*yīn líng quán*)	SP 6 (*sān yīn jiāo*)	PC 7 (*dà líng*)

Operation: After routine sterilization, moderate tapping is used. Tapping is applied to DU 14 (*dà zhuī*), BL 13 (*fèi shù*), BL 17 (*gé shù*) followed by cupping. Treatment is given once every two to three days and fifteen treatments make a course.

Point combination 2:

DU 14 (*dà zhuī*)	DU 13 (*táo dào*)	BL 18 (*gān shù*)
BL 20 (*pí shù*)	EX-B2 (*jiá jǐ*) from the 5th to 6th thoracic vertebra	EX-B2 (*jiá jǐ*) from the 1st to the 2nd lumbar vertebra

Point combination 3:

Lesion on the upper limbs, head and face:

LI 11 (*qŭ chí*)	SJ 6 (*zhī gōu*)	GB 20 (*fēng chí*)
LI 4 (*hé gŭ*)		

Secondary points: SP 10 (*xuè hăi*), SP 6 (*sān yīn jiāo*)

Lesion mostly on the face:

LI 20 (*yíng xiāng*)	ST 2 (*sì bái*)	SI 18 (*quán liáo*)

Lesion on the lower limbs:

SP 10 (*xuè hăi*)	SP 6 (*sān yīn jiāo*)	ST 36 (*zú sān lĭ*)

Secondary points: SJ 6 (*zhī gōu*), LI 11 (*qŭ chí*)

General lesion:

DU 14 (*dà zhuī*)	LI 11 (*qŭ chí*)	LI 4 (*hé gŭ*)
SP 10 (*xuè hăi*)	SP 6 (*sān yīn jiāo*)	

Operation: After routine sterilization, moderate tapping is used once every two to three days and fifteen treatments make a course.

[Nursing and Prevention]

(1) Have light meals, vegetables and fruits and do not eat spicy and irritating food.

(2) Keep a good mood and avoid stress.

5. Eczema

[Overview]

It is an allegic inflammatory dermatosis, divided into 3 groups, ie. acute, chronic and subacute eczema. It is characterized by polymorphic lesions, symmetric distribution, itching, repeated attack, easy to evolve to a chronic case.

[Cause and Mechanism of Disease]

(1) Dampness-heat immersion: It is caused by poor born gifts, improper diet, eating too much spicy and greasy food or liquor dependence, that impair the spleen and stomach, resulting in disturbed transportation and transformation, and interior generation of dampness-heat, accompanied by affliction from external wind. When the pathogenic factors reside in the skin, the condition occurs.

(2) Spleen deficiency and excessive dampness: It is caused by spleen deficiency, or over-strain and anxiety, which impairs the spleen and stomach and disturbs its transportation. When interiorly retained dampness attacks the skin and obstructs channels, the condition occurs.

(3) Blood deficiency with wind-dryness: It is caused by a chronic disease, that consumes yin and blood, or by kidney deficiency in the aged people, leading to deficiency of essence and blood, and stirring up of wind and malnutrition of the skin, then the condition occurs.

[Types of Syndromes]

(1) Dampness-heat immersion: Acute onset, symmetrical lesion, flush skin, small pimples, herpes and blister patches, extreme itching, oozing after scratching, erosion and scab, restlessness, thirst, brown urine, difficult bowels movement, red moist tongue with yellow greasy fur, and slippery rapid pulse.

(2) Spleen deficiency and excessive dampness: Long disease course, pale lesion, swelling and oozing relieved gradually, scaling, extreme itching, erosion, oozing and scabbing after scratching, accompanied by sluggishness, tastelessness in the mouth, anorexia, loose stools, tooth marks on the edge of an enlarged tongue with white greasy or thick greasy fur,and slow soggy pulse.

(3) Blood deficiency with wind-dryness: Repeated attack, long disease course, dark red or brown lesion, episodic itching, thickening skin, unsmooth surface, or chapping, scaling, lusterless complexion, dizziness, insomnia, pale red tongue with thin white fur, and thready weak pulse.

[Syndrome Differentiation and Treatment]

Treatment: To clear dampness-heat, nourish blood, remove dryness, extinguish wind and stop itching.

Point combination 1:

SP 6 (*sān yīn jiāo*)	ST 36 (*zú sān lǐ*)	SP 10 (*xuè hǎi*)

Secondary points:

Dampness-heat immmersion:

LI 11 (*qǔ chí*)	ST 44 (*nèi tíng*)	SP 9 (*yīn líng quán*)

Spleen deficiency and excessive dampness:

BL 20 (*pí shù*)	BL 21 (*wèi shù*)	RN 12 (*zhōng wǎn*)
GB 20 (*fēng chí*)		

Blood deficiency with wind-dryness:

BL 18 (*gān shù*)	BL 17 (*gé shù*)	LV 3 (*tài chōng*)
KI 3 (*tài xī*)		

Point combination 2: SP 10 (*xuè hǎi*), SP 6 (*sān yīn jiāo*)

Secondary points:

Eczema on the face:

SI 18 (*quán liáo*)	ST 4 (*dì cāng*)	ST 2 (*sì bái*)
ST 7 (*xià guān*)	ST 6 (*jiá chē*)	LI 4 (*hé gǔ*)
ST 41 (*jiě xī*)		

Eczema on the ear:

SJ 17 (*yì fēng*)	SI 19 (*tīng gōng*)	SJ 20 (*jiǎo sūn*)
SJ 5 (*wài guān*)	GB 40 (*qiū xū*)	

Eczema around the umbilicus:

ST 25 (*tiān shū*)	SP 15 (*dà héng*)	ST 26 (*wài líng*)
ST 36 (*zú sān lǐ*)		

Eczema on the hand:

SJ 4 (*yáng chí*)	LI 4 (*hé gǔ*)	SJ 5 (*wài guān*)
SI 5 (*yáng gǔ*)		

Eczema on the scrotum:

RN 2 (*qū gǔ*)	LV 10 (*zú wǔ lǐ*)	LV 3 (*tài chōng*)
LV 5 (*lǐ gōu*)		

Eczema on the leg:

BL 40 (*wěi zhōng*)	GB 34 (*yáng líng quán*)	ST 37 (*shàng jù xū*)
BL 59 (*fū yáng*)	ST 44 (*nèi tíng*)	

Operation: After routine sterilization, moderate tapping is used for the excess syndrome, while gentle tapping for the deficiency syndrome. If the points are located at the lesion, other points are selected. Treatment is given once every two to three days and fifteen treatments make a course.

[Nursing and Prevention]

(1) Never wash the lesion in an acute case with hot water or other irritating agents.

(2) Never scratch the lesion and avoid spicy greasy foods or seafood.

6. Albinism

[Overview]

It is caused by skin depigment, characterized by white patches on the skin without any subjective symptoms.

[Cause and Mechanism of Disease]

(1) Qi stagnation and blood stasis: This condition is caused by affliction from external wind-cold, which resides in the striated layer and obstructs the channels, or by stagnation of liver qi and unsmooth circulation of qi and blood, leading to blood stasis and malnutrition of the skin.

(2) Deficiency of essence and blood: This condition is caused by poor born gifts, or by a chronic disease, that consumes essence and blood, leading to deficiency of blood and malnutrition of the skin.

[Types of Syndromes]

Main manifestations: White patches on the skin with no subjective symptoms.

(1) Qi stagnation and blood stasis: White or light yellow lesion in the shape of spots or patches with unclear boundary, and a brown belt seen between the lesions and normal skin, scattered white patches, accompanied by distending pain in the chest and hypochondriac region, irascibility, dark red tongue or with ecchmosis, white fur and wiry pulse, or mental stress history with a short disease course.

(2) Deficiency of essence and blood: Pure white patches with clear boundary, accompanied by aching pain and weakness of the lower back and knees, dizziness, tinnitus, pale red tongue with thin white fur and deep thready pulse or family history with a long disease course.

[Syndrome Differentiation and Treatment]

Treatment: To move qi, activate blood circulation, nourish essence and blood.

Point combination 1:

LU 4 (*xiá bái*)	SP 10 (*xuè hǎi*)	SP 6 (*sān yīn jiāo*)
BL 13 (*fèi shù*)		

Secondary points:

Qi stagnation and blood stasis:

LI 4 (*hé gǔ*)	LV 3 (*tài chōng*)	BL 17 (*gé shù*)

Deficiency of essence and blood:

ST 36 (*zú sān lǐ*)	KI 3 (*tài xī*)	BL 20 (*pí shù*)
RN 6 (*qì hǎi*)		

Operation: After routine sterilization, moderate tapping is used for qi stagnation and blood stasis. Cupping is followed after tapping applied to BL 13 (*fèi shù*), BL 17 (*gé shù*) and LU 4 (*xiá bái*). Gentle tapping is used for deficiency of essence and blood. Treatment is given once every two to three days and ten treatments make a course.

Point combination 2: EX-UE (*xiá xià*) (on the lateral border of the biceps brachii muscle, slightly above the junction 1/3 from the middle and lower of the muscle), EX-UE (*diān fēng*) (on the lower border of the ventral side of the middle finger at the metacarpo-phalangeal joint, slightly above the cross striation of the joint)

Operation: After routine sterilization, tapping is applied until bleeding once a week. The two sides are alternately selected.

Point combination 3: Lesion in the lumbosacral region and relevant spinal segment (only for deficiency of qi and blood)

Operation: Tapping is applied once a day with a plum-blossom needle. After five treatments, an electro-plum-blossom needle is used with the application of 30% Extract of *Fructus Psoraleae* in the evening to the lesion.

Point combination 4: the lesion, LU 4 (*xiá bái*)

Operation: After routine sterilization, moderate tapping is applied to LU 4 (*xiá bái*) until presence of flush skin, followed by moxibustion. Each time select two to three white patches points and moderate tapping is applied to them until the skin becomes flushed. Treatment is given once every two to three days and ten treatments make a course.

7. Cutaneous Pruritus

[Overview]

It is a dermatosis having no primary skin injuries yet with abnormal sensation of the skin, characterized by paroxysmal itching, nail marks, bloody scab, stain or lickenification after scratching.

[Cause and Mechanism of Disease]

(1) External affliction from wind-heat: It is caused by constant excessive yang of the body. When wind-heat resides in the muscles, the condition occurs.

(2) Interior retention of dampness-heat: It is caused by improper diet, and eating too much greasy sweet food, which impair the spleen and stomach and disturb their normal transportation and transformation. Long retained dampness turns to heat and scorches the skin, causing occurrence of the condition.

(3) Blood deficiency with wind-dryness: This condition is caused by a chronic disease, which consumes qi and blood, resulting in stagnated blood in the muscles, or by innate insufficiency in the liver and kidney, and deficiency of blood, which triggers wind and dryness and malnutrition of the skin.

[Types of Syndromes]

(1) External affliction from wind-heat: Severe itching, relieved by cold, aggravated by heat, bloody scabs after scratching, restlessness, thirst, brown urine, constipation, thin yellow fur, and floating rapid pulse.

(2) Interior retention of dampness-heat: Skin itching, oozing after scratching, bitter taste in the mouth and dry throat, fullness in the abdomen, difficult bowels movement, red tongue with yellow greasy fur, and slippery rapid pulse.

(3) Blood deficiency with wind-dryness: Unhealed skin itching, worse at night, dry skin, nail marks after scratching, dizziness, tinnitus, restlessness, night sweating, red tongue with thin fur, and thready or thready rapid pulse.

[Syndrome Differentiation and Treatment]

Treatment: To disperse wind, clear heat, remove dampness, nourish blood and eliminate dryness.

Point Combination: SP 10 (*xuè hǎi*), SP 6 (*sān yīn jiāo*)

Secondary points:

External affliction from wind-heat:

DU 14 (*dà zhuī*)	BL 12 (*fēng mén*)	LI 11 (*qū chí*)
LU 5 (*chǐ zé*)		

Interior retention of dampness-heat:

ST 44 (*nèi tíng*)	SP 9 (*yīn líng quán*)	ST 36 (*zú sān lǐ*)
RN 12 (*zhōng wǎn*)	GB 31 (*fēng shì*)	

皮肤针疗法

DERMAL NEEDLING THERAPY

Blood deficiency with wind-dryness:

LV 3 (*tài chōng*)	LV 8 (*qŭ quán*)	KI 3 (*tài xī*)
RN 6 (*qì hăi*)		

Operation: After routine sterilization, moderate tapping is used for affliction from wind-heat and interior retention of dampness-heat. Cupping is followed after tapping applied to DU 14 (*dà zhuī*) and BL 12 (*fēng mén*). Gentle tapping is used for blood deficiency with wind-dryness. Treatment is given once every two to three days and fifteen treatments make a course.

[Nursing and Prevention]

(1) Cease liquor intake and eat less seafood. Have more vegetables, fruits and a light diet.

(2) Wear loose cotton or silk underwears. Do not wear wool clothes.

(3) Never scratch, rub and wash the lesion with hot water. Do not use alkaline washing agents to avoid irritations to the skin.

8. Acne

[Overview]

It is a chronic inflammatory disorder characterized by pilosebaceous pimples on the face, chest and back, mostly seen in young males and females. White substances present when squeezed.

[Cause and Mechanism of Disease]

(1) Hyperactivity of fire in the lung and stomach: It is caused by too much yang and heat of the body, or by overeating spicy food, leading to heat retained in the lung and stomach. When dry-heat goes along the channel and resides in the skin, the condition occurs.

(2) Damp-heat in the spleen and stomach: It is caused by overeating greasy sweet food, or by improper diet, which impairs the spleen and stomach and disturbs their normal transportation and transformation. Phlegm engenders from dampness and when it retains for days it turns to heat. The skin is scorches by them,causing the condition.

(3) Disorder of the Thoroughfare Vessel and *Ren* Vessel: This condition is caused by disorder of the Thoroughfare Vessel and *Ren* Vessel, stagnation of liver qi, leading to unsmooth flow of qi and dysfunction of the skin.

(4) Phlegm-dampness: It is caused by constant insufficiency in the spleen or improper diet, fatigue and anxiety, which impair the spleen and stomach and trigger disturbed transportation of the spleen. When dampness-phlegm gathers under the skin, the condition occurs.

[Types of Syndromes]

Main manifestations: Pimples on the face, chest and back, presence of white substances when squeezed, or pus on the top of a pimple.

(1) Hyperactivity of fire in the lung and stomach: Flushed face, bright red hard pimples with burning pain, or pustules, aversion to heat, dry throat, thirst, preference for cold drinks, brown urine, dry stools, red tongue with thin yellow fur, and rapid pulse.

(2) Damp-heat in the spleen and stomach: Oily face, red, swollen and painful eruptions or pustules, tubercles, anorexia, bloated abdomen, foul breath, difficult bowels movement, yellow greasy fur, and slippery rapid pulse.

(3) Disorder of the Thoroughfare Vessel and *Ren* Vessel: Periodical change of the condition, aggravated and relieved according to menstrual cycle, usually accompanied by menstrual irregularity, dysmenorrhea, pale red tongue with thin yellow fur and wiry pulse.

(4) Phlegm-dampness: Cyst formation, tubercles, poor appetite, lassitude, loose stools, enlarged tongue with tooth marks on its edge, white greasy fur, and soggy slow pulse.

[Syndrome Differentiation and Treatment]

Treatment: To disperse wind, clear heat, remove dampness and regulate the Thoroughfare Vessel and *Ren* Vessel.

Point combination 1:

EX-HN3 (*yìn táng*) (supranasal point)	LI 4 (*hé gŭ*)	SP 10 (*xuè hăi*)
SP 6 (*sān yīn jiāo*)		

Secondary points:

Wind-heat in the Lung Channel:

LU 5 (*chĭ zé*)	LU 10 (*yú jì*)	SJ 5 (*wài guān*)
DU 16 (*fēng fŭ*)		

Dampness-heat in the spleen and stomach:

ST 44 (*nèi tíng*)	ST 40 (*fēng lóng*)	RN 12 (*zhōng wăn*)
SP 9 (*yīn líng quán*)		

Disoder of the Thoroughfare Vessel and *Ren* Vessel:

LV 3 (*tài chōng*)	RN 6 (*qì hăi*)	SP 4 (*gōng sūn*)
KI 3 (*tài xī*)		

Phlegm-dampness:

ST 36 (*zú sān lĭ*)	RN 12 (*zhōng wăn*)	ST 25 (*tiān shū*)
ST 27 (*shàng jù xū*)		

Point combination 2:

ST 7 (*xià guān*)	ST 6 (*jiá chē*)	BL 2 (*cuán zhú*)
ST 36 (*zú sān lĭ*)	LI 4 (*hé gŭ*)	ST 40 (*fēng lóng*)
EX-CA (*guān xià*) (0.5 *cun* under RN 4 (*guān yuán*)	EX-CA (*líng gōng*) (2.5 *cun* lateral to EX-CA (*guān xià*)	SP 6 (*sān yīn jiāo*)

Point combination 3:

LI 4 (*hé gŭ*)	SI 3 (*hòu xī*)	PC 8 (*láo gōng*)

Point combination 4: Between the scapulas, seek the reactive spots close to the first lateral line of the Bladder Channel (as large as a head acupuncture top, grey in color, like a pimple often with a pilus)

Operation: After routine sterilization, moderate tapping is used once every two to three days and fifteen treatments make a course.

[Differential Dignosis]

(1) Rosacea is mostly seen in middle-aged people with the lesion on the nose, sometimes in the cheeks and forehead but no other portions are involved. The lesion is flush, congestive, usually accompanied by capillary hyperplasia, but without blaco-headed comedo.

(2) Occupational acne occurs in workers who contact coal tar, paraffin wax or engine oil. It is characterized by concentrated lesion, accompanied by follicular kerotosis, found on the face, dorsum of the hands, elbows and knees.

[Nursing and Prevention]

(1) Have a light diet, more vegetables and fruits and less spicy and irritating food.

(2) Keep a good mood and avoid worry beyond measure.

(3) Never squeeze the eruptions.

(4) Keep free bowels movement.

9. Chloasma

[Overview]

It is mainly seen on the face of women in pregnancy and menopause. There are no subjective symptoms. It is triggered by pigmentation due to estrin and progesterone in terms of Western medicine.

[Cause and Mechanism of Disease]

(1) Qi stagnation and blood stasis: This condition is caused by qi stagnation and blood stasis or moodiness, or long-term stress, leading to stagnation of liver qi and blood stasis, which obstructs the channels.

(2) Qi deficiency and blood stasis: It is caused by innate spleen deficiency, which impedes production of qi and blood, or by a chronic disease, which consumes qi and blood and triggers malnutrition of the skin, then the condition occurs.

(3) Deficiency of liver and kidney: It is caused by deficiency in the liver and kidney in aged people, or by indulgence in sexual activities and a chronic disease, which impair the kidney. Deficiency of essence, blood and undernourishment of the skin leads to the condition.

[Types of Syndromes]

Main manifestations: Smooth patches of pigmentation in different size on the face, mostly distributed on cheeks or around the eyes and mouth, absence of subjective symptoms.

(1) Qi stagnation and blood stasis: Tan and dim patches on the face, or fullness in the hypochondrium, irritability, depression, or too much stress or fatigue, dim lips and tongue with thin white fur, and wiry rough pulse.

(2) Deficiency of qi and blood: Yellowish brown or light yellow patches on the face, lassitude, weakness of limbs, insomnia, dream-disturbed sleep, poor appetite, loose stools, pale red tongue or with tooth marks on its edge, thin white fur, and deep thready pulse.

(3) Liver-kidney yin deficiency: Darkish complexion, dark brown patches, aching pain and weakness in the lower back and knees, dizziness, tinnitus, tidal fever, night sweating, red tender-soft tongue with scanty fur or no coating, and deep thready or thready rapid pulse.

[Syndrome Differentiation and Treatment]

Treatment: To nourish yin and blood, resolve blood stasis and expel chloasma.

Point combination 1: Lesion, LI 4 (*hé gǔ*)

Secondary points:

Qi stagnation and blood stasis:

LV 3 (*tài chōng*)	LV 14 (*qī mén*)	SP 6 (*sān yīn jiāo*)
BL 17 (*gé shù*)		

Deficiency of qi and blood:

ST 36 (*zú sān lǐ*)	RN 6 (*qì hǎi*)	BL 20 (*pí shù*)
BL 21 (*wèi shù*)		

Liver-kidney yin deficiency:

KI 3 (*tài xī*)	KI 10 (*yīn gǔ*)	BL 18 (*gān shù*)
BL 23 (*shèn shù*)		

Point combination 2:

GB 14 (*yáng bái*)	EX-HN5 (*tài yáng*)	SI 18 (*quán liáo*)
BL 20 (*pí shù*)	BL 23 (*shèn shù*)	BL 18 (*gān shù*)
SP 6 (*sān yīn jiāo*)		

Secondary points:

Qi stagnation and blood stasis: SP 10 (*xuè hǎi*)

Kidney deficiency: KI 3 (*tài xī*)

Operation: After routine sterilization, gentle tapping is used for the deficiency syndrome, while moderate tapping for the excess syndrome. Tapping is applied to the lesion till it turns to red. Cupping is applied to BL 17 (*gé shù*) after tapping. Treatment is given once every two to three days and ten treatments make a course.

[Nursing and Prevention]

(1) Keep a good mood and avoid stress and fatigue. Lead a regular life and have enough sleep.

(2) Choose right cosmetics and avoid long exposure to sunlight.

10. Baldness

[Overview]

It refers to alopecia or total alopecia. It is in the category of alopecia due to oil and wind in traditional Chinese medicine.

[Cause and Mechanism of Disease]

(1) Blood deficiency with wind-dryness: This condition is caused by a chronic or serious illness, which consumes qi and blood, or by deficiency of blood and malnutrition of the hair.

(2) Qi stagnation and blood stasis: It is caused by moodiness, or long-term stress, leading to stagnation of liver qi, *or* traumatic injury, resulting in impeded flow of qi and blood from blood stasis. When the hair is undernourished, the condition occurs.

[Types of Syndromes]

Main manifestations: Sudden falling off hair and eyebrow without any subjective symptoms.

(1) Blood deficiency with wind-dryness: Sudden hair falling off in patches, bald scalp, clear boundary, slight itching, pale complexion, insomnia, dizziness, pale red tongue with white fur and thready pulse.

(2) Qi stagnation and blood stasis: Sudden hair falling off in patches, dark dim scalp where hair falls off, dim complexion, petechiae on the tip and edge of the tongue and wiry pulse.

[Syndrome Differentiation and Treatment]

Treatment: To move qi, activate and nourish blood and promote hair growth.

Point combination 1:

SP 10 (*xuè hǎi*)	SP 6 (*sān yīn jiāo*)	KI 3 (*tài xī*)
EX-HN (*shēng fà*) (in the middle between GB 20 (*fēng chí*) and DU 16 (*fēng fǔ*)		

Secondary points:

Blood deficiency with wind-dryness:

BL 12 (*fēng mén*)	ST 36 (*zú sān lǐ*)	RN 6 (*qì hǎi*)

Qi stagnation and blood stasis:

GB 34 (*yáng líng quán*)	LV 2 (*xíng jiān*)	BL 17 (*gé shù*)
LV 3 (*tài chōng*)		

Operation: After routine sterilization, moderate tapping is used once a day and ten treatments make a course.

Point combination 2:

Alopecia region	Positive reactive spots on and bilateral to the spinal column	LU 9 (*tài yuān*)
PC 6 (*nèi guān*)		

Operation: Tapping is applied to the hair loss area from the boundary to the centre spirally. Moderate tapping is applied to the positive reactive spots and any other points. Treatment is given once a day and ten treatments make a course.

Point combination 3: alopecia region

Operation: After routine sterilization, tapping is applied until slight bleeding. Wipe the lesion with sterilized absorbent cotton and wash it with ginger juice until presence of a burning sensation. Moxibustion follows with tolerable heat for about three to five minutes. Treatment is given once a day.

Point combination 4:

DU 20 (*bǎi huì*)	EX-HN1 (*sì shén cōng*)	ST 8 (*tóu wéi*)
EX-HN (*shēng fà*)		

Secondary points:

Hypersteatosis: DU 23 (*shàng xīng*)

Head itching: DU 14 (*dà zhuī*)

Insomnia: EX (*ān mián*), EX-HN14 (*yì míng*)

Operation: After routine sterilization, bird-pecking tapping is used once a day and ten treatments make a course.

[Nursing and Prevention]

(1) Keep on the treatment and keep a good mood. Avoid stress and fatigue to prevent recurrence.

(2) Have a light diet and avoid greasy food.

Section 4 Gynecological and Pediatric Diseases

1. Advanced Menstruation

[Overview]

It refers to periods that come one week or more ahead of due time for more than two successive periods, similar to uterine bleeding from luteal phase defect due to ovulatory dysfunctional uterine bleeding and pelvic inflammation in

Western medicine.

[Cause and Mechanism of Disease]

(1) Bleeding due to blood heat: It is caused by agitation or rage, leading to stagnation of liver qi and generation of fire. When fire disturbs the Thoroughfare Vessel and *Ren* Vessel, or heat retains in the uterus, the condition occurs.

(2) Failure of the spleen to control blood: It is caused by fatigue and improper diet, which impair the spleen and stomach, resulting in spleen qi deficiency. When the spleen fails to control blood, the condition occurs.

[Types of Syndromes]

Main manifestations: Menstruation that comes one week or more ahead of due time or that comes twice in one month

(1) Bleeding due to blood heat: Excessive bright red menstrual blood, thick in quality with rotten fish smell, thirst, restlessness, irritation, brown urine, dry stools, red tongue with yellow fur, and slippery rapid pulse.

(2) Failure of the spleen to control blood: Pale red menstrual blood, thin in quality with no smell, sallow complexion, lassitude, anorexia, insomnia, pale enlarged tongue with thin white fur, and thready slow pulse.

[Syndrome Differentiation and Treatment]

Treatment: To clear heat, cool blood, invigorate the spleen, replenish qi and regulate menstruation.

Point combination 1:

SP 10 (*xuè hăi*)	SP 6 (*sān yīn jiāo*)	KI 8 (*jiāo xìn*)

Secondary points:

Bleeding due to blood heat:

LV 3 (*tài chōng*)	LV 2 (*xíng jiān*)	LV 1 (*dà dūn*)

Failure of the spleen to control blood:

ST 36 (*zú sān lĭ*)	BL 20 (*pí shù*)	RN 6 (*qì hăi*)

Fullness and pain in the chest and hypochondrium: PC 6 (*nèi guān*)

Restlessness: PC 5 (*jiān shĭ*), PC 7 (*dà líng*)

Menorrhagia: SP 1 (*yĭn bái*)

Point combination 2: The lower abdomen where the *Ren* Vessel, the Spleen Channel and the Stomach Channel pass

Operation: Each time select three to four points or the relevant channels. After routine sterilization, moderate tapping is used for the excess syndrome, while gentle tapping for the deficiency syndrome. Start treatment five to seven days before periods. Treatment is given once a day or every other day until the end of periods.

[Nursing and Prevention]

(1) Do not eat too much spicy food and keep a good mood.

(2) Keep on treatment and start it about one week before periods.

2. Delayed Menstruation

[Overview]

It refers to periods that come one week or more after due time for more than two successive periods, or periods that come in forty to fifty days.

[Cause and Mechanism of Disease]

(1) Cold retained in the uterus: This condition is caused by exposure to rain, or wading through water, or eating too much cold raw food, which triggers blood stasis.

(2) Stagnation of liver qi: It is caused by moodiness. When qi flow is impeded, the Thoroughfare Vessel and the *Ren* Vessel are blocked, the condition follows.

(3) Deficiency of qi and blood: This condition is caused by spleen deficiency and stomach, resulting in poor generation of qi and blood, which fails to supplement the Thoroughfare Vessel and *Ren* Vessel.

[Types of Syndromes]

Main manifestations: Periods that come more than seven days after due time, or that come in forty to fifty days

(1) Cold retained in the uterus: Scanty dark menstrual blood, thick in quality or with clots, chilled and painful lower abdomen, intolerance to cold and preference for warmth, thin white fur, and tight pulse.

(2) Stagnation of liver qi: Dark red menstrual blood, scanty with clots, impeded discharge of menstrual blood, moodiness, fullness in the chest and hypochondrium, mammary distending pain, thin white fur and wiry pulse.

(3) Deficiency of qi and blood: Scanty light red menstrual blood, thin in quality, a sensation of emptiness in the lower abdomen, pale or sallow complexion, dizziness, palpitation, insomnia, pale tongue with scanty coating, and thready feeble pulse.

[Syndrome Differentiation and Treatment]

Treatment: To disperse cold, resolve blood stasis, replenish qi, nourish blood, regulate the Thoroughfare Vessel and *Ren* Vessel

Point Combination:

SP 10 (*xuè hǎi*)	SP 6 (*sān yīn jiāo*)	KI 13 (*qì xué*)

Secondary points:

Cold retained in the uterus:

RN 4 (*guān yuán*)	ST 29 (*guī lái*)	RN 3 (*zhōng jí*)

Stagnation of liver qi:

LV 14 (*qī mén*)	RN 17 (*dàn zhōng*)	LV 3 (*tài chōng*)
LI 4 (*hé gǔ*)		

Deficiency of both qi and blood:

RN 6 (*qì hǎi*)	ST 36 (*zú sān lǐ*)	BL 20 (*pí shù*)
BL 21 (*wèi shù*)		

Operation: Each time select three to five points. After routine sterilization, moderate tapping is used for the excess syndrome, while gentle tapping for the deficiency syndrome. After tapping applied to RN 4 (*guān yuán*) and RN 3 (*zhōng jí*), mild moxibustion is followed for five to ten minutes for cold retained in the uterus. Start treatment five days before periods, once a day or every other day until the end of periods.

[Nursing and Prevention]

Do not expose to rain, wade through water, or eat too much raw cold food during periods.

3. Menstruation at Irregular Intervals

[Overview]

It refers to periods that come with an irregular cycle, more than one week or early or later, similar to menstrual irregularity due to uterine bleeding from ovulatory dysfunction in Western medicine. If it occurs in one year after menarche or climaterium without any symptoms, it is unnecessary to treat.

[Cause and Mechanism of Disease]

(1) Stagnation of liver qi: It is caused by rage and moodiness, leading to disorder of qi activity. When the Thoroughfare Vessel and *Ren* Vessel do not function well, the condition occurs.

(2) Kidney deficiency: It is caused by indulgence in sexual activities or more childbirth, or by constant deficiency of kidney qi in teenagers whose Thoroughfare Vessel and *Ren* Vessel are not sufficiently supplemented. There is dysfunction of blood storage and discharge, finally the condition occurs.

(3) Spleen deficiency: It is caused by worry beyond measure or improper diet that impairs spleen qi and impedes production of enough qi and blood. Dysfunction of the Thoroughfare Vessel and *Ren* Vessel results in abnormal storage and discharge of blood, finally, the condition occurs.

[Types of Syndromes]

Main manifestations: Advanced or delayed periods.

(1) Liver qi stagnation: Excessive or scanty menstrual blood, dark and purplish in color or with clots, mammary swelling and hypochondriac distending pain, frequent eructations, thin white fur, and wiry pulse.

(2) Kidney deficiency: Scanty pale red menstrual blood, thin in quality, dim complexion, dizziness, tinnitus, aching pain and weakness of the lower back and knees, pale tongue with white fur, and deep thready pulse.

(3) Spleen deficiency: Excessive pale red menstrual blood, thin in quality, lassitude, anorexia, fullness of the lower abdomen, pale red tongue with thin white fur,and slow pulse.

[Syndrome Differentiation and Treatment]

Treatment: To soothe the liver, regulate qi, reinforce the kidney, invigorate the spleen, regulate the Thoroughfare Vessel and *Ren* Vessel.

Point combination 1: RN 4 (*guān yuán*), SP 6 (*sān yīn jiāo*)

Secondary points:

Liver qi stagnation:

LV 14 (*qī mén*)	BL 18 (*gān shù*)	LV 3 (*tài chōng*)
GB 34 (*yáng líng quán*)		

Kidney deficiency:

KI 3 (*tài xī*)	BL 23 (*shèn shù*)	BL 18 (*gān shù*)
KI 5 (*shuǐ quán*)		

Spleen deficiency:

SP 4 (*gōng sūn*)	ST 36 (*zú sān lǐ*)	BL 20 (*pí shù*)
BL 21 (*wèi shù*)		

Lumbovertebral aching pain: BL 52 (*zhì shì*), BL 40 (*wěi zhōng*)

Point combination 2: 1.5 *cun* or 3 *cun* bilateral to the posterior midline of the spinal column, especially the sacrum and leg where the Spleen Channel, the

Kidney Channel and the Liver Channel pass

Operation: Each time select three to four points. After routine sterilization, moderate tapping is applied for the excess syndrome, while gentle tapping for the deficiency syndrome. Start treatment five days before periods or during periods. Treatment is given once every two days and ten treatments make a course.

[Nursing and Prevention]

Avoid mental stress, heavy physical labor and over-strain.

4. Dysmenorrhea

[Overview]

It refers to painful menstruation before or after periods. Periodic pain usually occurs in the lower abdomen with the lumbosacral portion involved. In severe cases, intense pain may trigger syncope.

[Cause and Mechanism of Disease]

(1) Qi stagnation and blood stasis: It is caused by rage that impedes smooth flow of liver qi. Stagnation of qi and blood in the Thoroughfare Vessel and *Ren* Vessel results in this condition.

(2) Retention of cold-dampness: It is caused by eating too much cold and raw food, or exposure to rain and cold during periods or after childbirth. When stagnated qi and blood retain in the Thoroughfare Vessel and *Ren* Vessel, the condition occurs.

(3) Retention of dampness-heat: It is caused by affliction from dampness-heat or retention of internal damp-heat, leading to qi and blood stagnation and the condition occurs.

(4) Insufficiency of qi and blood: This condition is caused by poor health or spleen deficiency and stomach, or a chronic or serious illness that consumes qi and blood, leading to malnutrition of the Thoroughfare Vessel and *Ren* Vessel.

[Types of Syndromes]

Main manifestations: Painful lower abdomen before or after and during periods, accompanied by vomiting.

(1) Qi stagnation and blood stasis: Distending pain in the lower abdomen during or before periods, dark red menstrual blood with clots, unsmooth discharge of menses, mammary swelling or hypochondriac distending pain, dark tongue or with petechiae, and wiry pulse.

(2) Retention of cold-dampness: Cold pain in the lower abdomen during or before periods, relieved by warmth, aggravated by pressure, scanty dark menstrual blood with clots, white greasy fur, and deep tight pulse.

(3) Retention of dampness-heat: Burning pain in the lower abdomen before or during periods, aggravated by pressure, excessive purplish menstrual blood, lasting for several days, thick in quality, excessive yellow thick, foul leucorrhea, dark urine, difficult bowels movement, red tongue with yellow greasy fur, and rapid slippery or rapid soft pulse.

(4) Insufficiency of qi and blood: Dull pain in the lower abdomen during or after periods, relieved by pressure, scanty pale red menstrual blood, thick in quality, pale tender-soft tongue with thick white fur, and thready pulse.

[Syndrome Differentiation and Treatment]

Treatment: To warm channels, regulate qi flow, replenish qi, nourish blood, regulate menstruation to stop pain.

Point combination 1:

RN 3 (*zhōng jí*)	SP 8 (*dì jī*)	BL 32 (*cì liáo*)
SP 6 (*sān yīn jiāo*)		

Secondary points:

Qi stagnation and blood stasis:

LV 3 (*tài chōng*)	SP 10 (*xuè hǎi*)	GB 34 (*yáng líng quán*)

Rentention of cold-dampness:

RN 4 (*guān yuán*)	ST 29 (*guī lái*)	ST 36 (*zú sān lǐ*)

Retention of dampness-heat:

DU 14 (*dà zhuī*)	LI 11 (*qū chí*)	SP 9 (*yīn líng quán*)

Insufficiency of qi and blood:

ST 36 (*zú sān lǐ*)	RN 6 (*qì hǎi*)	BL 20 (*pí shù*)
BL 23 (*shèn shù*)		

Point combination 2: Both sides of the spinal column, especially the sacral region, lower abdomen and leg where the Spleen Channel and the Liver Channel pass

Operation: Each time select three to four points. After routine sterilization, moderate tapping is applied for the excess syndrome, while gentle tapping for the deficiency syndrome. Start treatment one week before or during periods, once a day or every two days and ten treatments make a course.

[Nursing and Prevention]

(1) Investigate the cause of dysmenorrhea, primary or secondary. If it is secondary dysmenorrhea, treat the primary disease first.

(2) Avoid stress. Do not eat too much cold and raw food, wade through water or be exposed to cold during periods and lying-in.

5. Profuse Menstruation

[Overview]

It refers to a normal menstrual cycle where the volume of menstrual blood is obviously more than usual. Consult this section in the treatment of menorrhagia in ovulatory dysfunctional uterine bleeding or hysteromyoma and endometriosis.

[Cause and Mechanism of Disease]

(1) Spleen qi deficiency: It is caused by improper diet, fatigue or worry beyond measure, which impairs spleen qi, as a result, the spleen fails to control blood. When there is insecurity of the Thoroughfare Vessel and *Ren* Vessel, the condition occurs.

(2) Bleeding due to blood-heat: It is caused by affliction from heat, or retention of excessive heat, which disturbs the Thoroughfare Vessel and *Ren* Vessel. When blood is forced to overflow, the condition occurs.

(3) Stagnation of blood stasis: It is caused by rage that impairs the liver and triggers stagnation of liver qi and blood stasis. As a result, when blood overflows from the Thoroughfare Vessel and *Ren* Vessel, the condition occurs.

[Types of Syndromes]

Main manifestations: More volume of menstrual blood obviously than that in the past menstrual periods.

(1) Spleen qi deficiency: Excessive menstrual blood, pale red in color, thin in quality, pale complexion, lassitude, drooping sensation of the lower abdomen, pale tongue with tooth marks on its edge, thin white fur, and slow pulse.

(2) Bleeding due to blood-heat: Excessive menstrual blood, bright red or dark red in color, thick in quality, or with stinking smell, thirst, restlessness, brown urine, dry stools, red tongue with yellow fur, and rapid or rapid slippery pulse.

(3) Stagnation of blood stasis: Excessive menstrual blood, purplish in color, thick in quality with clots, or stabbing pain or distending pain in the lower abdomen, dark tongue or with petechiae, white thin fur, and rough pulse.

[Syndrome Differentiation and Treatment]

Treatment: Stop bleeding and regulate menstruation

Point combination 1:

RN 3 (*zhōng jí*)	SP 8 (*dì jī*)	BL 32 (*cì liáo*)
SP 6 (*sān yīn jiāo*)		

Secondary points:

Qi stagnation and blood stasis:

LV 3 (*tài chōng*)	SP 10 (*xuè hǎi*)	GB 34 (*yáng líng quán*)

Retention of cold-dampness:

RN 4 (*guān yuán*)	ST 29 (*guī lái*)	ST 36 (*zú sān lǐ*)

Retention of dampness-heat:

DU 14 (*dà zhuī*)	LI 11 (*qǔ chí*)	SP 9 (*yīn líng quán*)

Insufficiency of qi and blood:

ST 36 (*zú sān lǐ*)	RN 6 (*qì hǎi*)	BL 20 (*pí shù*)
BL 23 (*shèn shù*)		

Point Combination 2:

SP 1 (*yǐn bái*)	LV 1 (*dà dūn*)	SP 4 (*gōng sūn*)

Point combination 3: The lumbosacral portion where the Bladder Channel passes

Operation: Each time select three to five points. After routine sterilization, moderate tapping is applied for the excess syndrome, while gentle tapping for the deficiency syndrome. For the cold-dampness syndrome moxibustion is applied to RN 4 (*guān yuán*) and ST 36 (*zú sān lǐ*) for five to ten minutes after tapping; for the dampness-heat syndrome tapping is applied to DU 14 (*dà zhuī*) followed by cupping. Treatment is given once every two to three days and ten treatments make a course.

6. Scanty Menstruation

[Overview]

It refers to a normal menstrual cycle where the volume of menstrual blood is obviously less than usual, and periods less than two days. Consult this section in the treatment of hypomenorrhea in hypogonadism, endometrial tuberculosis, inflammation or uterine hypoplasia.

[Cause and Mechanism of Disease]

(1) Kidney deficiency: This condition is caused by poor born gifts, or indulgence in sexual activities, or a chronic disease, or frequent abortion, leading to consumption of essence and blood, and the sea of blood is not sufficiently supplemented.

(2) Spleen deficiency: It is caused by improper diet, fatigue, worry beyond measure, that impair the spleen and produces less qi and blood, or by a chronic disease or massive loss of blood. When the Thoroughfare Vessel and *Ren* Vessel are not supplemented, the condition occurs.

(3) Blood cold: It is caused by affliction from cold during periods or after childbirth, or by eating too much raw cold food, leading to cold retained in the Thoroughfare Vessel and *Ren* Vessel and impeded flow of blood.

[Types of Syndromes]

Main manifestations: Menstrual blood obviously less than usual, periods for only two days or much less.

(1) Kidney deficiency: Scanty and dark menstrual blood, thin in quality, aching pain and weakness of the lower back and knee, dizziness, tinnitus, night polyuria, pale red tongue, white thin fur, and deep thready pulse.

(2) Spleen deficiency: Scanty menstrual blood, short duration, pale red in color, thin in quality, sallow complexion, palpitation and dizziness, insomnia, dream-disturbed sleep, pale red tongue with white thin fur, and thready slow pulse.

(3) Blood cold: Scanty dark red menstrual blood with clots, cold pain in the lower abdomen, aggravated by pressure or cold, relieved by warmth, dark tongue with white fur, and deep tight pulse.

[Syndrome Differentiation and Treatment]

Treatment: To reinforce the kidney and the spleen, warm the channels, disperse cold and regulate menstruation.

Point combination 1:

Kidney deficiency:

RN 4 (*guān yuán*)	BL 23 (*shèn shù*)	BL 18 (*gān shù*)
KI 3 (*tài xī*)	KI 7 (*fù liū*)	

Spleen deficiency:

ST 36 (*zú sān lǐ*)	RN 6 (*qì hǎi*)	RN 12 (*zhōng wǎn*)
SP 4 (*gōng sūn*)	SP 6 (*sān yīn jiāo*)	

皮肤针疗法

DERMAL NEEDLING THERAPY

Blood cold:

RN 4 (*guān yuán*)	RN 5 (*shí mén*)	SP 10 (*xuè hǎi*)
DU 4 (*mìng mén*)	BL 17 (*gé shù*)	

Point combination 2: The inferior part of umbilicus where the *Ren* Vessel passes, the lumbosacral portion where the Bladder Channel passes

Operation: Each time select three to five points. After routine sterilization, moderate tapping is applied for the excess syndrome, while gentle tapping for the deficiency syndrome. For cold in blood moxibustion is applied to RN 8 (*shén què*) for five to ten minutes after tapping. Treatment is given once every two to three days and ten treatments make a course.

7. Amenorrhea

[Overview]

It refers to absence of the menses over 18 years old in females, or abnormal stoppage of the menses for more than 6 months after menstruation coming.

[Cause and Mechanism of Disease]

(1) Deficiency syndrome: It is due to innate deficiency or juvenile insufficient essence, or a chronic disease or indulgence in sexual activities, which impairs kidney essence and triggers deficiency in the Thoroughfare Vessel and *Ren* Vessel, or it is due to fatigue, worry beyond measure, that impairs the spleen and stomach, leading to insufficiency of qi and blood, less blood in the sea of blood.

(2) Excess syndrome: It is due to depression, leading to failure of liver qi to flow smoothly and impeded flow of qi and blood and obstruction of the Thoroughfare Vessel and *Ren* Vessel, or it is due to exposure to rain and cold during periods or after childbirth, or eating too much raw and cold food, leading to cold retained in the Thoroughfare Vessel and *Ren* Vessel and impeded flow of blood from cold.

[Types of Syndromes]

Main manifestations: Absence of the menses or cessation of the menses

(1) Deficiency syndrome: Gradually reduced volume of menstrual blood, absence of the menses, pale complexion, loss of appetite, loose stools, dizziness, palpitation, lassitude, pale red tongue and deep thready pulse.

(2) Excess syndrome: Absence of the menses, distending pain and cold in the lower abdomen, pain aggravated by pressure, or distending pain in the chest and hypochondrium, restlessness, irritability, dark red tongue, and wiry or tight

rough pulse.

[Syndrome Differentiation and Treatment]

Treatment: To reinforce the liver and kidney, resolve stasis and regulate menstruation.

Point combination 1:

Deficiency of kidney essence:

BL 23 (*shèn shù*)	RN 4 (*guān yuán*)	BL 18 (*gān shù*)
SP 6 (*sān yīn jiāo*)		

Defficiency of qi and blood:

ST 36 (*zú sān lǐ*)	SP 6 (*sān yīn jiāo*)	RN 6 (*qì hǎi*)
BL 20 (*pí shù*)	BL 21 (*wèi shù*)	

Qi stagnation and blood stasis:

LV 14 (*qī mén*)	BL 18 (*gān shù*)	RN 17 (*dàn zhōng*)
LV 3 (*tài chōng*)	GB 41 (*zú lín qì*)	

Cold congealing with blood stasis:

RN 4 (*guān yuán*)	DU 4 (*mìng mén*)	ST 36 (*zú sān lǐ*)
BL 32 (*cì liáo*)	BL 26 (*guān yuán shù*)	

Point combination 2: DU 1 (*cháng qiáng*), BL 31,32,33,34 (*eight liáo*)

Point combination 3:

LI 4 (*hé gǔ*)	LV 3 (*tài chōng*)	SP 6 (*sān yīn jiāo*)

(for the excess syndrome)

Operation: Each time select three to five points. After routine sterilization, moderate tapping is applied for the excess syndrome, while gentle tapping for the deficiency syndrome. For cold retention moxibustion is applied to RN 4 (*guān yuán*) and DU 4 (*mìng mén*) for five to ten minutes after tapping. Treatment is given once every two to three days and ten treatments make a course.

Point combination 4: Both sides of the spinal column, lower abdomen, groin, especially the lumbosacral vertebrae and both sides of them

Operation: Gentle tapping is used. First tap the lateral three lines on both sides of the spinal column twice, and then focus on the lumbosacral vertebrae and the five lines on both sides for five times, finally tapping is applied to the lower abdomen and groin. Treatment is given once a day and ten treatments make a course.

[Differential Diagnosis]

It should be differentiated from early pregnancy. Pregnant immunologic test in pregnancy is positive, but it is negative in absence of the menses.

[Nursing and Prevention]

(1) Remove psychological burden and any harmful stimulus to patients.

(2) Do not eat too much cold food, wade through water or be exposed to rain during periods.

8. Functional Uterine Bleeding

[Overview]

It refers to sudden profuse uterine bleeding or incessant dribbling of blood not in the regular menstrual period. When it lasts for two weeks, it is metrorrhagia and metrostaxis.

[Cause and Mechanism of Disease]

(1) Kidney deficiency: This condition is caused by insufficient juvenile kidney qi, or gradual diminished kidney qi during the climacteric period, leading to insecurity of essence storage, or by kidney yin deficiency, giving rise to interior heat, which pushes blood to move recklessly.

(2) Spleen deficiency: It is caused by worry beyond measure, which impairs the spleen, or by constant spleen qi deficiency, leading to failure of the spleen to control blood. Then disorders of the Thoroughfare Vessel and *Ren* Vessel trigger the condition.

(3) Blood heat: It is caused by moodiness. When it retains longer, heat is generated. Or it is due to preference for spicy food, leading to interior intense heat, impairment of the Thoroughfare Vessel and *Ren* Vessel and escape of blood, causing occurrence of the condition.

(4) Blood stasis: It is caused by moodiness, leading to impeded flow of liver qi and blood stasis, or by interior excessive yin-cold and failure of the Thoroughfare Vessel and *Ren* Vessel to be warmed. When there are cold retention and blood stasis, blood escapes, and the condition occurs.

[Types of Syndromes]

Main manifestations: Profuse uterine bleeding other than normal menstruation or incessant dribbling of blood.

(1) Kidney deficiency:

(i) Kidney yang deficiency: Profuse uterine bleeding or incessant dribbling of blood, pale red blood, thin in quality, aversion to cold and cold limbs, loose stools, pale red tongue with white fur, and deep thready pulse.

(ii) Kidney yin deficiency: Bright red blood, thick in quality, dizziness, tinnitus, tidal fever, night sweating, aching pain and weakness of the lower back and knees, red tongue with scanty coating,and thready rapid pulse.

(2) Spleen deficiency: Profuse bleeding, or incessant dribbling of blood, pale red in color, thin in quality, lassitude, lethargy, dream-disturbed sleep, insomnia, poor appetite, loose stools, pale red enlarged tongue with thin white fur, and thready slow pulse.

(3) Blood heat: Profuse bleeding, or incessant dribbling of blood, purplish in color, thick in quality with rotten fish smell, restlessness, irritability, oppressed feeling in the chest, hypochondriac pain, bitter taste in the mouth, dry throat, constipation, brown urine, red tongue with yellow fur and wiry pulse.

(4) Blood stasis: Profuse or scanty bleeding, incessant dribbling of blood, purplish in color with clots, or pain in the lower abdomen aggravated by pressure, dark tongue or with petechiae or ecchymoses, with white fur and rough or wiry pulse.

[Syndrome Differentiation and Treatment]

Treatment: To reinforce the spleen and kidney, cool blood and arrest profuse bleeding.

Point combination 1:

SP 10 (*xuè hǎi*)	SP 6 (*sān yīn jiāo*)	SP 8 (*dì jī*)

Secondary points:

Kidney yin deficiency:

KI 2 (*rán gǔ*)	KI 3 (*tài xī*)	KI 8 (*jiāo xìn*)

Spleen deficiency:

SP 1 (*yǐn bái*)	ST 36 (*zú sān lǐ*)	BL 20 (*pí shù*)
RN 6 (*qì hǎi*)		

Blood heat:

LV 1 (*dà dūn*)	GB 43 (*xiá xī*)	LV 14 (*qī mén*)
DU 14 (*dà zhuī*)		

Blood stasis:

LV 3 (*tài chōng*)	LV 14 (*qī mén*)	BL 46 (*gé shù*)

Point combination 2: SP 1 (*yǐn bái*), LV 1 (*dà dūn*).

Point combination 3: The lower abdomen where the *Ren* Vessel, the Spleen Channel and the Kidney Channel pass.

Operation: Each time select three to five points or channels. After routine sterilization, moderate tapping is applied for the excess syndrome, while gentle tapping for the deficiency syndrome. For blood heat cupping is applied to DU 14 (*dà zhuī*) after tapping. Treatment is given once every two days and ten treatments make a course.

[Nursing and Prevention]

(1) If repeated uterine bleeding occurs in menopausal women, find out the cause with relevant gynecologic examinations.

(2) Take emergency measures when collapse occurs in profuse uterine bleeding.

(3) Avoid fatigue to prevent deterioration.

9. Vaginitis

[Overview]

It is frequently seen in such gynecologic diseases, such as cervicitis, pelvic inflammation, etc.

[Cause and Mechanism of Disease]

(1) Dampness-heat: It is caused by liver qi stagnation, invasion of the spleen by liver fire, leading to collection of dampness. When dampness-heat pours the *Ren* Vessel and Belt Vessel are impaired, and vaginitis occurs.

(2) Spleen deficiency: It is caused by fatigue and worry beyond measure, or improper diet, which impairs the spleen and stomach, leading to dysfunction of transformation and transportation. Dampness pours and impairs the *Ren* Vessel and Belt Vessel, then the condition occurs.

(3) Kidney deficiency: This condition is caused by innate kidney deficiency, or indulgence in sexual activities, which impairs kidney qi and kidney's storage function of essence, leading to insecurity of the Thoroughfare Vessel and Belt Vessel.

[Types of Syndromes]

Main manifestations: Excessive leucorrhea with abnormal quality, color and smell.

(1) Dampness-heat: Dribbling morbid leucorrhea, yellow or red and white in color, thick in quality with rotten fish smell, heat sensation, bitter taste in the mouth, brown urine, constipation, red tongue with yellow greasy fur, and slippery or slippery rapid pulse.

(2) Spleen deficiency: Dribbling morbid leucorrhea, thin in quality like nasal discharge, white in color, cold limbs, lassitude, loss of appetite, loose stools, tooth marks on the tongue edge with white fur and soggy pulse.

(3) Kidney deficiency: Dribbling morbid leucorrhea, thin in quality like water, white in color with no smell, chills and cold limbs, aching pain and weakness of the lower back and knees, thin white fur, and deep pulse.

[Syndrome Differentiation and Treatment]

Treatment: To clear heat, remove dampness, warm the kidney, invigorate the spleen, strengthen the function of the *Ren* Vessel to stop vaginal discharge.

Point combination 1:

RN 3 (*zhōng jí*)	GB 26 (*dài mài*)	BL 30 (*bái huán shù*)

Secondary points:

Dampness-heat:

BL 34 (*xià liáo*)	SP 9 (*yīn líng quán*)	LV 2 (*xíng jiān*)
DU 14 (*dà zhuī*)		

Spleen deficiency:

ST 36 (*zú sān lǐ*)	RN 6 (*qì hǎi*)	BL 20 (*pí shù*)
SP 6 (*sān yīn jiāo*)		

Kidney deficiency:

RN 4 (*guān yuán*)	BL 23 (*shèn shù*)	DU 20 (*bǎi huì*)
KI 3 (*tài xī*)		

Point combination 2: RN 2 (*qū gǔ*)

Point combination 3: The lumbosacral portion where the Bladder Channel passes and EX-B2 (*jiá jǐ*) of the lumbosacral portion, the lower abdomen where the Spleen Channel, Kidney Channel and Belt Vessel pass

Operation: Each time select three to five points or two to four channels. After routine sterilization, moderate tapping is applied for the excess syndrome, while gentle tapping for the deficiency syndrome. Treatment is given once every two days and ten treatments make a course.

[Nursing and Prevention]

(1) If yellow and red vaginal discharge presents, it is necessary to do gynecologic examinations to tell it from cervical carcinoma.

(2) Control sexual life, pay attention to sanitation during periods and keep the vulva clean.

10. Pruritus Vulvae

[Overview]

It is characterized by pruritus of women's vulva or vagina, restlessness in severe cases, seen in many systemic or local diseases, such as diabetes, trichomonal vaginitis, colpomycosis, senile vaginitis, leucoplakia of vulva, eczema of vulva and so on; the treatment of these conditions can be referred to in this section.

[Cause and Mechanism of Disease]

(1) Depressed rage damaging liver: It is caused by rage that impairs the liver and triggers stagnation of liver qi, heat and dampness. When dampness-heat pours along the Liver Channel and macerates the vulva, the condition occurs.

(2) Invasion by insect toxins: This condition is due to insect toxins, or parasites from dampness-heat, which invades the vulva.

(3) Insufficiency of essence and blood: This condition is caused by insufficiency of essence and blood with indulgence in sexual activities, or being worn out with age, leading to deficiency of kidney essence and liver blood, and malnutrition of the vulva.

[Types of Syndromes]

Main manifestations: Pruritus of vulva or vagina, or extreme itching and restlessness.

(1) Downward pouring of dampness-heat: Pruritus of vulva or with pain, or accompanied by yellow thick leucorrhea, sticky bitter taste in the mouth, distress in the chest, yellow greasy fur,and slippery rapid pulse.

(2) Invasion by insect toxins: Pruritus of vulva like insect crawling, extreme itching, burning pain, excessive foamy leucorrhea, yellow in color, or white in color like bean dregs, foul smell, bitter taste in the mouth, dry throat, red tongue with yellow greasy fur, and smooth rapid pulse.

(3) Insufficiency of essence and blood: Dry vulva, itching with burning feeling, worse at night, feverish sensation in the chest, palms and soles, tidal

fever, night sweating, red tongue with scanty fur, and thready rapid pulse.

[Syndrome Differentiation and Treatment]

Treatment: To clear heat, remove dampness, relieve toxicity, replenish yin, eliminate dryness and stop itching.

Point combination 1:

SP 6 (*sān yīn jiāo*)	LV 5 (*lǐ gōu*)	RN 3 (*zhōng jí*)

Secondary points:

Downward pouring of dampness-heat:

SP 9 (*yīn líng quán*)	PC 7 (*dà líng*)	LV 2 (*xíng jiān*)
LV 8 (*qū quán*)		

Invasion by insect toxins:

LV 8 (*qū quán*)	DU 14 (*dà zhuī*)	EX-LE3 (*bǎi chóng wō*)

Insufficiency of essence and blood:

KI 3 (*tài xī*)	KI 7 (*fù liū*)	KI 2 (*rán gǔ*)

Point combination 3:

LI 11 (*qū chí*)	HT 8 (*shào fǔ*)	SP 6 (*sān yīn jiāo*)
LV 5 (*lǐ gōu*)		

Secondary points:

Exessive leucorrhea:

RN 6 (*qì hǎi*)	SP 10 (*xuè hǎi*)	GB 26 (*dài mài*)

Leucoplakia of vulva: RN 2 (*qū gǔ*)

It is used in simple pruritus of valvae, trichomonal vaginitis or colpomycosis, or leukoplakia of vulva.

Point combination 4: The groin, lower abdomen where the *Ren* Vessel, the Kidney Channel and the Spleen Channel pass

Operation: Each time select three to five points or two to three channels. After routine sterilization, moderate tapping is used for the excess syndrome and strong tapping is applied to LV 5 (*lǐ gōu*), while gentle tapping for the deficiency syndrome. Treatment is given once every two days and ten treatments make a course.

[Differential Diagnosis]

Pruritus of valvae occurs if drug rash or urticaria is found in the vulva. When it is due to drug rash, the patient must have taken related drugs. If urticaria wheal is found, all of which should be distinguished from pruritus of valva.

[Nursing and Prevention]

(1) Keep the vulva sanitary.

(2) Treat the primary cause of pruritus of valvae, such as diabetes.

11. Climacteric Syndrome

[Overview]

Climacteric syndrome refers to the relevant symptoms with menopause occurring before and after menopausal periods, characterized by burning and flushed cheeks, sweating, irritability, lassitude, dizziness, tinnitus, palpitation and amnesia.

[Cause and Mechanism of Disease]

(1) Liver-kidney yin deficiency: It is caused by before and after menopause, diminished sex-stimulating essence and insufficient essence and blood, leading to deficiency in the sea of blood and malnutrition of the liver. It results in hyperactivity of liver yang and the climacteric syndrome.

(2) Kidney yang deficiency: It is caused by constant deficiency of yang, or exhaustion of kidney yang, leading to malnutrition of the Thoroughfare Vessel and *Ren* Vessel, and dysfunction of the *zang-fu* organs, finally the climacteric syndrome occurs.

[Types of Syndromes]

(1) Liver-kidney yin deficiency: Burning sensation and sweating, irritability, quick temper, suspicion, worries, insomnia, amnesia, dizziness, tinnitus, distending pain in the hypochondrium, preference for sighing, dry stools, red tongue with scanty coating and wiry or thready rapid pulse.

(2) Kidney yang deficiency: Listlessness, depression, suspicion, edema of the face and limbs, aversion to cold, cold limbs, aching pain and weakness of the lower back and knees, fullness in the abdomen, loose stools, clear and profuse urine, pale red tongue with thin white fur, and deep, thready forceless pulse.

[Syndrome Differentiation and Treatment]

(1) Liver-kidney yin deficiency

Treatment: To nourish the liver and kidney

Point combination 1:

BL 23 (*shèn shù*)	BL 18 (*gān shù*)	LV 3 (*tài chōng*)
LV 8 (*qū quán*)	KI 3 (*tài xī*)	

Secondary points:

Pain in the hypochondrium: PC 6 (*nèi tíng*), LV 14 (*qī mén*)

Dizziness: RN 16 (*fēng fǔ*), GB 39 (*xuán zhōng*)

Tinnitus: SJ 21 (*ěr mén*), SJ 3 (*zhōng zhǔ*)

Insomnia:

HT 7 (*shén mén*)	PC 7 (*dà líng*)	SP 6 (*sān yīn jiāo*)

(2) Kidney yang deficiency

Treatment: To warm kidney yang

point combination 2:

RN 4 (*guān yuán*)	RN 4 (*mìng mén*)	BL 23 (*shèn shù*)
ST 36 (*zú sān lǐ*)	SP 6 (*sān yīn jiāo*)	

Point combination 3: Lines of 1.5 *cun* and 3 *cun* lateral to the midline on the back where the Bladder Channel passes, EX-B2 (*jiá jǐ*)

Operation: Each time select three to five points or one to two channels. After routine sterilization, gentle tapping is used. Treatment is given once every two days and ten treatments make a course.

[Differential Diagnosis]

(1) If the climacteric syndrome is accompanied by palpitation, shortness of breath and painful chest, it is essential to tell it from cardiovascular disease through examination.

(2) If irregular uterine bleeding presents, it is essential to tell it from uterine cancer.

[Nursing and Prevention]

(1) Keep a good mood and do the best to avoid harmful psychological stimulus. Never think that one has the climacteric syndrome to prevent deterioration.

(2) Take part in healthy activities, including physical exercises, entertainments and so on.

12. Postpartum Retention of Urine

[Overview]

It refers to postpartum dribbling urination or anuresis with painful and acute bloated lower abdomen.

[Cause and Mechanism of Disease]

(1) Qi deficiency: It is caused by qi deficiency after childbirth with massive loss of blood, leading to collapse of qi, blockage of the water passage and impeded bladder qi movement.

(2) Kidney deficiency: It is caused by kidney deficiency from childbirth and declined kidney yang. Declined qi movement results in this condition.

(3) Qi stagnation: It is caused by prolonged labor, leading to impeded circulation of qi and blood, disturbance of bladder qi movement.

[Types of Syndromes]

Main manifestations: Pastpartum difficult urination, bloated or painful lower abdomen

(1) Qi deficiency: Dribbling urination or difficult urination, drooping and painful lower abdomen, pale complexion, short breath, lassitude, enlarged pale red tongue with white fur, and thready weak pulse.

(2) Kidney deficiency: Dribbling urination or acraturesis after childbirth, listlessness, dim complexion, aching pain and weakness of the lower back and knees, pale red tongue with thin white fur, and deep slow thready pulse.

(3) Qi stagnation: Difficult urination, acute pain in the lower abdomen, or having cesarean section with posterior incision.

[Syndrome Differentiation and Treatment]

Treatment: To reinforce the kidney, replenish and move qi, resolve stasis and promote urination.

Point combination 1: RN 3 (*zhōng jí*), BL 28 (*páng guāng shù*)

Secondary points:

Qi deficiency:

DU 20 (*bǎi huì*)	RN 6 (*qì hǎi*)	LU 5 (*chǐ zé*)
ST 36 (*zú sān lǐ*)		

Kidney deficiency:

KI 3 (*tài xī*)	RN 4 (*guān yuán*)	BL 23 (*shèn shù*)
GB 25 (*jīng mén*)		

Qi stagnation:

BL 39 (*wěi yáng*)	RN 17 (*dàn zhōng*)	LV 3 (*tài chōng*)
LI 4 (*hé gǔ*)		

Point combination 2: RN 3 (*zhōng jí*), SP 6 (*sān yīn jiāo*)

Secondary points:

RN 6 (*qì hǎi*)	BL 22 (*sān jiāo shù*)	BL 23 (*shèn shù*)

Point combination 3: EX-B2 (*jiá jǐ*) and the Bladder Channel on the lumbosacral portion, lower abdomen where the *Ren* Vessel and Kidney Channel pass.

Operation: Each time select three to five points or two to three channels. After routine sterilization, gentle tapping is applied for the deficiency syndrome, while moderate tapping for the excess syndrome. Treatment is given once one to two days and ten treatments make a course.

[Differential Diagnosis]

It should be differentiated from retention of urine in urinary infection, which is characterized by hot and painful sensation in urination, but it has no such complaints.

13. Hypogalactia

[Overview]

It refers to deficiency of milk secretion or no milk secretion during lactation.

[Cause and Mechanism of Disease]

(1) Deficiency of both qi and blood: This condition is caused by innate deficiency of qi and blood, and loss of blood and qi in childbirth, leading to deficiency of qi and blood, or by hypofunctioning of the spleen and stomach, leading to less production of qi and blood, where the source of breast milk is not sufficient.

(2) Liver depression and qi stagnation: This condition is caused by stagnation of liver qi or moodiness after childbirth, leading to disharmony between qi and blood, obstruction of the channels, and unsmooth secretion of milk.

[Types of Syndromes]

(1) Deficiency of both qi and blood: Insufficiency of breast milk, thin in quality, even absence of breast milk, absence of distending pain in the breasts, pale lusterless complexion, dry skin, loss of appetite, loose stools, pale tongue with thin white fur, and thready weak pulse.

(2) Liver depression and qi stagnation: Scanty milk secretion after childbirth, or unsmooth secretion, distending pain in the breasts, fullness in the chest and hypochondrium, thin white fur and wiry pulse.

[Syndrome Differentiation and Treatment]

Treatment: To replenish qi and blood, regulate qi to promote lactation.

Point combination 1:

RN 17 (*dàn zhōng*)	ST 18 (*rŭ gēn*)	SI 1 (*shào zé*)

Secondary points:

Deficiency of both qi and blood:

ST 36 (*zú sān lĭ*)	BL 20 (*pí shù*)	BL 21 (*wèi shù*)
LV 13 (*zhāng mén*)		

Liver depression and qi stagnation:

LV 14 (*qī mén*)	GB 34 (*yáng líng quán*)	LV 3 (*tài chōng*)

Point combination 2: RN 17 (*dàn zhōng*), ST 18 (*rŭ gēn*)

Operation: Each time select three to five points. After routine sterilization, gentle tapping is applied for the deficiency syndrome, while moderate tapping for the excess syndrome. Treatment is given once one to two days and ten treatments make a course.

Point combination 3:

SI 1 (*shào zé*)	RN 17 (*dàn zhōng*)	RN 12 (*zhōng wăn*)
ST 18 (*rŭ gēn*)	ST 36 (*zú sān lĭ*)	BL 20 (*pí shù*)
BL 18 (*gān shù*)	BL 21 (*wèi shù*)	EX-B2 (*jiá jĭ*) (C5~C9, L1~L9)
the circum-breasts		

Operation: After routine sterilization, gentle tapping is applied around the breasts. Three to five points are selected. Gentle tapping is applied for the deficiency syndrome, while moderate tapping for the excess syndrome. Treatment is given once a day and ten treatments make a course.

[Nursing and Prevention]

(1) Supply more nutrition during the period of treatment. Eat more pig knuckles and crucian carp soup.

(2) Determine if the feeding method is correct and feed the baby at regular time.

(3) When the mother and baby are separated temporarily, pump milk out where there is mammary swelling.

14. Sterility

[Overview]

It refers to inability of the female to conceive over two years after marriage, but her husband has normal reproduction function, which is known as primary sterility. When women with a pregnant history fail to conceive without the use of contraceptives, such condition is called secondary sterility.

[Cause and Mechanism of Disease]

(1) Kidney deficiency: It is caused by poor born gifts, or by indulgence in sexual activities, or a serious or chronic disease, which consumes kidney essence and leads to deficiency in the Thoroughfare Vessel and *Ren* Vessel and undernourishment of uterus; or by declined fire of the gate of life, resulting in failure of the uterus to be warmed and to absorb sperms, then the condition occurs.

(2) Liver depression: This condition is caused by moodiness, leading to disturbance of qi movement, disharmony between qi and blood, and failure of the Thoroughfare Vessel and *Ren* Vessel to be nourished.

(3) Phlegm-dampness: It is caused by obesity or eating too much greasy and sweet food, leading to interior retention of phlegm-dampness and impeded qi movement. When the uterus is obstructed, the condition occurs.

[Types of Syndromes]

Main manifestations: Sterility after marriage for years without contraception.

(1) Kidney deficiency: Sterility after marriage for years, excessive or scanty menstrual blood, dizziness, tinnitus, aching pain and weakness in the lower back and knees, or aversion to cold, cold lower abdomen, severe lower back pain, excessive vaginal discharge, white in color, thin in quality, and thready weak or deep slow pulse.

(2) Liver depression: Sterility after marriage for years, menstrual irregularity, mammary distending pain before periods, fullness in the chest and hypochondrium, frequent eructation, depression or irritability, dark red tongue with white fur, and wiry or rough pulse.

(3) Phlegm-dampness: Sterility after marriage for years, obesity, delayed menstruation, excessive menstrual blood, fullness in the chest and stomach, fatigue and lassitude, pale red tongue with white greasy fur, and slippery pulse.

[Syndrome Differentiation and Treatment]

Treatment: To warm the kidney, replenish essence, soothe the liver, remove dampness and resolve phlegm.

Point combination 1:

EX-CA1 (*zǐ gōng*) (3 *cun* lateral to RN 3 (*zhōng jí*))	RN 4 (*guān yuán*)	SP 6 (*sān yīn jiāo*)

Secondary points:

Kidney essence deficiency:

BL 23 (*shèn shù*)	BL 18 (*gān shù*)	KI 7 (*fù liū*)
KI 10 (*yīn gǔ*)		

Fire of life gate decline:

DU 4 (*mìng mén*)	BL 26 (*guān yuán shù*)	BL 32 (*cì liáo*)
ST 36 (*zú sān lǐ*)		

Liver depression and qi stagnation:

BL 18 (*gān shù*)	LV 14 (*qī mén*)	LV 3 (*tài chōng*)
GB 34 (*yáng líng quán*)		

Interior excessive phlegm-dampness:

SP 9 (*yīn líng quán*)	RN 12 (*zhōng wǎn*)	LU 7 (*liè quē*)

Point combination 2: The lumbosacral portion where the Bladder Channel passes, the inguinal region groin, the lower abdomen where the *Ren* Vessel and the Kidney Channel pass.

Operation: Each time select three to five points or two channels. After routine sterilization, gentle tapping is used. Treatment is given once every two to three days and ten treatments make a course.

15. Enuresis

[Overview]

It refers to urinary incontinence in children over the age of three, at which urinary control should have been achieved with specific reference to that occurring during sleep at night. Enuresis occurring in school-age children because of playing games too much at daytime and drinking much water before sleep is not at a morbid state.

[Cause and Mechanism of Disease]

(1) Cold-deficiency of lower-jiao: It is caused by insufficient born gifts and kidney qi in children, leading to cold and deficiency in the lower-*jiao*, which fails to warm the bladder. It results in disturbance of bladder qi movement and dysfunction of storage, which fails to control the water passage, causing the occurrence of this condition.

(2) Lung-spleen qi deficiency: It is causecd by innate spleen-stomach weakness, or improper diet, which impairs the spleen, or by prolonged coughing, which impairs the lung. Spleen-lung qi deficiency hinders spleen essence to fill and regulate the bladder. When the water passage is not controlled, the condition occurs.

[Types of Syndromes]

(1) Cold-deficiency of lower-*jiao*: Enuresis in sleep, clear, profuse frequent urine, pale complexion, lassitude, aversion to cold, preference for warmth, enlarged tender-soft tongue, thin white fur and deep pulse.

(2) Lung-spleen qi deficiency: Enuresis in sleep, usually occurring after a serious or chronic disease, poor appetite, loose stools, tooth marks on the tongue edge with thin white fur, and soggy pulse.

[Syndrome Differentiation and Treatment]

Treatment: To warm and reinforce the spleen and kidney, replenish qi and reduce urine.

Point combination 1:

RN 3 (*zhōng jí*)	BL 28 (*páng guāng shù*)	RN 6 (*qì hǎi*)

Secondary points:

Cold-deficiency of lower-*jiao*:

RN 4 (*guān yuán*)	BL 23 (*shèn shù*)	KI 3 (*tài xī*)

Lung-spleen qi deficiency:

ST 36 (*zú sān lǐ*)	SP 6 (*sān yīn jiāo*)	BL 20 (*pí shù*)
BL 13 (*fèi shù*)		

Point combination 2: RN 6 (*qì hǎi*), LV 1 (*dà dūn*)

Point combination 3:

RN 3 (*zhōng jí*)	RN 4 (*guān yuán*)	RN 6 (*qì hǎi*)
RN 2 (*qǔ gǔ*)	ST 36 (*zú sān lǐ*)	SP 6 (*sān yīn jiāo*)
KI 3 (*tài xī*)		

Point combination 4: Both sides of the spinal column, especially the lumbosacral portion, and lower abdomen where the *Ren* Vessel passes, the forearm where the Lung Channel passes, the leg where the Spleen Channel and Kidney Channel pass

Operation: After routine sterilization, gentle tapping is applied until skin is flushed. Treatment is given once every two to three days and ten treatments make a course.

[Nursing and Prevention]

(1) Control water drinking before sleep and wake the child to pass water.

(2) Treat enuresis as early as possible to prevent mental burden in the future.

(3) Find the cause of the disease. If it is caused by organic diseases, treat the primary disease first.

16. Infantile Cerebral Palsy

[Overview]

It is a motor disorder appearing in young children, characterized by dysfunction of limbs and mental retardation, resulting from brain damage due to many reasons in medicine. It is in the category of "five kinds of retardation" and "five kinds of flaccidity" in traditional Chinese medicine.

[Cause and Mechanism of Disease]

(1) Liver-kidney deficiency: This disorder is caused by poor born gifts, leading to deficiency of essence and blood, which fails to supplement tendons and bones, resulting in flaccidity.

(2) Deficiency of both qi and blood: This disorder is caused by poor born gifts, or lack of proper care after birth, leading to deficiency in the brain, undernourishment of the heart and lusterless hairs.

(3) Blood stasis and phlegm obstructing vessels: It is caused by innate spleen-stomach deficiency or lack of proper care after birth, leading to failure of the spleen to transport and to production of phlegm from collected dampness, which obstructs the orifices. When the brain is not nourished, motor disorders occur.

[Types of Syndromes]

Main manifestations: Motor disorders, mental retardation

(1) Liver-kidney deficiency: Delayed development of the ability of sitting, standing, walking, tooth growing and talking, fatigue and preference for lying, lifelessness, incontinence of urine and feces, pale red tongue with thin white fur, and deep thready pulse.

(2) **Deficiency of both qi and blood:** Flaccidity of limbs, or flaccidity of the neck, mental retardation, pale complexion, indigestion, pale red tongue and lips with white fur, and slow pulse.

(3) **Blood stasis and phlegm obstructing vessels:** Lifelessness, aphasia, dementia, flaccidity of limbs, pale tongue or with ecchymosis and white greasy or yellow greasy fur,and wiry slippery or rough pulse.

[Syndrome Differentiation and Treatment]

Treatment: To reinforce the liver and kidney, replenish qi and blood, and resolve phlegm.

Point combination 1:

DU 20 (*bǎi huì*)	GB 39 (*xuán zhōng*)	DU 24 (*shén tíng*)
SP 6 (*sān yīn jiāo*)	RN 16 (*fēng fǔ*)	

Secondary points:

Liver-kidney deficiency:

LV 3 (*tài chōng*)	KI 3 (*tài xī*)	L 23 (*shèn shù*)
BL 18 (*gān shù*)		

Deficiency of both qi and blood: ST 36 (*zú sān lǐ*), RN 12 (*zhōng wǎn*)

Blood stasis and phlegm obstructing vessels: BL 17 (*gé shù*), ST 40 (*fēng lóng*)

Flaccidity of the neck: BL 23 (*shēn zhù*), DU 14 (*dà zhuī*)

Flaccidity of the upper limbs: EX-B2 (*jiá jǐ*) (T1~T7)

Flaccidity of the lower limbs: EX-B2 (*jiá jǐ*) (L1~L5)

Point combination 2: The top and back of the head, both sides of the spinal column, especially the nape, chest, the lumbosacral portion and forearm where the Large Intestine Channel, the Small Intestine Channel and the *Sanjiao* Channel pass, and the leg where the Stomach Channel, the Bladder Channel and the Gallbladder Channel pass.

Operation: After routine sterilization, gentle tapping is applied until the skin is flushed. Treatment is given once every two to three days and ten treatments make a course.

17. Child Indigestion

[Overview]

It is a chronic gastrointestinal disease, characterized by poor appetite, undigested food in stools, bloated abdomen, diarrhea or constipation.

[Cause and Mechanism of Disease]

(1) Food retention: This condition is caused by improper diet or feeding, or by eating too many raw cold, greasy and sweet foods, which impairs the spleen and stomach, leading to dysfunction of them.

(2) Spleen-stomach deficiency: It is caused by innate spleen-stomach deficiency and disturbance of transportation and transformation and digestion, where undigested food triggers this condition.

[Types of Syndromes]

Main manifestations: Anorexia, bloated abdomen, eructation, vomiting, diarrhea or constipation.

(1) Food retention: Poor appetite, disturbed sleep at night, vomiting acid rotten food, or undigested food, foul smell stools or loose stools, thick white fur or yellow greasy fur, and slippery pulse.

(2) Spleen-stomach deficiency: Loss of appetite, bloated abdomen, relieved by pressure, sallow complexion, lassitude, vomiting acid and rotten residue of food, loose stools or with undigested food, thin white fur, and thready weak pulse.

[Syndrome Differentiation and Treatment]

Treatment: To invigorate the spleen, harmonize the stomach and promote digestion.

Point combination 1:

ST 36 (*zú sān lǐ*)	ST 27 (*shàng jù xū*)	SP 6 (*sān yīn jiāo*)

Secondary points:

Food retention: RN 12 (*zhōng wǎn*), ST 20 (*chéng mǎn*)

Spleen-stomach deficiency:

BL 20 (*pí shù*)	BL 21 (*wèi shù*)	BL 50 (*wèi cāng*)

Diarrhea or constipation: ST 25 (*tiān shū*), LI 4 (*hé gǔ*)

Point combination 2:

BL 20 (*pí shù*)	BL 21 (*wèi shù*)	EX-B2 (*jiá jǐ*) (T7~L5)

Point combination 3: Both sides of the spinal column, especially the lower thoracic portion where the Bladder Channel passes, the upper abdomen where the *Ren* Vessel passes, the leg where the Spleen Channel and the Stomach Channel pass

Operation: After routine sterilization, gentle tapping is applied for 20 minutes and treatment is given once a day.

[Nursing and Prevention]

Properly feed the infants at regular time and do not give them much raw and cold food; do not expose to cold.

Section 5 Otolaryngological Diseases

1. Stye

[Overview]

It is an acute suppurative inflammation of the eyelid glandular tissues, characterized by red, swollen and painful eyelid. When one involving the sebaceous gland is called external stye, the other one that is marked by swelling on the conjunctival surface of the lid is called internal stye.

[Cause and Mechanism of Disease]

(1) Wind attacking channel and collateral: It is due to invasion of the channels by wind-heat, or wind-cold that turns to heat, leading to retention of heat toxins in eyelids, which scorches body fluids into a stye.

(2) Dampness-heat of spleen and stomach: It is due to eating too much spicy food and liquor addiction, leading to accumulation of dampness-heat in the spleen and stomach and stagnation of qi and blood. When stagnated qi and blood reside in the eyelid, the condition occurs.

(3) Spleen-stomach deficiency: It is due to poor health, or to improper diet and fatigue that impair the spleen and stomach and trigger dysfunction in transportation and transformation. When dampness resides in the eyelid, the condition occurs.

[Types of Syndromes]

Main manifestations: Red, swollen and painful eyelid.

(1) Wind attacking channel and collateral: Slightly red eyelid, itching, a little pain and swelling, headache, dry mouth, slightly red tongue with thin fur, and floating rapid pulse.

(2) Dampness-heat of spleen and stomach: Red, swollen and painful eyelid, subsided in a few days in mild cases; a yellow pus spot seen in severe cases, pus oozing after eruption, recovery in a few days, accompanied by fever, sticky taste in the mouth, constipation, yellow greasy fur,and slippery or slippery rapid pulse.

(3) Spleen-stomach deficiency: Itching pain of the eyelid, a little red swelling, no pus formation, repeated attack, or accompanied by indigestion, anorexia, loose stools, peeling fur, and soggy pulse.

[Syndrome Differentiation and Treatment]

Treatment: To disperse wind, clear heat and remove dampness

Point combination 1: *Ashi* points, LI 4 (*hé gŭ*)

Secondary points:

Wind attacking channel and collateral: GB 20 (*fēng chí*), DU 14 (*dà zhuī*)

Dampness-heat of spleen and stomach: ST 44 (*nèi tíng*), SP 9 (*yīn líng quán*)

Spleen-stomach weakness: RN 12 (*zhōng wăn*), ST 36 (*zú sān lĭ*)

Upper eyelid: SJ 23 (*sī zhú kōng*), EX-HN4 (*yú yāo*)

Lower eyelid: ST 1 (*chéng qì*), ST 2 (*sì bái*)

Point combination 2: BL 18 (*gān shù*), EX-HN5 (*tài yáng*)

Point combination 3: Ear Apex (HT 6.7i)

Point combination 4: LI 11 (*qŭ chí*) (opposite to the diseased eye), DU 14 (*dà zhuī*) (applicable to the excess-heat syndrome)

Point Combination 5: Both sides of the cervical vertebrea, swollen area of the eye, the forearm where the Large Intestine Channel, the Small Intestine Channel and the *Sanjiao* Channel pass, for the deficiency syndrome, adding the leg where the Stomach Channel and Spleen Channel pass.

Operation: After routine sterilization, moderate tapping is applied for the excess syndrome, while gentle tapping for the deficiency syndrome. Collateral-puncturing and cupping are applied to DU 14 (*dà zhuī*), and at the ear apex three to four drops of blood are squeezed out after tapping. Moderate tapping is applied to LI 11 (*qŭ chí*). Gentle tapping is applied to the *Ashi* points around the affected eye until the skin flushes with a warm sensation. Treatment is given once a day and five treatments make a course.

[Differential Dignosis]

(1) Stye: Red, swollen and painful hard eyelid, tenderness, unclear boundary of the mass.

(2) Tarsal gland cyst: Localized bulginess of the eyelid, hard, smooth, clear boundary, absence of pain.

[Nursing and Prevention]

(1) Don't eat spicy food in the course of illness.

(2) The dermal needling therapy is effective to stye without pus. In case of pus formation surgical operation is needed. Never squeeze it by yourself.

(3) Cultivate good sanitary habit, don't rub your eyes with hands, eat less greasy and sweet food.

2. Acute Conjunctivitis

[Overview]

It is one of commonly encountered ophthamologic diseases, characterized by red eyes, pain, photophobia and lacrimation, usually found in spring and summer. It is epidemic and infectious.

[Cause and Mechanism of Disease]

(1) Invasion of external seasonal toxins: The condition is due to invasion of the eyes by seasonal pathogenic or wind-heat, leading to obstruction of the channels and qi stagnation and blood stasis.

(2) Excessive fire of liver-gallbladder: It is due to depression and moodiness, leading to stagnation of liver qi and fire. When excessive liver and gallbladder fire goes along the channels, channel qi is blocked, and then the condition occurs.

[Types of Syndromes]

(1) Invasion of external seasonal toxins: Red swollen eyes, photophobia and lacrimation, excessive eye secretion, headache, aversion to wind, fever and floating pulse.

(2) Excessive fire of liver-gallbladder: Red swollen and painful eyes, photophobia and lacrimation, bitter taste in the mouth, dry throat, restlessness, irritability, constipation, brown urine, and wiry pulse.

[Syndrome Differentiation and Treatment]

Treatment: To clear heat, release toxicity, alleviate swelling and stop pain.

Point combination 1:

EX-HN5 (*tài yáng*)	BL 1 (*jīng míng*)	ST 44 (*nèi tíng*)
LI 11 (*qŭ chí*)	LI 4 (*hé gŭ*)	

(applicable to cases with seasonal toxins)

Treatment: To clear liver-gallbladder fire, alleviatie swelling and stop pain

Point combination 2:

GB 1 (*tóng zĭ liáo*)	LI 4 (*hé gŭ*)	LV 3 (*tài chōng*)
GB 43 (*xiá xī*)	GB 20 (*fēng chí*)	

(for excessive liver and gallbladder fire)

Secondary points:

Fever: DU 14 (*dà zhuī*), LI 11 (*qŭ chí*)

Bitter taste in mouth: SJ 6 (*zhī gōu*), GB 34 (*yáng líng quán*)

Constipation: ST 25 (*tiān shū*), ST 27 (*shàng jù xū*)

Operation: After routine sterilization, moderate tapping is applied. Collateral-puncturing and cupping are applied to DU 14 (*dà zhuī*) after tapping. Treatment is given once a day and five treatments make a course.

Point combination 3: Ear Apex, vein of back ear

Point combination 4: Symmetric tender spots on the ear lobe (If there are no tender spots, use the eye region.)

Point Combination 5: Both sides of the vertical vertebrea, around the orbit, the forearm where the Large Intestine Channel, the Small Intestine Channel and the *Sanjiao* Channel pass, and the leg where the Stomach Channel and the Liver Channels pass.

Operation: After routine sterilization, moderate or strong tapping is used until presence of spot bleeding. Treatment is given once one to two days and three treatments make a course.

[Differential Diagnosis]

Distinguish it from epidemic keratoconjunctivitis. They are both called "epidemic conjunctivitis."

(1) Acute conjunctivitis is characterized by conjunctival congestion and excessive mucous or mucopurulent secretion.

(2) Epidemic keratoconjunctivitis is characterized by conjunctival congestion and edema, excessive follicles, scanty watery secretion. Superficial petechial infiltration of the cornea is seen in majority of patients and the treatment for this can be referred to in this section.

[Nursing and Prevention]

(1) Forbid putting on an eye patch because it may trigger accumulation of the secretion in the eye, leading to higher temperature of the conjunctiva and more heat toxins, which induces deterioraton. Don't eat spicy food and seafood.

(2) Don't rub your eyes with dirty hands and restrict sharing with others' basin and towel. Have the patient's basin and towels sterilized.

3. Nearsightedness

[Overview]

It is characterized by seeing nearby objects clearly and distant ones vaguely owing to refractive error.

[Cause and Mechanism of Disease]

(1) Deficiency of both qi and blood: It is usually caused by poor innate essence and lack of proper postnatal care, resulting in yin deficiency in the liver and kidney, and both qi and blood deficiency that fails to nourish the eyes.

(2) Stasis of channels and vessel: It is caused by improper posture in reading, dim light, continuous reading or writing for hours at incorrect posture, resulting in blockage of the channels and collaterals, failure of qi to run to eyes and unsmooth circulation of qi and blood, which deprives the eyes of nourishment.

[Types of Syndromes]

Main manifestations: Clear sight in seeing nearby objects and vague sight in seeing distant ones.

(1) Deficiency of both qi and blood: Accompanied by amnesia, insomnia, aching pain and weakness of the lower back, lassitude, dryness in eyes, distending and heaviness sensation in the head, dizziness, pale tongue with thin and white fur and thready pulse.

(2) Stasis of channels and vessel: Accompanied by distending or stabbing pain in eyes, headache, dark tongue with white fur, and wiry or choppy pulse.

[Syndrome Differentiation and Treatment]

Treatment: To nourish blood and clear channels and collaterals to improve vision.

Point combination 1:

GB 14 (*yáng bái*)	GB 1 (*tóng zǐ liáo*)	BL 1 (*jīng míng*)
EX-HN5 (*tài yáng*)		

Secondary points:

Deficiency of both qi and blood:

BL 20 (*pí shù*)	BL 18 (*gān shù*)	BL 23 (*shèn shù*)
ST 36 (*zú sān lǐ*)	KI 3 (*tài xī*)	LV 3 (*tài chōng*)

Stasis of channels and vessel:

BL 17 (*gé shù*)	LV 3 (*tài chōng*)	LI 4 (*hé gǔ*)

Point combination 2:

GB 1 (*tóng zǐ liáo*)	ST 1 (*chéng qì*)	BL 1 (*jīng míng*)
GB 20 (*fēng chí*)	LI 4 (*hé gǔ*)	LV 3 (*tài chōng*)
ST 36 (*zú sān lǐ*)	GB 37 (*guāng míng*)	

Point combination 3:

ST 1 (*chéng qì*)	GB 20 (*fēng chí*)	EX-HN14 (*yì míng*)

Point combination 4: EX-HN (*huì guāng*) (in the postero-lateral neck, on the horizontal intersection between the line to the cricoid cartilage backward and postauricular process's vertical line), EX-LE (*míng chá*) (8 *cun* vertically up to the lateral malleolus, close to the anterior margin of the splinter bone), EX-HN (*xiāo yì*) (in the inferior middle point of the suborbital margin).

Point combination 5: Eye 1 (on the anterior-inferior intertragic notch); Eye 2 (on the postero-inferior intratragic notch); Eye (on the anterior and middle aspect of the ear lobe, or Ear Lobe 4)

Point combination 6: Nuchal region on both sides of the spinal column, temporalis part, parietal region, LI 4 (*hé gǔ*) and LV 3 (*tài chōng*)

Operation: After sterilization, moderate tapping is applied once every two days and five treatments make a course.

[Nursing and Prevention]

(1) Most cases of nearsightedness are caused by improper use of eyes and a few are due to congenital defect, so it is important to have correct posture in reading and writing, and discard bad habits.

(2) Do eye exercise after much reading to prevent nearsightedness.

(3) Perform acupressure or massage to the points.

(4) Do not watch TV and play computer games during treatment.

4. Acute Congestive Glaucoma

[Overview]

This category discusses "bluish glaucoma" or "greenish glaucoma" in traditional Chinese medicine.

[Cause and Mechanism of Disease]

(1) Excess of liver-gallbladder fire: It is caused by yang excess and emotional stress, resulting in blazing of liver-gallbladder fire with wind-phlegm that disturbs the eyes.

(2) Deficiency fire flaming upward: It is caused by liver-kidney yin deficiency in the debilitated aged people, or indulgence in sexual activities that impairs body fluids, or yin deficiency with yang hyperactivity and inner production of deficiency-fire, which blazes along the channel and injures the eyes.

[Types of Syndromes]

Main manifestations: Sudden onset in both eyes of the aged and middle-aged people, severe headache, distending pain of eyeballs as if they would rush out of the orbits, vision with red-green circles when looking at light, quick decline of vision, failure to recognize people, blurred vision except dark and light, irritability, nausea and vomiting.

(1) Excess of liver-gallbladder fire: Accompanied by severe headache with a distending feeling, blurred vision, vision with red-green circles when looking at light, irritability, bitter taste and dryness in the mouth, constipation, wiry pulse, usually triggered by excitement.

(2) Deficiency fire flaming upward: Accompanied by headache with distending sensation, blurred vision, dryness of the eyes, dizziness, tinnitus, tidal fever, night sweating, red tongue with scanty fur and rapid pulse, triggered by great fatigue.

[Syndrome Differentiation and Treatment]

Treatment: To clear liver-gallbladder heat and nourish yin to improve vision.

Point combination 1:

BL 1 (*jīng míng*)	ST 1 (*chéng qì*)	GB 1 (*tóng zǐ liáo*)
EX-HN5 (*tài yáng*)	GB 8 (*shuài gǔ*)	LV 3 (*tài chōng*)
LI 4 (*hé gǔ*)		

Secondary points:

Excess of liver-gallbladder fire:

LV 2 (*xíng jiān*)	GB 43 (*xiá xī*)	SJ 6 (*zhī gōu*)

Deficiency fire flaming upward:

KI 7 (*fù liū*)	LV 8 (*qū quán*)	KI 2 (*rán gǔ*)

Point combination 2: Both sides of the cervical vertebrae, around the orbit, the forearm where the *Sanjiao* Channel passes, and the lower leg where the Gallbladder Channel and the Liver Channel pass

Operation: After routine sterilization, gentle or moderate tapping is used and gentle tapping is applied to KI 17 (*fù liū*) and LV 8 (*qū quán*). Treatment is given once every two days and five treatments make a course.

[Differential Diagnosis]

Make a differential diagnosis between this disorder and acute iridocyclitis.

(1) Acute congestive glaucoma: Diminished vision, vision with red-green circles when looking at light, platycoria, and elevation of intraocular pressure

(2) Iridocyclitis: Diminished vision, myosis and normal or lower intraocular pressure

[Nursing and Prevention]

(1) This therapy is used in combination with other therapies. On the onset of disease, it is important to give some duration of time for treatment to reduce the risk of blindness.

(2) It is a severe ophthalmologic disease and it is essential to make preventive measures. Try to be in a good mood and avoid rage.

5. Optic Atrophy

[Overview]

It develops from optic neuritis or occurs as a secondary disease from primary encephalitis with manifestations of diminished vision and contraction of the visual field. It is in the category of "vision obstruction" and "bluish blindness" in traditional Chinese medicine.

[Cause and Mechanism of Disease]

(1) Liver depression and qi stagnation: It is caused by of emotional stress, unsmooth flow of qi and blood and obstruction of channels.

(2) Liver blood deficiency: It is caused by poor born gifts, or insufficient essence and blood, or a chronic disease, or loss of blood and injury to body fluids, leading to failure of the eyes to be nourished.

(3) Deficiency of both heart and spleen: It is caused by improper diet, fatigue, or worry beyond measure that impairs the heart and spleen, resulting in failure of the eyes to be nourished owing to deficiency of qi and blood.

[Types of Syndromes]

Main manifestations: Diminished vision, contraction of the visual field, or blindness in severe cases.

(1) Liver depression and qi stagnation: Blurred vision, irascibility, hypochondriac pain, depression, sighing, bitter taste in the mouth, pale-red tongue with white and thin fur, and wiry pulse.

(2) Liver blood deficiency: Blurred vision, dryness of eyes, pallor, insomnia, palpitation, dizziness, lassitude, pale tongue with white and thin fur, and thready weak pulse.

(3) Deficiency of both heart and spleen: Blurred vision, insomnia, dream-disturbed sleep, weakness of limbs, poor appetite and loose stools, pale and enlarged tongue with tooth marks, and soggy moderate pulse.

[Syndrome Differentiation and Treatment]

Treatment: To soothe the liver to remove stagnancy of liver qi, and nourish blood to improve vision.

Point combination 1:

BL 1 (*jīng míng*)	EX-HN14 (*yì míng*)	GB 20 (*fēng chí*)
EX-HN7 (*qiú hòu*)		

Secondary points:

Liver depression and qi stagnation:

RN 17 (*dàn zhōng*)	LV 3 (*tài chōng*)	GB 34 (*yáng líng quán*)
LV 14 (*qī mén*)		

Liver blood deficiency:

LV 8 (*qū quán*)	BL 18 (*gān shù*)	BL 23 (*shèn shù*)
BL 20 (*pí shù*)		

Deficiency of both heart and spleen:

BL 20 (*pí shù*)	ST 36 (*zú sān lǐ*)	SP 3 (*tài bái*)
HT 7 (*shén mén*)		

Point combination 2:

GB 20 (*fēng chí*)	EX-HN14 (*yì míng*)	LI 4 (*hé gǔ*)
BL 2 (*cuán zhú*)	ST 36 (*zú sān lǐ*)	GB 37 (*guāng míng*)

Point combination 3:

(1) Both sides of the cervical vertebrae: 0.5~1 *cun* from the spinous process of the cervical vertebrae (C2~C7)

(2) The first line of the Bladder Channel on the back: 1.5 *cun* from the spinous process of the 1st thoracic vertebra to the 5th lumbar vertebra

(3) Around the orbit: The projection image on the body surface of the orbicular muscle of the eye and on the leg along the course of the Gallbladder Channel, the Spleen Channel and the Liver Channel (ie, from SJ 23 (*sī zhú kōng*) to EX-HN4 (*yú yāo*), BL 2 (*cuán zhú*), BL 1 (*jīng míng*), ST 1 (*chéng qì*), EX-HN7 (*qiú hòu*), GB 1 (*tóng zǐ liáo*).

(4) The leg where the Gallbladder Channel passes (from GB 34 (*yáng líng quán*) to SP 5 (*shāng qiū*)) and the traveling course of the Liver Channel (from LV 8 (*qū quán*) to KI 3 (*tài xī*).

Operation: After routine sterilization, gentle and moderate tapping is used once every two days and five treatments make a course.

[Differential Diagnosis]

Make a differential diagnosis between this disorder and optic atrophy which is usually caused by cerebral tumors, trauma, tabes, alcoholism or cinchonism, etc.

(1) Primary optic atrophy: White papilla of the optic nerves with clear edge and sieve plate.

(2) Secondary optic atrophy: Grayish white or wax yellow turbid papilla of the optic nerves with unclear edge and sieve plate.

[Nursing and Prevention]

(1) It is in combination with other therapies to strengthen the curative effect.

(2) This section can be referred to in the treatment of secondary optic atrophy. But primary disease should be dealt with simultaneously.

6. Color Blindness and Color Weakness

[Overview]

Color blindness and color weakness are dichromatopsia, usually due to congenital defect. Color blindness is divided into three categories: protanopia, deuteranopia and achromatism. Color weakness refers to poor ability to see red and green color. Both of them are in the category of "syndrome of mistaking red for white" in traditional Chinese medicine.

[Cause and Mechanism of Disease]

The two conditions are due to poor born gifts, liver-kidney deficiency, insufficient essence and blood, resulting in failure of essence and blood to go upward to nourish the eyes.

[Types of Syndromes]

Red, green blindness or color blindness, accompanied by lassitude, pallor, aching pain and weakness of the lower back and knees, blurred vision, pale tongue with white fur, and thready pulse.

[Syndrome Differentiation and Treatment]

Treatment: To reinforce the liver and kidney

Point combination 1:

BL 1 (*jīng míng*)	ST 1 (*chéng qì*)	GB 1 (*tóng zǐ liáo*)
EX-HN7 (*qiū hòu*)	ST 2 (*sì bái*)	LV 3 (*tài chōng*)
KI 3 (*tài xī*)	ST 36 (*zú sān lǐ*)	

Point combination 2:

GB 20 (*fēng chí*)	BL 2 (*cuán zhú*)	EX-HN5 (*tài yáng*)
ST 36 (*zú sān lǐ*)	ST 2 (*sì bái*)	LI 4 (*hé gǔ*)
GB 37 (*guāng míng*)	SJ 23 (*sī zhú kōng*)	EX-HN4 (*yú yāo*)
ST 1 (*chéng qì*)	KI 3 (*tài xī*)	SP 6 (*sān yīn jiāo*)

The three groups of points are used alternately.

Point combination 3: Both sides of the cervical vertebrae, around the orbits, where the Gallbladder Channel, Kidney Channel and the Liver Channel pass

Operation: After routine sterilization, gentle tapping is used once every two days and ten treatments make a course.

7. Acute Rhinitis

[Overview]

It is characterized by stuffy running nose and sneezing, or loss of smell. It occurs in all seasons and is often seen in winter and spring. It has a short course and recovers in several days. It is in the category of "nasal obstruction due to wind" in traditional Chinese medicine.

[Cause and Mechanism of Disease]

(1) Invading of external wind-cold: It is caused by insufficiency of healthy qi, loose striated layer and insecurity of defensive qi, resulting in an invasion to the body by wind-cold. Another cause is that the lung is fettered by cold, thus failing to purify, causing pathogenic toxins gathering in the nose to give rise to stuffy nose due to invasion by exogenous wind.

(2) Invading of external wind-heat: The nose is the window of the lung, which is closely related to skin and hair. Insecurity of defensive qi results in invasion of the lung through the mouth and nose by wind-heat, leading to failure of lung qi to diffuse.

[Types of Syndromes]

Main manifestations: Stuffy and running nose, and sneezing.

(1) Invading of external wind-cold: Stuffy and running nose with thin, white nasal discharge, aversion to cold, absence of thirst, general aching pain, thin and white fur, and floating tight pulse.

(2) Invading of external wind-heat: Stuffy and running nose with yellow sticky discharge, nasal itching, hot breath, headache, difficult expectoration of phlegm, fever, aversion to cold, sore dry throat, red tongue edge and tip with thin yellow fur,and floating rapid pulse.

[Syndrome Differentiation and Treatment]

Treatment: To disperse wind, release the exterior and ease nasal congestion.

Point combination 1:

LI 20 (*yíng xiāng*)	DU 23 (*shàng xīng*)	LI 14 (*hé gǔ*)
LU 7 (*liè quē*)	SJ 5 (*wài guān*)	

Secondary points:

Wind-heat:

LI 11 (*qū chí*)	LI 1 (*shāng yáng*)	DU 14 (*dà zhuī*)

Wind-cold:

BL 12 (*fēng mén*)	BL 13 (*fèi shù*)	GB 20 (*fēng chí*)

Point combination 2

LI 20 (*yíng xiāng*)	EX-HN3 (*yìn táng*)	LI 4 (*hé gǔ*)
GB 20 (*fēng chí*)		

Point combination 3: Both sides of the cervical vertebrae, the first line of the Bladder Channel on the back, the lateral sides of the nose and the forearm where the Large Intestine Channel and the Lung Channel pass.

Operation: After routine sterilization, moderate tapping is used once a day and five treatments make a course.

[Differential Diagnosis]

It is the premonitory symptoms of epidemic encephalitis, encephalitis B, measles and diphtheria, which are similar to the clinical manifestations of acute rhinitis. That's why differential diagnosis should be made in consideration of the epidemic season, condition and clinical features, in combination with lab tests and examination.

[Nursing and Prevention]

(1) Patients should have proper rest, drink enough water, and eat digestible food.

(2) Do not blow nose with force on stuffy nose so as to prevent toxins entering the ear and trigger ear diseases.

(3) Give treatment in time to prevent an interior syndrome from an exterior syndrome which gives rise to other disorders or to chronic rhinitis.

8. Chronic Rhinitis

[Overview]

Its main manifestations are recurrent stuffy nose, mild or severe, prolonged stuffed nostrils. In severe cases, sense of smell is lost.

[Cause and Mechanism of Disease]

It is caused by insufficiency of lung qi, insecurity of defensive qi, prone to invasion of the body by exogenous pathogenic factors, which results in impairment of the purification and down-sending function of the lung, deficiency of healthy qi and residence of pathogenic factors, or improper diet and fatigue, which injures the spleen and stomach and affects normal transportation and transformation, and impedes sending usables up and sending unusables down. Finally, dampness resides in the nose, causing stuffy nose.

[Types of Syndrome]

Main manifestations: Recurrent stuffy nose, mild or severe, loss of sense of smell, profuse nasal discharge, accompanied by distending headache, pallor, pale tongue, and thready pulse.

[Syndrome Differentiation and Treatment]

Treatment: To replenish lung qi and ease the nose

Point combination 1:

LI 20 (*yíng xiāng*)	LI 4 (*hé gŭ*)	DU 23 (*shàng xīng*)
LU 8 (*jīng qú*)		

Secondary points:

Headache: GB 20 (*fēng chí*), EX-HN3 (*yìn táng*)

Pallor: ST 36 (*zú sān lĭ*), SP 6 (*sān yīn jiāo*)

Point combination 2: Both sides of the cervical vertebrae, the first line of the Bladder Channel on the back, the lateral side of the nose, the forearm where the Large Intestine Channel and the Lung Channel pass, and the leg where the Stomach Channel passes.

Operation: After routine sterilization, gentle tapping is used, once every two days and five treatments make a course.

[Nursing and Prevention]

(1) Do exercises to build up health, avoid wind-cold, take preventive measures and treat common cold.

(2) Avoid using vasoconstrictors for nasal drip, do not blow nose with force so

as to prevent invasion of the ear by toxins and trigger ear diseases.

(3) Massage the points on the nasal region by oneself every day to strengthen the therapeutic effect.

9. Allergic Rhinitis

[Overview]

It is a commonly seen nasal disorder, characterized by sudden and repeated attack of nasal itching, sneezing with thin nasal running and stuffy nose.

[Cause and Mechanism of Disease]

(1) **Lung qi deficiency:** It is caused by insufficiency of lung qi, loose striae layer, insecurity of defensive qi, resulting in invasion of the lung by wind-cold, leading to failure of lung qi to descend and retention of body fluids, which obstructs the nose and gives rise to allergic rhinitis.

(2) **Spleen-kidney qi deficiency:** It is caused by deficiency of lung, spleen and kidney qi due to poor born gifts and improper care after birth, leading to spleen-kidney deficiency and failure of the refined essence to send up to the lung, resulting in insufficiency of lung qi, dysfunction of the lung to send qi down and retention of fluids in the nose, thus the condition occurs.

[Types of Syndromes]

Main manifestations: Paroxysmal nasal itching and stuffy nose, frequent sneezing and running nose

(1) **Lung qi deficiency:** Accompanied by spontaneous sweating, aversion to wind, disinclination to talk, low voice, pale tongue with thin and white fur, and deep pulse.

(2) **Spleen-kidney qi deficiency:** Accompanied by bloated abdomen, anorexia, lassitude, aching pain and weakness of the lower back and knees, aversion to cold and cold limbs, loose stools, pale tongue with tooth marks on its edge, thin white fur and slow moderate pulse.

[Syndrome Differentiation and Treatment]

Treatment: To regulate the nutrient and defensive aspects, invigorate the spleen and kidney to ease stuffy nose.

Point combination 1: EX-HN8 (*shàng yíng xiāng*), GB 20 (*fēng chí*)

Secondary points:

Lung qi deficiency:

BL 13 (*fèi shù*)	RN 6 (*qì hăi*)	LI 4 (*hé gŭ*)
BL 12 (*fēng mén*)		

CHAPTER 2

Treatment

Spleen-kidney qi deficiency:

BL 20 (*pí shù*)	BL 23 (*shèn shù*)	ST 36 (*zú sān lǐ*)

Point combination 2:

LI 20 (*yíng xiāng*)	EX-HN8 (*shàng yíng xiāng*)	GB 20 (*fēng chí*)
LI 4 (*hé gǔ*)	ST 36 (*zú sān lǐ*)	RN 6 (*qì hǎi*)

Point combination 3:

LI 20 (*yíng xiāng*)	DU 23 (*shàng xīng*)	BL 12 (*fēng mén*)
BL 13 (*fèi shù*)	BL 23 (*shèn shù*)	

Point combination 4: Both sides of the cervical vertebrae, the first line of the Bladder Channel on the back, the lateral side of the nose, the forearm where the Large Intestine Channel and the Lung Channel pass, the leg where the Stomach Channel passes.

Operation: After routine sterilization, gentle tapping is used, once every two days and five treatments make a course.

[Nursing and Prevention]

(1) Make known of the sensitizers and try to avoid them as far as possible.

(2) Avoid wind-cold and take exercise to build up health.

(3) Do not eat too much cold, raw, greasy and sweet food and seafood.

10. Nasal Sinusitis

[Overview]

It is characterized by prolonged running nose with turbid discharge, usually accompanied by headache, stuffy nose, diminished sense of smell, etc., and it is a frequently seen nasal disorder, in the category of "rhinorrhea with turbid discharge" in traditional Chinese medicine.

[Cause and Mechanism of Disease]

(1) Wind-heat invading lung: It is due to invasion of the lung by wind-heat, which obstructs the Lung Channel and impedes its descending and diffusing function. Pathogenic heat goes upward along the Lung Channel and scorches the nose, and the condition occurs.

(2) Heat stagnation in gallbladder channel: It is due to rage that impairs the liver and leads to unsmooth flow of gallbladder qi. Stagnant qi turns to fire, which goes along the channel and injures the nasal sinus, thus the condition occurs.

(3) Spleen deficiency and dampness prevailing: Since the spleen and stomach are exteriorly-interiorly related and the Stomach Channel passes the lateral side of the nose, overeating greasy, sweet and spicy foods leads to internal production of dampness-heat, affecting the spleen and stomach. Then their function of transportation and transformation is disturbed, and they fail to send the usables up and the unusables down. Finally, dampness-heat goes upward along the channels and resides in the nasal sinus, thus the condition occurs.

[Types of Syndromes]

(1) Wind-heat invading lung: Massive nasal discharge, sticky, yellow or white in color, stuffy nose, loss of the sense of smell, fever, aversion to cold, headache, cough, red tongue with white or light yellow fur, and floating rapid pulse.

(2) Heat stagnation in gallbladder channel: Massive yellow fetid sticky nasal discharge, stuffy nose, diminished sense of smell, lassitude, bloated and painful chest and hypochondrium, bitter taste in the mouth and dry throat, dizziness, tinnitus, irritability and hot temper, red tongue with yellow fur, and wiry or wiry rapid pulse.

(3) Spleen deficiency and dampness prevailing: Stuffy nose with massive thick discharge, diminished sense of smell, lassitude, bloated stomach, anorexia, loose stools, pale and enlarged tongue with thin white fur, and soggy, moderate pulse.

[Syndrome Differentiation and Treatment]

Treatment: To diffuse lung qi and purge heat, invigorate the spleen, resolve dampness, ease the nose and expel pus.

Point combination 1:

LU 7 (*liè quē*)	LI 4 (*hé gŭ*)	LI 20 (*yíng xiāng*)
BL 2 (*cuán zhú*)	EX-HN4 (*yú yāo*)	

Secondary points:

Wind-heat invading lung:

LU 5 (*chĭ zé*)	LI 11 (*qŭ chí*)	GB 20 (*fēng chí*)

Heat stagnation in gallbladder channel:

GB 34 (*yáng líng quán*)	GB 43 (*xiá xī*)	SJ 2 (*yè mén*)

Spleen deficiency and dampness prevailing:

ST 36 (*zú sān lĭ*)	SP 9 (*yīn líng quán*)	ST 40 (*fēng lóng*)

Point combination 2:

EX-HN3 (*yìn táng*)	LI 20 (*yíng xiāng*)	LI 4 (*hé gǔ*)

Point combination 3: Both sides of the cervical vertebrae, the lateral side the of nose, the forearm where the Large Intestine Channel and Lung Channel pass, and the leg where the Stomach Channel passes

Operation: After routine sterilization, moderate tapping is used for the excess syndrome while gentle tapping for the deficiency syndrome, once every two days and ten treatments make a course.

[Differential Diagnosis]

It is necessary to differentiate this condition from nasitis.

(1) Nasitis: No purulent discharge from the nasal meatus or olfactory tubercle.

(2) Nasal sinusitis: The symptoms mentioned above can be seen in local examination. Nasal sinusitis can be determined with a roentgenogram.

[Nursing and Prevention]

(1) Keep the nasal meatus free. Ask the patients to bow and incline the head to let nasal discharge out.

(2) Pay attention to the method of blowing nose, do not do it with force so as to prevent invasion of the ear by toxins, causing ear disorders.

(3) Avoid pungent, hot and greasy food. Quit smoking and alcohol dependence.

(4) Take exercises to keep fit and prevent common cold.

11. Hearing Difficulty and Tinnitus

[Overview]

The two conditions may occur alone or together and they are the symptoms of multiple ear diseases, or it is a single disorder.

[Cause and Mechanism of Disease]

(1) Wind invading: It is due to invasion of the body by wind-heat, or wind-cold which turns to fire and attacks the ear, resulting in obstruction of the ear, thus the two conditions occur.

(2) Blazing of liver-gallbladder fire: It is caused by emotional problems, or impairment of the liver from rage, or stagnated liver qi which turns to fire, and goes up along the channel to disturb the ear, thus the two conditions occur.

(3) Depletion of kidney essence: It is caused by wearing out with age, and hypofunctioning of the liver and kidney, or indulgence in sexual activities, or chronic diseases, leading to consumption of kidney essence and malnutrition of the brain and ears, which gives rise to these conditions.

[Types of Syndromes]

(1) Wind invading: Sudden onset, hearing difficulty or deafness, distending sensation in the ear, tinnitus, unrelieved by pressing the ear, accompanied by headache, fever, thin, white or yellow fur, and floating pulse.

(2) Blazing of liver-gallbladder fire: Sudden deafness, mild or severe, aggravated after rage, hearing difficulty or continual ringing in the ear with sound of tide or wind and thunder, unrelieved by pressing the ear, or bitter taste in the mouth, dry throat, irritability and hot temper, hypochondriac pain, yellow urine, constipation, red tongue with yellow fur, and wiry rapid pulse.

(3) Depletion of kidney essence: Protracted deafness, tinnitus with a shrill chirping noise, relieved in the daytime but aggravated at night, sudden stop or onset, alleviated by pressing the ear and aggravated on tiredness, accompanied by dizziness, aching pain and weakness of the lower back and knees, tidal fever, night sweating, heat sensation in the chest, palms and soles, red tongue with scanty fur, and thready weak pulse.

[Syndrome Differentiation and Treatment]

Treatment: To disperse wind, purge fire, replenish essence and enrich blood.

Point combination 1:

SJ 21 (*ěr mén*)	SI 19 (*tīng gōng*)	SJ 17 (*yì fēng*)
SJ 3 (*zhōng zhǔ*)		

Secondary points:

Invasion by wind:

GB 20 (*fēng chí*)	SJ 5 (*wài guān*)	LI 6 (*piān lì*)

Excessive liver and gallbladder fire:

LV 2 (*xíng jiān*)	GB 43 (*xiá xī*)	GB 40 (*qiū xū*)

Deficiency of essence and blood:

KI 3 (*tài xī*)	BL 23 (*shèn shù*)	BL 18 (*gān shù*)
GB 39 (*xuán zhōng*)		

Point combination 2:

BL 23 (*shèn shù*)	SJ 20 (*jiǎo sūn*)	SJ 5 (*wài guān*)
KI 3 (*tài xī*)	GB 2 (*tīng huì*)	

Point combination 3: Around the ear and the leg where the Gallbladder Channel and the Kidney Channel pass

Operation: After routine sterilization, moderate tapping is used for the excess syndrome and gentle tapping for the deficiency syndrome, once every two days and ten treatments make a course.

[Nursing and Prevention]

(1) These conditions are caused by wind and should be treated in time.

(2) When these conditions are caused by hyperactivity of liver and gallbladder fire, remove emotional problems, keep an easy mind and avoid unhealthy mental stress.

(3) Soak feet in hot water before sleep at night and it can relieve tinnitus. In addition, do not drink strong tea, coffee, cocoa, or liquor.

(4) Concern traffic safety when one has hearing difficulty.

12. Sore Throat

[Overview]

It is commonly seen in acute or chronic pharyngitis, tonsillitis and laryngitis, characterized by red swollen and painful throat and difficult swallowing. It is in the category of "throat blockage" or "tonsillitis" in traditional Chinese medicine.

[Cause and Mechanism of Disease]

(1) Wind-heat invading: It is due to improper care in daily life, sudden weather change leading to insecurity of lung qi, attack of the lung by wind-heat via the mouth and nose. When pathogenic factors reside in the throat, the condition occurs.

(2) Exuberance of lung-stomach heat: It is due to overeating spicy food or liquor addiction. When the heat goes up along the channel to the throat, the condition occurs.

(3) Deficiency-fire flaming upward: It is due to constant yin deficiency of the body, or impaired body fluids from a chronic disease, leading to rise of deficiency-fire along the channel, which scorches the throat, thus the condition occurs.

[Types of Syndromes]

(1) Wind-heat invading: Dry, burning sensation and slight pain of the throat, uneasy swallowing at the initial stage, followed by burning pain of the throat, and feeling a foreign body in the throat, fever, aversion to cold, headache, thirst and preference for cold drinks, thin, yellow fur, and floating rapid pulse.

(2) Exuberance of lung-stomach heat: Sore throat, pain aggravated during swallowing, fever, thirst, foul breath, coughing with expectorations of yellow, thick phlegm and hoarseness, yellow urine, dry stools, yellow or yellow dry fur, or slippery and rapid pulse.

(3) Deficiency-fire flaming upward: Discomfort in the throat with slightly pain, dry and itching, pink throat, dry cough or retching, tidal fever, night sweatng, dizziness, tinnitus, red tongue with scanty fur, and rapid pulse.

[Syndrome Differentiation and Treatment]

Treatment: To dissipate wind and clear heat, purge lung and stomach fire, replenish yin and extinguish fire.

Point combination 1:

LU 11 (*shào shāng*)	LU 7 (*liè quē*)	LI 4 (*hé gŭ*)
LU 5 (*chǐ zé*)		

Secondary points:

Wind-heat invading:

DU 14 (*dà zhuī*)	BL 12 (*fēng mén*)	LI 11 (*qū chí*)

Exuberance of lung-stomach heat:

LU 10 (*yú jì*)	ST 44 (*nèi tíng*)	LI 2 (*èr jiān*)

Deficiency-fire flaming upward:

KI 3 (*tài xī*)	KI 6 (*zhào hǎi*)	LU 10 (*yú jì*)

Point combination 2:

ST 6 (*jiá chē*)	SI 17 (*tiān róng*)	LI 4 (*hé gŭ*)
LI 11 (*qŭ chí*)		

Point combination 3: Both sides of the cervical vertebrae, the first line of the Bladder Channel on the back, 1.5 *cun* lateral to the middle line; the forearm where the Large Intestine Channel and the Lung Channel pass, the leg where the Stomach Channel passes, and the Kidney Channel for the deficiency syndrome.

Operation: After routine sterilization, moderate tapping is used for the excess syndrome, while gentle tapping for the deficiency syndrome, once a day or every two days and five treatments make a course.

[Differential Diagnosis]

Sore throat can also be seen in some infectious diseases, such as measles,

CHAPTER 2

Treatment

scarlet fever, etc. The condition should be differentiated according to the epidemic season and disease characteristics.

[Nursing and Prevention]

(1) Avoid fried, roasted or spicy food and drink enough water.

(2) Have a good rest, avoid over-fatigue to prevent deficiency-fire disturbing upward.

(3) Avoid excessive talking and dust, quit smoking and liquor addiction.

13. Toothache

[Overview]

It is a common symptom in stomatopathy, either dental or periodontal diseases. Toothache occurring in dental caries, pulpitis or periodontitis, is treated as described in this section.

[Cause and Mechanism of Disease]

(1) Wind-heat invading: It is due to invasion of the body by wind-heat, which impairs the teeth and gums, and leads to accumulation of heat and stagnation of qi and blood in channels, thus the condition occurs.

(2) Accumulated heat in stomach and intestines: It is due to preference for pungent, spicy food that brings about internal production of fire-heat, or due to constant stomach heat and attack by wind-heat. Stomach heat goes up along the channel and disturbs the gum and impairs blood vessels, thus the condition occurs.

(3) Deficiency-fire flaming upward: It is due to a chronic disease or indulgence in sexual activities or kidney deficiency in the aged, or kidney yin deficiency and hyperactivity of fire, which injures the gum, thus the condition occurs.

[Types of Syndromes]

(1) Wind-heat invading: Paroxysmal toothache when exposed to wind, alleviated by cold and aggravated by heat, accompanied by red swollen gums, chills and fever, thirst, dry throat, red tongue, with thin white and dry fur, and floating rapid pulse.

(2) Exuberance of lung-stomach heat: Severe toothache involving cheeks, red swollen painful gums, or oozing of blood and pus, thirst, drinking much water, dry throat, foul breath, yellow urine, constipation, red tongue with yellow fur, and slippery rapid pulse.

(3) Deficiency-fire flaming upward: Mild pain occasionally aggravated in the afternoon, slightly red and swollen gums, or gingival atrophy, loose teeth, aching pain and weakness of the lower back and knees, dizziness, tinnitus, dry mouth without a desire for drinking water, red tender-soft tongue with scanty or no coating, and thready rapid pulse.

[Syndrome Differentiation and Treatment]

Treatment: To disperse wind and clear heat, purge stomach fire, replenish yin and bring down fire.

Point combination 1:

ST 6 (*jiá chē*)	ST 7 (*xià guān*)	LI 4 (*hé gǔ*)

Secondary points:

Wind-heat invading: LI 11 (*qū chí*), SJ 5 (*wài guān*)

Exuberance of lung-stomach heat:

ST 44 (*nèi tíng*)	LI 2 (*èr jiān*)	DU 14 (*dà zhuī*)

Flaming of deficiency fire:

KI 3 (*tài xī*)	KI 2 (*rán gǔ*)	LV 2 (*xíng jiān*)

Point combination 2:

SI 18 (*quán liáo*)	RN 24 (*chéng jiāng*)	ST 6 (*jiá chē*)
ST 7 (*xià guān*)	LI 4 (*hé gǔ*)	

Point combination 3: The forearm where the Large Intestine Channel passes, and leg where the Stomach Channel passes.

Operation: After routine sterilization, moderate tapping is used for toothache due to wind-heat invading or exuberance of lung-stomach heat, or tapping is applied to LI 11 (*qū chí*) or DU 14 (*dà zhuī*) until bleeding. Gentle tapping is used along the channel for toothache caused by deficiency-fire flaming upward, once a day or every two days and five treatments make a course.

[Differential Diagnosis]

It should be differentiated from trigeminal neuralgia, which has evident trigger points. There is a lancinating pain. It is necessary to do careful examination, and see if there is any dental disorder. In this section, toothache is triggered by dental conditions.

[Nursing and Prevention]

(1) Have a habit of brushing teeth in the morning and at night, keep oral cavity clean, and take less sweet and sour food and prevent dental caries.

(2) Treat toothache in time, investigate the cause and give treatment.

14. Ulcerative Stomatitis

[Overview]

It refers to superficial ulcerative spots as large as a bean in the sarcolemma of the mouth. It is usually divided into two types: excess and deficiency. The former is similar to aphtha, while the latter like recurrent ulcer of the mouth. It is in the category of "aphthae", or "oral sore" in traditional Chinese medicine.

[Cause and Mechanism]

(1) Accumulated heat in heart and spleen: It is due to overeating pungent food or liquor addiction that brings about fire-heat in the heart and spleen. Then the fire goes along the related channels and attacks the mouth. The sarcolemma is fumigated and putrefacted, or it is due to unclean or ruptured mouth which leads to invasion of the body by toxins and putrefaction of the sarcolemma of the mouth, thus the condition occurs.

(2) Yin deficiency with effulgent fire: It is due to, yin deficiency at birth or consumption of kidney yin in a chronic disease that impairs the heart and kidney, or blazing of fire from yin deficiency, that injures the sarcolemma of the mouth, thus the condition occurs.

[Types of Syndromes]

(1) Accumulated heat in heart and spleen: Ulcerative spots on lips, inner cheeks, gums or tongue, as large as soy beans or mung beans. They are in dots of various sizes. There are multiple ulcerative spots which sometimes present in patches. The ulcerous surface is yellowish white, depressed in the centre with peripheral fresh red mucosa, accompanied by burning pain, thirst, foul breath, concentrated urine, dry stools, red tongue with yellow fur, and slippery rapid pulse.

(2) Yin deficiency with effulgent fire: There are a few ulcerative spots. The ulcerous surface is grayish white with peripheral pale red or pale mucosa. Recurrence is seen, difficult to cure. Other symptoms are red tender-soft dry tongue with scanty coating,and thready rapid pulse.

[Syndrome Differentiation and Treatment]

Treatment: To clear heat and relieve toxicity, replenish yin and bring down fire, subside swelling and kill pain

Point combination 1:

ST 44 (*nèi tíng*)	ST 6 (*jiá chē*)	LI 4 (*hé gŭ*)

Secondary points:

Accumulated heat in heart and spleen:

SP 8 (*dì jī*)	PC 7 (*dà líng*)	ST 44 (*nèi tíng*)

Yin deficiency with effulgent fire:

KI 2 (*rán gǔ*)	KI 1 (*yǒng quán*)	LV 3 (*tài chōng*)

Point combination 2: Both sides of the cervical vertebrae, 0.5 *cun* lateral to the middle line; the forearm where the Heart Channel passes, the Spleen Channel for the excess syndrome, and the Kidney Channel for the deficiency syndrome

Operation: After routine sterilization, moderate tapping is used for the excess syndrome and gentle tapping for the deficiency syndrome, once a day and five treatments make a course.

[Nursing and Prevention]

(1) Avoid pungent, greasy food and quit smoking and liquor addiction.

(2) It is appropriate to eat substances that can invigorate the spleen and drain dampness, for example, congee or soup with *Semen Coicis*, water chestnut, *Semen Euryales*, and *Semen Phaseoli*.

Index by Point Names

D

E

L

O

P

R

S

T

Index by Disease Names and Symptoms

皮肤针疗法

DERMAL NEEDLING THERAPY

C

D

E

F

G

H

N

O

P

R

S

图书在版编目（CIP）数据

皮肤针疗法（英文）/张学丽等编著. —北京：人民卫生出版社，2008.10

ISBN 978-7-117-10636-8

Ⅰ.皮… Ⅱ.张… Ⅲ.皮肤针疗法-英文
Ⅳ.R245.31

中国版本图书馆CIP数据核字（2008）第144077号

皮肤针疗法（英文）

编　　著：张学丽　刘　颖
出版发行：人民卫生出版社（中继线+8610-6761-6688）
地　　址：中国北京市丰台区方庄芳群园三区3号楼
邮　　编：100078
网　　址：http://www.pmph.com
E - mail：pmph@pmph.com
发　　行：pmphsales@gmail.com
购书热线：+8610-6769-1034（电话及传真）
开　　本：787×1092　1/16
版　　次：2008年10月第1版　2008年10月第1版第1次印刷
标准书号：ISBN 978-7-117-10636-8/R·10637